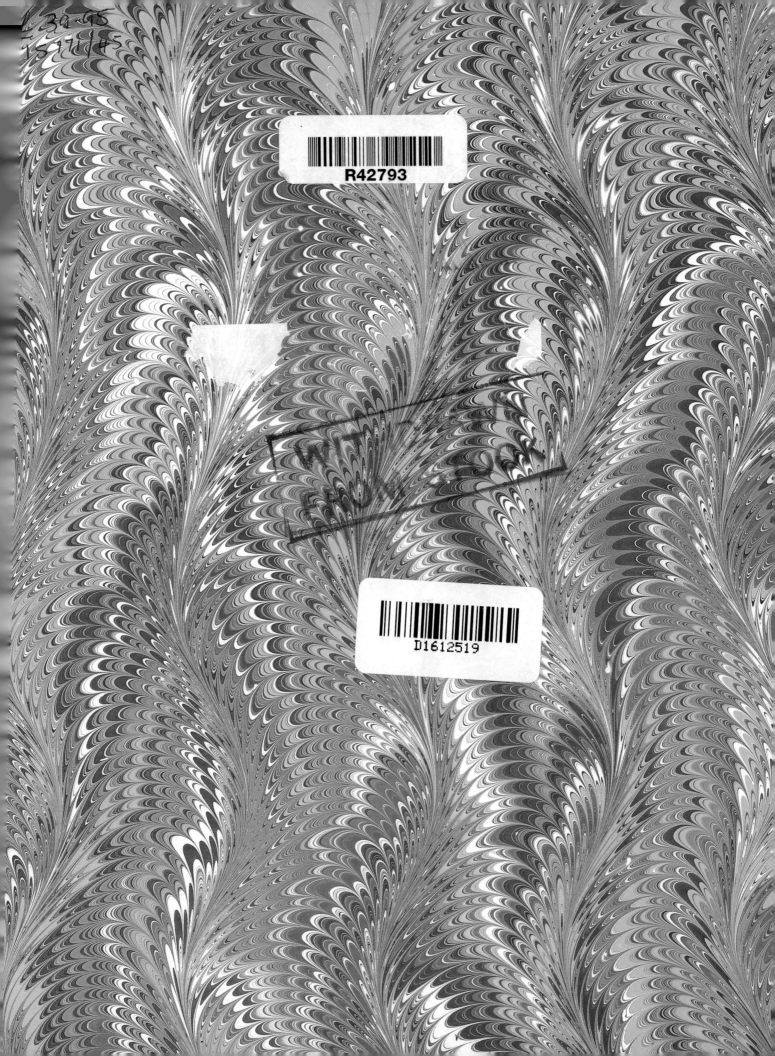

# Collectible Fashions
## of the Turbulent 30s

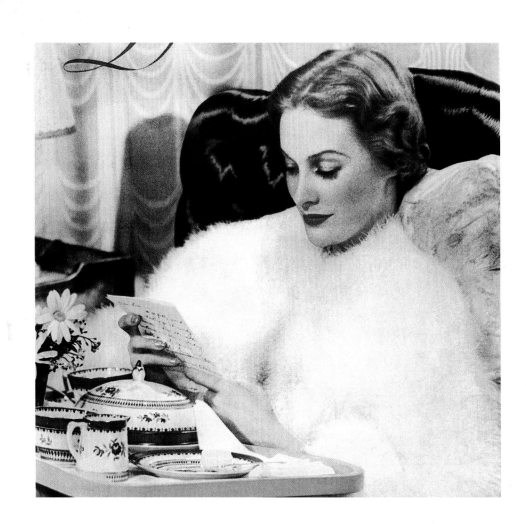

# Collectible Fashions
## of the Turbulent 30s

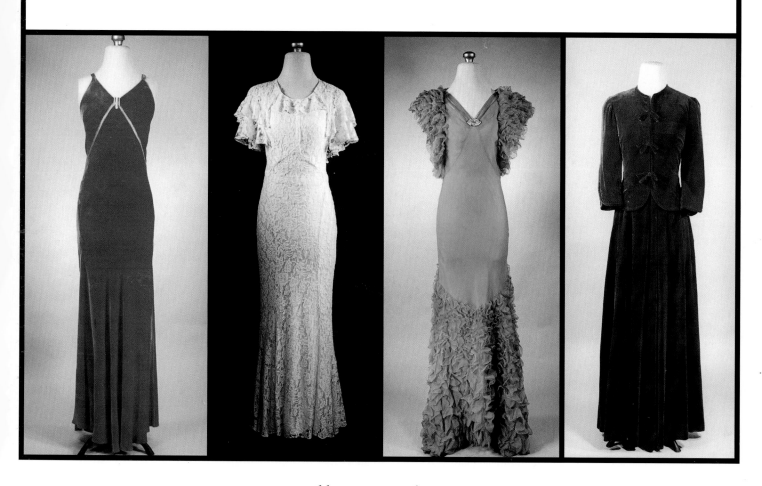

Ellie Laubner

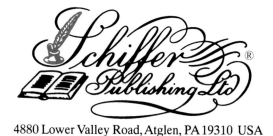

4880 Lower Valley Road, Atglen, PA 19310 USA

## Dedication

To my wonderful husband, Paul, for his patience
and understanding. Thank you for encouraging me
to pursue a dream.

Book Design by Anne Davidsen
Type set in Bernhard Modern /Aldine721

ISBN: 0-7643-0867-X
Printed in China
1 2 3 4

Back cover photo: *Town & Country*, 1934.

Published by Schiffer Publishing Ltd.
4880 Lower Valley Road
Atglen, PA 19310
Phone: (610) 593-1777; Fax: (610) 593-2002
E-mail: Schifferbk@aol.com
Please visit our web site catalog at
**www.schifferbooks.com**

This book may be purchased from the publisher.
Include $3.95 for shipping.
Please try your bookstore first.
We are interested in hearing from authors
with book ideas on related subjects.
You may write for a free catalog.

In Europe, Schiffer books are distributed by
Bushwood Books
6 Marksbury Rd.
Kew Gardens
Surrey TW9 4JF England
Phone: 44 (0)208 392-8585; Fax: 44 (0)208 392-9876
E-mail: Bushwd@aol.com

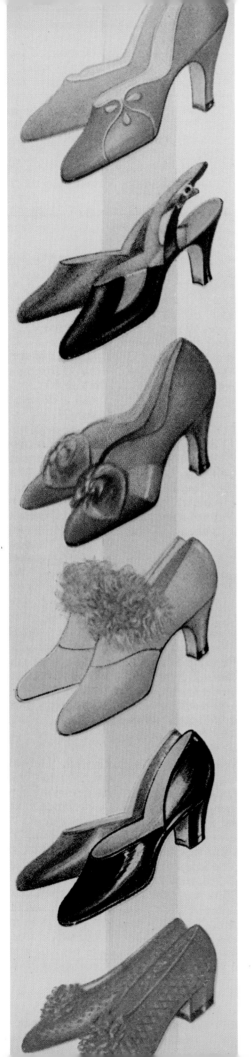

# Contents

# Preface

The history of mankind has always influenced the trends in fashion. The predominant styles of the 20th century are a reflection of the events, wars, economy, new technology, morals, customs, prominent individuals, fashion designers, and the prevailing mood of the period. There is also a strong correlation between fashion and the decorative arts, architecture, and interior design of an era. Therefore, once you are able to "read" them, fashions from the past can give you clues to the social and cultural history of the period in which they were worn. Those studying the history of costume will find it more interesting and easier to understand and remember if they can relate the styles of a period to the events which influenced them. The objects pictured on the following pages chronicle the 1930s, a period of economic instability in our nation's history, and the many lighthearted diversions designed to relieve or temporarily escape the doldrums of the Depression.

This is a "cross-over" book which will appeal to a variety of readers. The comprehensive text and hundreds of color photographs will keep dealers and collectors of vintage clothing and accessories well informed. It will also prove a valuable resource for period costumers and a source of inspiration for contemporary fashion designers. Cultural historians will enjoy the interplay between fashion and history.

The format of this book was designed primarily to meet the needs of two types of readers. First, are those with a genuine interest in all facets of vintage fashion. These readers usually study the book cover to cover, absorbing all they can about clothing and accessories of the decade. Second, are those researching a particular garment or accessory. These readers will find that the text has been organized by chapter and further by heading and subheading, affording easy access to the desired information. The author hopes that everyone else with an interest in fashion will also find this book useful and entertaining.

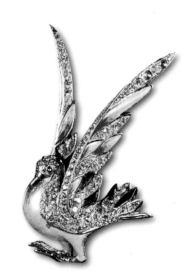

Women's fashions were extremely diverse and subject to numerous style changes within the decade. To adequately discuss the many facets of women's wear, it was necessary to devote eleven chapters to the task. One chapter was devoted to men's wear and one to children's wear as these fashions were less diverse and changes in style were less frequent.

France has been the arbiter of fashion since the days of Louis XIV; therefore, many terms throughout this text are in the French language. The glossary, located at the back of the book, contains the definitions and phonetic pronunciations of French words, along with other terms specific to this discipline.

The values of objects pictured in this book have been placed in the captions for your convenience. Prices vary greatly according to the craftsmanship, overall design, size, color, condition, rarity, and the intrinsic value of the materials. Current fashion trends and the location of the market are also determining factors. The price ranges offered here reflect these variations and are merely a guide.

# Chapter 1

# Historical Overview

Fashion has always been a mirror of what transpired during any given period and the decade of the 1930s was no exception. The following events, technology, art movements, designers, and Hollywood films helped to shape the decade known as the thirties and influenced the fashions worn during this period.

## The Economy

The 1920s had been a period of great prosperity and conspicuous spending. Just when many people were learning to enjoy their new found wealth, however, the good life came to an abrupt end. Millions of Americans had been buying shares of stock on credit, forcing stock prices well above their true value. When analysts issued warnings about the unstable financial conditions, people lost confidence in the economy and a state of panic developed. Investors hastily sold off millions of shares of stock and stormed the banks in an attempt to withdraw their savings. This led to the stock market crash on October 4, 1929, which sent the country reeling into a new decade with a very ominous future. Many people lost their lifes' savings overnight and twelve million workers were out of a job.

## Fashion

The depression which followed the crash created a need to economize at all levels of society. The degree to which this economizing was necessary, however, was relative to the individual. For those fortunate members of the leisure class who survived the crash, it might simply mean canceling the order for that extravagant diamond bracelet or doing without a new fur coat. For them the effects of the depression were not as overwhelming and many could go on about their daily lives in their usual fashion. For some, the harsh effects of the depression began to subside towards the middle of the decade. For those on the lower end of the economic scale, however, life became a constant struggle to make ends meet. "Hand-me-downs" and mended clothing became the order of the day. Unfortunately, the depression widened the gap between the "haves" and the "have-nots." Although the haves represented only a small minority of the population, their influence on fashion was considerable. This book will focus on the fashions worn by upper and middle class men, women, and children during the 1930s.

Since the depression effected the fashion industry on every level, cost became a primary concern from *haute couture* to ready-to-wear. In order to survive, the *couture* houses of Paris responded to the faltering economy with a number of prudent measures. Designers abandoned the expensive bead work so popular during the 1920s. Instead, they focused their attention on sophisticated cut and fluid lines to create designs with a graceful, timeless elegance.

During the teens and twenties, American buyers attended Paris shows and returned to the U.S. with original *couture* fashions which they either resold or copied for the mass market at lower prices. After the crash, however, United States customs discouraged foreign imports by placing duties on original *couture* creations. This rendered Paris originals too expensive for many small retailers to import. To cut their losses French fashion houses produced inexpensive *toiles* (muslin or linen patterns of original designs) which they were permitted to sell duty free to American retailers. To increase their volume of sales, most *couture* houses developed their own *prêt-à-porter* (ready-to-wear) lines and created boutiques in which to sell them. Some resourceful designers made use of inexpensive fabrics which, in the past, were considered too humble for *couture* creations. Chanel and Patou produced striking summer evening wear using economical cottons such as eyelet, organdy, piqué, and lace.

In an effort to cut costs and lower prices manufacturers like Berth Roberts, Fifth Avenue Modes, and Betty Wales Creations offered garments to "finish-at-home." The following excerpts from a 1935 Berth Roberts pamphlet explained this new concept: "...any model which you select, will be made exactly in accordance with your own individual measurements... expert tailors complete every bit of the difficult sewing for you; they make the collars, cuffs, belts, etc. and finish all the work on the intricate new necklines, shoulders, and sleeves and... your garment comes to you in a few completely-made parts...all that's left for you to sew are the seams and the hem."

In order to update their wardrobes with new longer dresses, many working-class women had no choice but to make their own clothing. Recognizing this trend, the yard goods section of the 1931 Sears, Roebuck and Co. catalog used catch phrases such as "In the spirit of smart economy." Readers were encouraged to "Save by making your coat or suit." Thousands of women took up knitting and crocheting to create inexpensive yet stylish dresses, sweaters, hats, gloves, and even handbags.

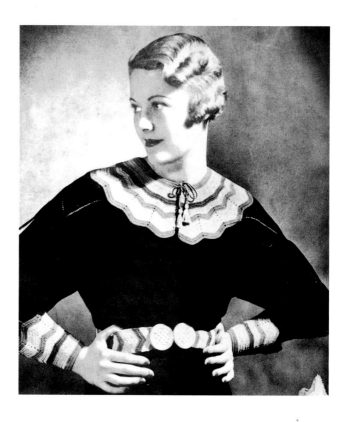

This cover from the Bucilla crochet manual (1934) features a collar with matching belt and cuffs, typical of the hand-crocheted items made during the 1930s. *Courtesy of Elaine Cruse.*

By the 1930s, department stores were well established in all the major cities. These stores offered a choice of fashions to suit every budget. Their *couture* departments featured imported French fashions from designers like Schiaparelli, Vionnet, Chanel, Louiseboulanger, Alix, Worth, Mainbocher, Lelong, Molyneux, Paquin, and Rouff. Private fashion shows of *couture* designs were presented daily for wealthy clientele. Customers could also take advantage of the store's custom dressmaking and tailoring departments. For those on a more modest budget, there were *prêt-à-porter* fashions, many of which were less expensive copies of French *couture* creations. And finally, the piece-goods departments carried fabric and patterns for the do-it-yourselfers.

Many Americans who had grown accustomed to domestic servants during the 1920s could no longer afford this luxury. There was, therefore, a trend toward fabrics which needed less care. Garments made from printed fabrics became desirable as they were less likely to appear soiled than solid colors.

### Politics

Undaunted by crippling polio, Franklin Delano Roosevelt was elected president in 1933 and served for four terms, longer than any other president. During the first 100 days of his administration, Roosevelt implemented his "New Deal" recovery reforms by introducing to Congress mass legislation to establish over 36 new government agencies. These agencies had the power to regulate banks, assist farmers, establish a social security system, promote conservation, develop adequate housing, and provide new jobs for the unemployed through public works projects.

One of the programs designed to promote economic recovery was the NRA (National Recovery Administration), founded in 1933. This agency had the authority to set the lowest prices,

minimum wages, and mandatory quality standards. Any manufacturer who conformed to the NRA codes was permitted to fasten the blue NRA recovery-eagle label on its merchandise and use the recovery logo in its advertising. The NRA was deemed unconstitutional by the Supreme Court on May 27, 1935, therefore, any garments containing an NRA label were produced between 1933 and 1935.

Roosevelt's wife, Eleanor, was well prepared to play an active role as First Lady and she became well known for her humanitarian efforts. She traveled around the country gathering information to keep the president well informed. In addition, she gave numerous lectures and wrote a syndicated daily

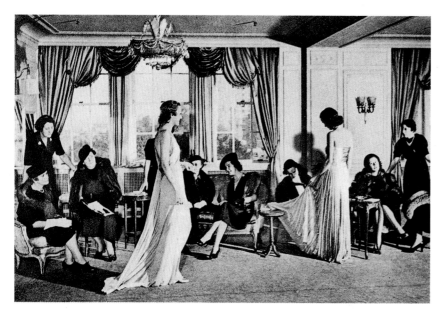

This photograph from *Picture* magazine (2/38) captures wealthy, fur-decked customers watching one of the daily private fashion shows in a salon at Bergdorf Goodman, New York. *Left*: backless gown by Lelong. *Right*: pleated gold-*lamé* halter-style gown by Vionnet.

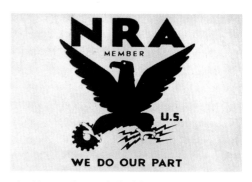

The blue eagle, symbol of the NRA (National Recovery Administration), which was in existence from 1933 to 1934.

8

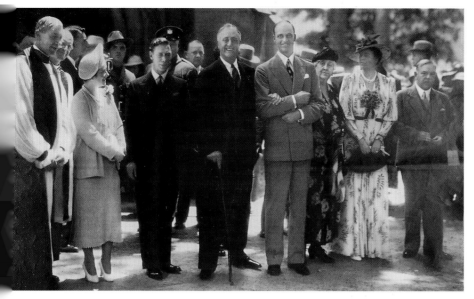

The *Sunday News* (6/2/39) published this photo of King George VI and Queen Elizabeth visiting with President Franklin D. Roosevelt and his wife Eleanor at their home in Hyde Park, New York. The purpose of the visit was to solicit America's support against Germany during World War II.

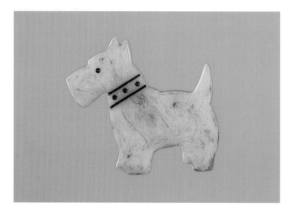

Bakelite Scottie pin in the likeness of President Roosevelt's dog "Fala." $40-$50.

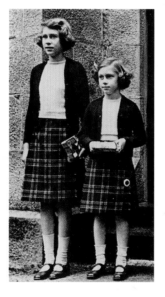

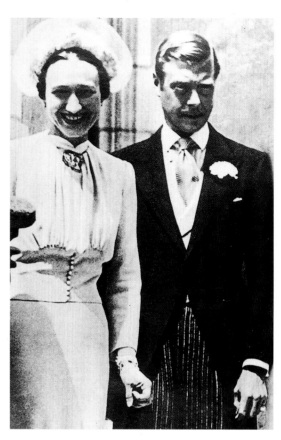

**Above:** *Picture* ran this photo (2/38) of the Duke and Duchess of Windsor on their wedding day, June 3, 1937. She wears a full-length blue jacket dress designed by Mainbocher and halo-shaped headpiece of pink and blue feathers. The Duke wears a morning suit with striped trousers.

**Left:** *Vogue* published this photo (8/1/39) of the English princesses Elizabeth and Margaret wearing matching sweaters and Scottish kilts. The Queen "Mum" invariably dressed her daughters in matching outfits.

newspaper column. Together the Roosevelts led the country through 12 years of adversity created not only by the depression but by the Second World War.

FDR's Scottish terrier, "Fala," became the country's mascot and Americans' fondness for the little dog triggered a "Scottiemania." Scottie pins, bracelets, charms, buttons, napkin rings, book ends, appliqués, and much more were mass produced during the 1930s and 1940s.

### English Royals

Upon the death of King George V of England on January 20, 1936, his eldest son Edward VIII ascended the throne. When Edward announced his intention to marry the American divorcee, Wallis Simpson, he was informed by government officials that she was totally unacceptable. After due deliberation, Edward announced to the British people that he could not undertake his duties as king without the help and support of the

woman he loved. He abdicated the throne and married Wallis Simpson in a civil ceremony at the *Château de Condé* in France on June 3, 1937. They were given the titles Duke and Duchess of Windsor and lived the remainder of their lives (with the exception of the war years) in exile in Paris.

The Duke and Duchess became one of the most celebrated couples of the decade and were considered by many to be great connoisseurs of good taste and fine fashion. The duchess was a fastidious dresser and wore the very best *haute couture* fashions from such designers as Balmain, Schiaparelli, Mainbocher, Molyneux, and Lelong. Many of her shoes were custom made by Roger Vivier, her hats by Caroline Reboux, her bags by Hermés, and her jewels by Cartier and Van Cleef & Arpels.

With no training for the role, Edward's younger brother Albert was duly crowned George VI and his wife, Elizabeth Bowes-Lyon, became Queen Elizabeth. This unexpected turn of events placed their eldest daughter, Elizabeth, the next in line to the throne.

## High Society

By 1931, many wealthy Americans had recovered sufficiently from the jolt of the crash to resume their endless rounds of parties, sports, entertainment, and travel. Like a flock of exotic birds, the wealthy descended upon the playgrounds of the world, to see and be seen by other members of their social circles. Many pampered elite sailed to and from Europe in the height of elegance aboard the newly commissioned luxury liners the Normandy (1935) and the Queen Mary (1936).

Americans finally came to the realization that Prohibition had not solved the drinking problem in this country; in reality it had made matters worse. So, in 1933, prohibition was repealed and "speakeasies" of the "Roaring Twenties" were converted into chic restaurants and nightclubs frequented by the fashionable "café society."

It was a tradition in high society for 18 year old daughters to make their debut into polite society at lavish "coming-out" parties given in their honor by their parents. To celebrate this much anticipated rite of passage, an appropriate *ingénue*-style" gown was ordered from one of the leading *couture* houses.

This gown could be made of shimmering satin, billowy organdy, or *bouffant* layers of tulle. Accounts and photographs of the many parties, dinners, and cotillions of the débutante season were the subject of immense public interest and were eagerly followed in newspapers and magazines. Brenda Frazier, American heiress and one of the most popular débutantes of the decade, made her debut in 1938. Brenda set a trend for strapless evening gowns in the late '30s.

In the hope of meeting some eligible young English lords, the more assertive American mothers arranged to take their daughters abroad and introduce them into London society. The highlight of the trip was their presentation to the King and Queen in the throne room of Buckingham Palace. For this formal occasion, the prescribed code of dress required a long white formal gown with a six-foot train and a white veil with three white ostrich plumes fastened at the back of the head.

## Hollywood

As *This Fabulous Century: 1930 - 1940* (Time and Life Books, Inc. 1969: 180) succinctly put it: "No one who spent time at the movies during the 1930s would ever have known that the nation was down in the dumps." Hollywood movies of the 1930s contained cheerful, optimistic "food for the spirit." Knee-slapping comedies, carefree musicals, and lighthearted romances (all with happy endings) offered the ultimate escape from the harsh realities of life.

Who could resist the graceful strides of Fred Astaire and Ginger Rogers gliding effortlessly over a mirrored floor...he in white tie and tails, she in a gown of frothy white ostrich feathers which fluttered with her every move? Women swooned over Clark Gable, America's favorite leading man, as he tamed a feisty

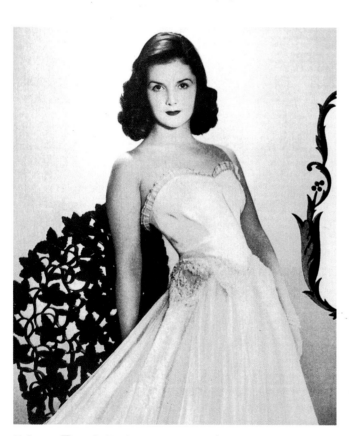

Debutante Brenda Frazier wearing a strapless evening gown which she helped to popularize, 1939.

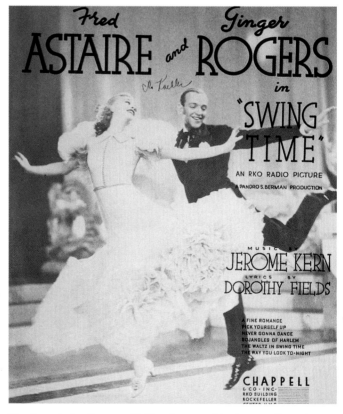

Sheet music for the song "A Fine Romance" by Jerome Kern, which was featured in the movie *Swing Time* (1936) starring Fred Astaire and Ginger Rogers. Her gown (similar to the Letty Lynton dress) is accented at the sleeves and hem with mounds of crisp organdy ruffles.

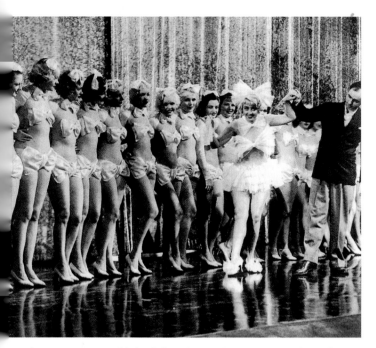

*Film Fun* (1934) published this photo of actress Joan Blondell assisted by dance director Busby Berkeley, as a row of chorus girls look on. Their costumes, for the movie *Dames*, consisted of bodysuits and large butterfly bows.

Claudette Colbert in the romantic-comedy, *It Happened One Night*. Child star, Shirley Temple, became the top box office attraction from 1935 to 1938 and mothers everywhere dressed their daughters in Shirley Temple-style dresses and bouncy ringlets. Parents and children alike enjoyed *Snow White and the Seven Dwarfs*, Walt Disney's first feature-length cartoon.

Busby Berkeley, the master choreographer of 1930s movies, staged extravagant song and dance routines featuring scores of elegant chorus girls dancing in unison through intricate formations. Girls in glamorous bathing costumes became part of a towering water fountain in *Footlight Parade* (1933). His staggering imagination was evident in the spectacular "Shuffle Off to Buffalo" number from *42nd Street* (1933). Dancers, wearing snug little hats and gowns of billowy white organdy, danced about the sleeping cars of a life-sized train which split in half during the number. The piano sequence from the *Gold Diggers of 1935* featured 50 beautiful girls playing 50 white grand pianos arranged in two long rows that stretched as far as the eye could see. Berkeley's desire to glorify women was evident in the human-harps from *Fashion Follies* (1934) and the fiddling fairies in *Gold Diggers of 1933*. Aerial views of his kaleidoscopic dance routines were featured in many of his films and became his well-recognized trademark.

During the 1920s, movie stars were required to provide their own clothing on screen. In 1929, Paris decreed that hems drop below the calf for daytime and to the instep for evening. This sudden change caught the movie studios off guard leaving them with brand new releases featuring short, out-dated dresses.

To prevent this unfortunate situation from recurring, movie moguls hired their own fashion designers. Gilbert Adrian was hired by MGM in 1928 and soon became its top designer. He created glamorous fashions designed to project each star's film persona. For "blonde bombshell," Jean Harlow, he designed slinky bias-cut gowns and satin *négligées* dripping with ostrich feathers. He created the "slouch" hat (a head-concealing version of the *cloche*) for the aloof Greta Garbo and suits with broad masculine shoulders for the assertive roles played by Joan Crawford. Through the efforts of designers like Adrian, Hollywood films provided a never-ending stream of sophisticated fashions which eager viewers quickly emulated.

Selling copies of fashions worn in Hollywood films became a lucrative business. Retailers with Hollywood connections received sketches of the fashions worn in soon-to-be-released movies. The retailers then placed orders for these styles with their manufacturers who mass produced less expensive copies and shipped them to the stores before the movies were released. These Hollywood styles were then promoted in movie magazines, newsreels, and advertising campaigns. The popular "Letty Lynton" dress, worn by Joan Crawford in the 1932 movie of the same name, was a good example of this profitable relationship. Designed by Adrian, this crisp white organdy dress featured multiple rows of billowy ruffles over the sleeves and hem. R.H. Macy in New York alone sold half a million copies of the dress.

Sears, Roebuck and Co. also realized the marketing potential associated with Hollywood stars and often commissioned actresses like Joan Crawford, Claudette Colbert, and Shirley Temple to model fashions for their mail-order catalogs. These garments usually contained a label bearing the star's signature. As Hollywood became more influential, it began to vie with Paris for the role of fashion arbiter.

## Music

In 1934, musician Benny Goodman formed a band and began playing a new kind of jazz called "swing." Teenagers went wild over this spirited music and soon other so-called "big bands" were formed by Glenn Miller, Tommy and Jimmy Dorsey, Artie Shaw, and Count Basie. The lively beat inspired fast swinging dances like the "Lindy Hop," the "Big Apple," and the "Jitterbug." A dance ensemble soon developed which included a sweater or blouse, a full "swing" skirt, and white socks and saddle shoes.

## Radio

Radio not only featured the melodious sounds of the big bands, it broadcast comedy shows like Amos & Andy, Burns & Allen, Fibber McGee & Molly, and the Jack Benny Show. Families would gather around the radio in the evening to listen to their favorite shows.

## World's Fairs

The two world's fairs held during the 1930s were instrumental in introducing new technological advances and the latest styles in architecture and the decorative arts. The theme of the Chicago World's Fair in 1933 was "A Century of Progress," represented by the giant red star Arcturus whirling through the heavens. The architecture of the fair pavilions and the interior design of the sample homes were dominated by the sleek modern lines of Art Deco.

The theme of the New York World's Fair in 1939 was "The World of Tomorrow," symbolized by a futuristic 700-foot tall needle called a Trylon and a 200-foot globe-like Perisphere. Television, robots, and nylon stockings were among the tech

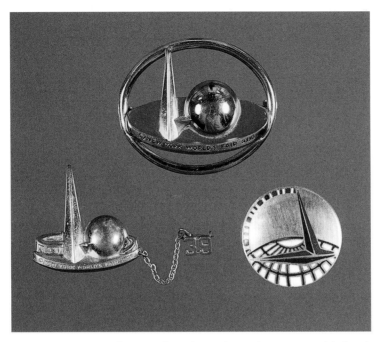

World's Fair pins featuring the trylon and perisphere. *Top:* Gold-plated brass, blue enamel. Marked: New York World's Fair N.Y.W.F. *Left:* Gold-plated brass. Marked: New York World's Fair 1939. A smaller '39 pin attached with chain. *Right:* Modernistic version of the 1939 fair logo decorated in *champlevé* enameling. Marked: LeVelle & Co. Phila, PA. Sterling. *Courtesy of F. Paul Laubner.* $40-$80.

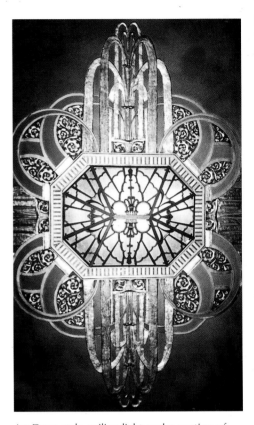

Art Deco-style ceiling light and a portion of the stylized gilt fountains, arches, and Deco roses which embellish the ceiling of the 19th Street Theater in Allentown, Pennsylvania. *Photo by William Childs.*

nological advances introduced at this fair. Souvenirs incorporating World's Fair logos included jewelry, powder compacts, cigarette cases, ash trays, key rings, scarves, and buttons. These items are now called "cross-over" collectibles as they are sought after by both fashion collectors and World's Fair enthusiasts alike. (For a World's Fair scarf see Sportswear, Chapter 6.)

## Art Movements

*Art Deco.* In 1925, the *Parisian Exposition International des Arts Décoratifs et Industriels Modernes,* an international exhibition of modern decorative arts, introduced to the world a new modern form of art, later called "Art Deco." This new movement had a profound effect on all the decorative arts from 1925 to 1935.

Art Deco was characterized by hard-edged geometric shapes, concentric circles, semi-circles, parallel lines (both straight and curved which appeared in the form of "railroad stitching" on many 1930s garments), broad sweeping lines (resembling comet trails), sunrays, star bursts (as in star-cut crystal jewelry), step patterns, converging lines, zigzags, lightning bolts and fountains. These designs were most often used in a symmetrical format. Flowers and leaves were portrayed in a stylized fashion, i.e. the "Deco rose." All motifs, whether natural or abstract, were bold and simplified.

Art Deco was actually an eclectic synthesis of many forces including the elements of several modern art movements, as well as motifs and materials from numerous ancient civilizations. It incorporated clean lines from Purism, geometric interpretation and stylization from Cubism, and dynamic color combinations from Fauvism. It also assimilated sumptuous fabrics from the

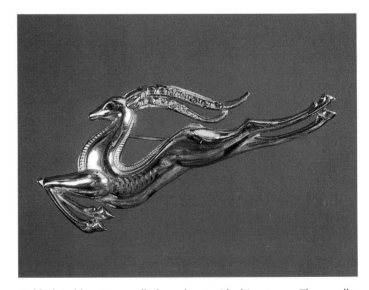

Gold-plated leaping-gazelle brooch set with rhinestones. The gazelle was a motif frequently used during the 1920s and 1930s to symbolize speed. *Courtesy of Suzanne M. Checksfield.* $95-$125.

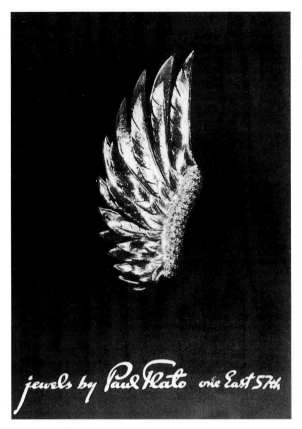

*Harper's Bazaar* advertisement (11/37) for a gold Mercury-wing brooch by renowned jewelry designer, Paul Flato.

Middle East; materials such as jade, carnelian, ivory, and lacquer from China; zigzag patterns from Native American art, and step patterns from the Aztec, Mayan (pyramid), and Assyrian (ziggurat) architecture. Even the bold *sans-serif* letters of the Art Deco-style alphabet reflected the geometric quality of this new art movement.

Newer, faster modes of transportation inspired a preoccupation with speed, and streamlined designs began to emerge in architecture, home furnishings, textiles, and jewelry. "Built for speed" motifs like planes, trains, leaping gazelles, antelopes, whippets, greyhounds, and Mercury's wings were common symbols of this new fast-paced society.

Skyscrapers like New York's Chrysler Building (1930), the Empire State Building (1931), and Rockefeller Center (1931-33) are prime examples of Art Deco-style architecture. The Chrysler Building, in particular, has wonderful triangular windows forming a multiple Deco sunburst-effect often referred to as "zigzag modern."

Art Deco interiors were characterized by curved walls, indirect lighting, fan-shaped lighting fixtures, geometric-shaped furniture, and round porthole-shaped windows and mirrors. Furniture was often finished with Chinese-red and black lacquer or grained veneer creating zigzag-marquetry. Carpets, draperies, wall hangings, and throw pillows were covered in geometric patterns. Sleek chrome railings with rounded corners were a popular feature in homes as well as public buildings.

Sculptures of slender nymph-like female nudes frolicked about every household masquerading as stems on glassware or bases for table lamps. They cavorted across clocks and bookends, and held aloft ashtrays, pipe rests, candles, and compotes. They were often portrayed kneeling, or standing with one leg raised as if engaged in an impromptu dance.

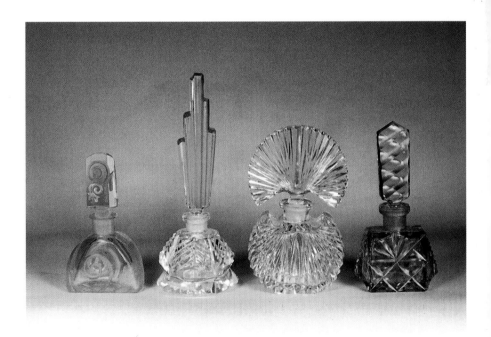

Art Deco Czechoslovakian-glass perfume bottles. Note: architectural styling of second bottle from the left. Marked: Czechoslovakia. *Courtesy of Roxanne Stuart.* $125-$175.

The Chrysler Building in New York City is a prime example of Art Deco-style architecture. It features streamlined design and "zigzag-moderne" window configuration.

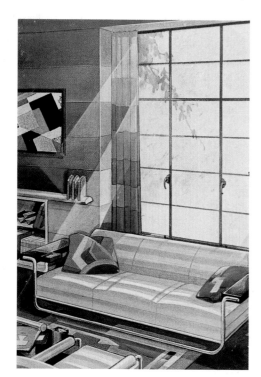

*House & Garden* advertisement (7/30) featuring an Art Deco-style living room containing chrome-plated tube-frame furniture plus pillows, draperies, wall hanging, and carpet decorated in geometric shapes.

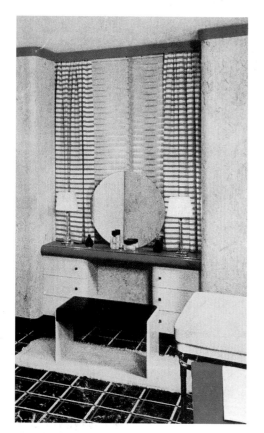

This photograph from *Woman's Home Companion* (10/37) displays an Art Deco-style red and black bathroom containing a woman's dressing table and round mirror.

This Barrett Harden Company advertisement displays a typical Art Deco nymph-like ashtray by Frankart. *Courtesy of Charlette Martin, (Charlette's Web Country Store).*

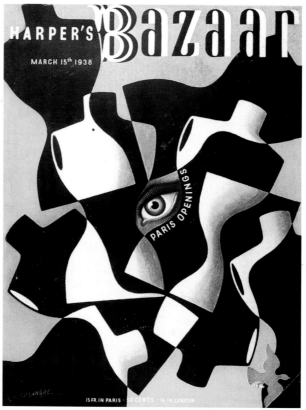

The cover of *Harper's Bazaar* (3/15/38) featuring a Surrealistic painting of an eye surrounded by dress forms. The renowned artist, A. M. Cassandre, painted many such covers for *Harper's* during the 1930s.

Art Deco jewelry, vanity cases, and smoking accessories featured futuristic industrial materials such as Bakelite, chrome, and aluminum. A new "machine esthetics" developed as machines became more involved in the world of decorative arts. Engine-turnings (machine engravings) were a popular form of industrial ornamentation frequently used to decorate metal objects of the 1920s-30s. Machines could engrave these intricate designs in a fraction of the time required for hand engraving.

***Surrealism.*** This hallucinatory form of modern art was based on the artist's wild imagination and the bizarre manifestations of his/her subconscious. It was introduced shortly after World War I, but did not reach its height of popularity until the mid-'30s. Atypical effects were created by moving a familiar object from its customary surroundings to a totally foreign environment or by juxtaposing it with dissimilar objects. Familiar items were also altered to resemble things totally unrelated. The effects were incongruous and deliberately designed to shock or, at the very least, cause a "double-take."

## Haute Couture

Elsa Schiaparelli was born into an aristocratic family and at an early age she began to absorb the splendid artistry and cultural heritage of her native Rome. She was also exposed to the wonders of astronomy through an uncle who allowed her to look through his telescope. Schiaparelli often drew on these childhood images when planning her collections.

Schiaparelli began her fashion career, in 1927, by designing black sweaters with the image of white bows knitted into the pattern. These *faux* bows looked three-dimensional so she named them her *trompe-l'oeil* (trick of the eye) sweaters.

In 1929, Schiaparelli opened her own *couture* house on the Rue de la Paix, where her business grew from just a few knitters in 1929 to 2,000 employees in 1936. Since she had no formal training with the needle and thread, she employed talented craftsmen and seamstresses to execute her designs. Schiaparelli was a great fan of Surrealism. With the help of artist friends like Salvador Dali, Jean Cocteau, Christian Bérard, and Marcel Vertè, she incorporated Surrealism in her *couture* collections. Her outrageous designs included a "shoe hat," "desk suit," "bird cage hat," and an "inkwell hat." With her creative mind and unique sense of mischief, Schiaparelli made Surrealism in fashion extremely chic.

The success of this playful use of art in fashion may be attributed to people's eagerness for amusing diversions during a period of hard times. The eerie dream-like landscapes which appeared in Surrealist paintings were also used as backdrops for window displays and fashion photography during the 1930s.

Schiaparelli's designs influenced many aspects of fashion and her unconventional designs are discussed in various chapters throughout the book.

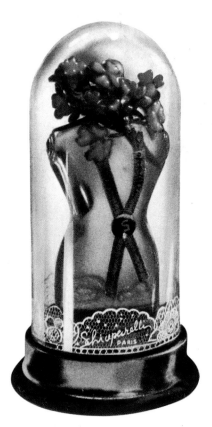

This advertisement for Schiaparelli's perfume, "Shocking," appeared in *Harper's Bazaar* (12/37). It was packaged in a dress-form-shaped bottle embellished with a crisscrossed tape measure and multicolored glass flowers, under a hand-etched Bohemian-crystal dome.

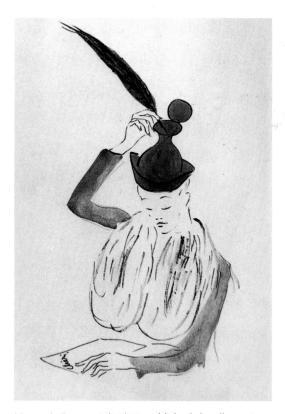

*Harper's Bazaar* (3/15/38) published this illustration by Marcel Vertès featuring Schiaparelli's zany "inkwell" hat complete with quill pen.

Less flamboyant than Schiaparelli, but none the less influential, was French *couturiere* Madeleine Vionnet. In 1927, she developed the bias cut, which revolutionized the principles of dressmaking and dominated fashion design for nearly a decade. Cutting on the bias created a natural elasticity in the fabric which made it easier to drape and mold to the figure. This technique was used to produce the clinging supremely-sensual styles so typical of 1930s evening wear. Vionnet's other contributions to couture include the cowl and halter necklines. (For more information on Vionnet and the bias cut, see Day Wear, Chapter 3).

**World War II and Beyond**

As Hitler's troops marched into Austria and Poland in the late 1930s, the world began to brace itself for yet another world war. During the occupation of Paris in 1940, many designers closed their doors and fled to England or to the United States. American designers could no longer rely on Paris for fashion inspiration and soon began to develop their own unique styles.

Fashions have a way of repeating themselves every thirty or forty years, consequently many 1930s fashions were revived during the late 1960s and 1970s. Wide-leg pants for men and women were resurrected under the new name, "bell-bottoms." Halter and cowl necklines, cape sleeves, bare midriffs, espadrilles, platform shoes, and wedgies were all revived for women during the 1970s. Men's plaid suits, wide lapels, dark shirts with light ties, and monk and moccasin-toe shoes also reappeared at this time.

# Chapter 2

# Lingerie

The word lingerie is derived from the French word *linge*, which means linen. It refers to ladies' intimate apparel including undergarments, sleepwear, and lounge wear which in the distant past had been made of linen.

## UNDERGARMENTS

The flat-chested, boyish silhouette of the 1920s was replaced by the soft sinuous curves of the natural feminine figure of the 1930s. The ideal woman was still slender but more mature with high, gently curving breasts and hips, and a flat stomach. For those women with a slim figure, undergarments were soft and comfortable, leaving the figure undistorted.

The bias cut, introduced by Madeleine Vionnet in 1927, dominated the fashion scene into the late 1930s. This cutting technique produced figure hugging garments which clung sensually to the body. These garments required smooth bias-cut lingerie such as brassieres, panties, combinations, and slips which could provide a sleek smooth contour. Three-dimensional ruffles or ribbon bows were not used on undergarments from 1930 to 1937-38 since they would produce unsightly lumps in the bias-cut garment above. In fact, the slinky backless gowns of the late 1920s and early 1930s were often worn with no undergarments at all (except perhaps a band-aid over each nipple). Undergarments were described as either "tailored" (devoid of ornamentation) or "trimmed" (embroidered, appliquéd, or edged with lace). If they were so inclined, women could embroider their own undies by using handy transfers included in needle-work magazines.

The straight-cut top—which characterized 1920s bandeaux, vests, combinations, and slips—was gradually replaced by the "California" or "V-shaped" top. The silk ribbon straps of the 1920s and early 1930s were soon replaced by adjustable tape straps.

*Fabrics.* The most elegant, admired, and consequently the most expensive undergarments were those made of silk satin, silk crepe de chine, or glove silk. As Alison Carter succinctly put it in her book *Underwear The Fashion History:* "...pure silk [was] for best or for the better-off." (1992:94) Silk undergarments were often embellished with appliqués, embroidery, pull-work, and ecru lace inserts or trim.

The inexpensive synthetic fiber called "rayon" dominated the industry during the depression. It became the mainstay for mass-produced undergarments worn by middle class and elderly women. Rayon was made of cellulose which was obtained from plants. It could be knit or woven into soft fabric with good drapability and its high absorbency made it easy to dye. Prior to 1930, rayon could be distinguished from silk by its tell-tale sheen;

however, technical advances now made it possible to produced a rayon which was "beautifully dull" or "permanently dull." This new rayon was also touted as "run-proof."

A monumental breakthrough in modern corsetry was introduced by the United States Rubber Company in 1931. This new elastic yarn, called "Lastex," had a rubber core wrapped with cotton, rayon, or silk fiber. Lastex could be woven or knit into fabric with high elasticity and "two-way s-t-r-e-t-c-h" which revolutionized the undergarment industry.

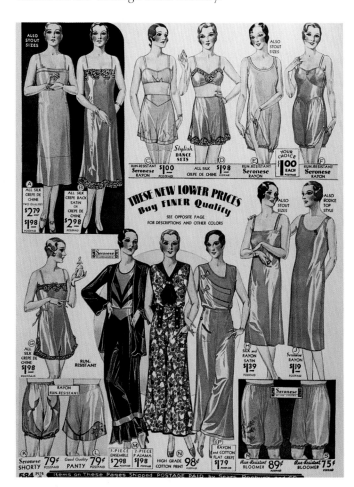

Sears, Roebuck and Co. page (1931) devoted to colorful lingerie. *(A,B)* Straight-top slips. *(C,D)* Dance sets including brassieres and panties. *(E,F)* Tailored bloomer knee suits. *(G)* Combination (teddy). *(H,J)* Tailored slips. *(K)* Rayon shorty bloomers. *(L)* Panties. *(M,N,P)* 2 and 3-piece lounging pajamas with tuck-in tops, Art Deco-style appliqués. *(R,S)* Bloomers.

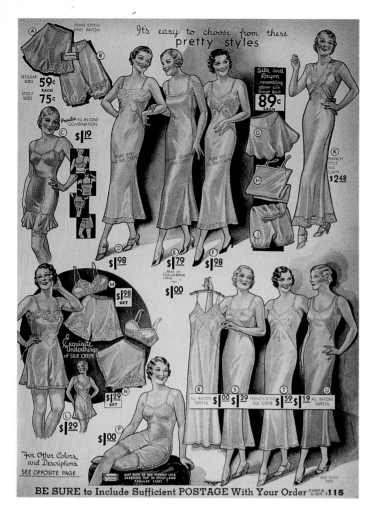

Advertisement from the Sears, Roebuck and Co. catalog (1933-34) for pastel lingerie. (A,G) Panties. (B,J) Bloomers. (C,L) Combinations. (D,E,S) Straight-top slips. (F,R,T) V-top slips. (H) Vest. (K) Nightgown. (M,N) Dance sets. (P) Bloomer knee suit.

**Colors.** The most popular colors for undergarments were pastels such as flesh, tea rose (light pink with a slight tint of orange), peach, Nile green (medium green), pale blue, buttercup, lavender, and occasionally white. Black and navy were added during the second half of the decade.

**Trapunto.** This decorative form of quilting was used on clothing and handbags during the late 1930s and 1940s. Unlike conventional quilting, which is often used for warmth, trapunto was created primarily for ornamentation. In traditional quilting, a layer of padding is sandwiched between the two layers of fabric. All three layers are the same size and shape. Running stitches are then made through all three layers covering the entire piece. In trapunto, the garment part to be decorated was made of only two thicknesses of fabric, the top and the backing. A small section of the chosen design was outlined with small running stitches through both layers. A tiny slit was then made in the backing, inside the outlined area. A small amount of cotton batting was then inserted into the slit, thus puffing up the small outlined area. This procedure was repeated with each small section of the design. Only the desired portions of the design were raised, leaving the remaining background area flat. Since it was difficult to stuff large sections uniformly, the designs best suited to this type of quilting were those with numerous small sections. Trapunto added dimension to the design, which was the most effective on solid-color fabric. This form of decoration was also used on dresses, coats, suits, and "sculptured" handbags. (For more examples of trapunto see Chapters 4, 7, and 9.)

## Brassiere

Brassieres were slowly evolving from the flattening bandeaux of the 1920s, to the uplifting supporters and conical shapers of the 1940s. They were designed for the slender, youthful figure and were created to "elevate, separate, and define" the breasts. Brassieres covered the bust only, and early models contained either vertical gathers or an adjustable drawstring between the breasts for shaping. Later versions contained tucks or darts to form shallow cups resembling a pre-teen training bra. Some cups were cut in two horizontal or vertical sections. By mid-decade, a triangular elastic gore was added between the breasts for a smooth fit. These styles were made of soft fabrics such as rayon satin, rayon jersey, silk crepe de chine, cotton-backed satin, lace, or rayon mesh. The most popular colors for brassieres were flesh, tea rose, and peach.

A long-line brassiere was devised for the fuller figure. It was designed not only to control the bust, but to slenderize the diaphragm and therefore required firmer fabric such as rayon patterned cotton brocade, rayon and cotton faille, rayon jacquard, coutil, and cotton madras. These styles had either "built-up" shoulders or fancy patterned-cotton tape straps.

The return to a shapelier figure was evident in the 1933-1934 Sears, Roebuck and Co. catalog which advertised the "Form Bust" brassiere. The captions read "Why be flat-chested? Do you lack the fascinating curves of the smart full-busted figure? If so, then you need a 'Form Bust' - a style that fills you out to firm, rounded shape." The "underdeveloped" bust could be augmented or fleshed out, in this case, by the use of removable Kapok pads (falsies) which fit into the inside pockets of the brassiere. These were later replaced by "lightweight bust pads made of an "Aerofoam" core (whipped latex) covered by six tiers of gathered net. In 1939, "light airy perforated rubber bust pads, covered with soft rayon" were advertised.

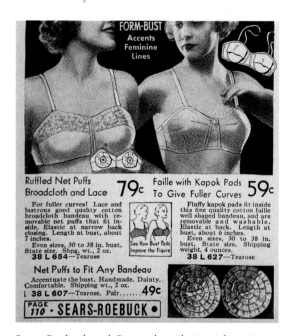

Sears, Roebuck and Co. catalog ad (1936) featuring two "Form Bust" bandeaux (brassieres). *Left:* Lace and broadcloth with removable net puffs (falsies). *Right:* Faille with built-in pockets for Kapok removable pads.

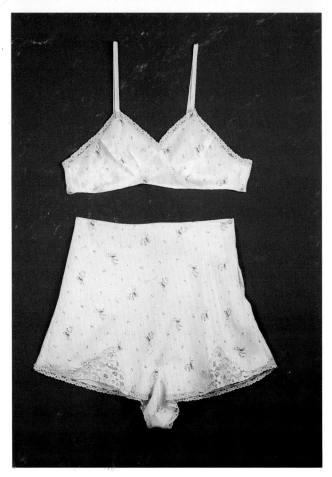

"Dance set" of gossamer-fine silk in pale-pink mini-floral print decorated with lace inserts and trim. $25-$40.

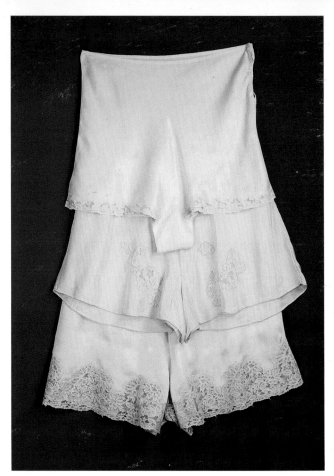

Silk tap panties with banded waists and two buttoned side plackets. *Top:* Flesh silk satin with lace trim. *Center:* Peach silk with matching lace inserts. *Bottom:* White silk-satin with ecru lace. $20-$25.

The strapless bra was introduced in 1938 as a foundation for the new strapless evening gowns. Strapless styles, however, were soon put on the back burner until after the war.

In 1935, the Warner Company devised a new standardized system for determining cup sizes. Four different sets of cup measurements were identified by the letters A, B, C, and D. This system was very successful and is still used today.

**Panties**

The term panty referred to the wide-leg underpants which ended at mid-thigh. They were also referred to as "tap pants" as they resemble the short pants worn by tap dancers in 1930s movies. They were produced in three waist styles: all elastic, narrow hem, or a waist-yoke front and an elastic back. The yoke was usually cut on the straight of the fabric, while the legs were cut on the bias, allowing the fabric to fall in graceful fluted folds. The most desirable panties were made of silk crepe or silk satin with inserts of lace or delicate appliqués. Less expensive run-proof rayon-knit panties were produced in trimmed or tailored variations. Some were made of rayon containing dull and shiny satin stripes. "Step-ins" (a carry-over from the 1920s) were similar to the pantie; however, they had a notch at the hem on either side. "Dance sets," consisting of a brassiere and matching panties or step-ins, were worn primarily by slender, young women during the 1920s and '30s.

**Bloomers**

Bloomers were a carry-over from the 1920s and were phased out in the late '30s. They were loose-fitting underpants which were gathered with elastic just above the knee. The waist was

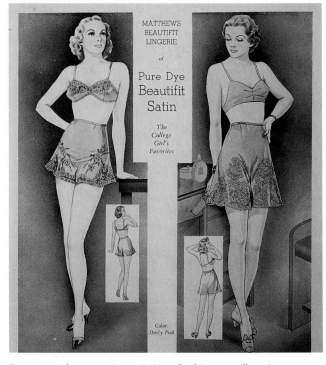

Dansettes (dance sets) consisting of a bias-cut silk satin brassiere and tap panties decorated with Alençon lace and embroidery, 1937-38.

all elastic or contained a pointed yoke front and an elastic back. "Brief bloomers," "shorty bloomers," or "bloomerettes" ended at mid-thigh. Bloomers were made of "run-proof" rayon knit, silk crepe, silk satin, or sateen.

## Panty Briefs

The leg openings on briefs, introduced in the early 1930s, were cut above the thigh and were favored by younger women. The 1937 Sears, Roebuck and Co. catalog advertised their rayon briefs as "skin-smooth," "without the shadow of a wrinkle," and promised "they cling to the body like a second skin." This style is still in use today.

## Bloomer Knee Suit

The "bloomer knee suit," also known as a "bloomer combination" (camiknickers during the 1920s), was a combination of the vest and bloomers. The bloomers contained side plackets which buttoned at the elasticized knee. Some varieties also had hooks and eyes on the side of the vest portion. This fashion had all but disappeared by the end of the decade.

## Combination

The combination, also known as a "step-in-chemise" or "teddy," was a combination of the chemise or vest, and panties or step-ins. A carry-over from the 1920s, this garment resembled a short slip with a narrow crotch. The tubular combinations of the '20s were cut on the straight of the fabric, with a straight drawstring neckline. Combinations of the mid-to-late 1930s, however, were cut on the bias for a more figure-hugging fit over the bust and waist. To further define the waist, a half girdle was attached at the side seams and tied at the back, thus drawing the fabric in to the waist. (Sashes of this kind were also common on nightgowns and pajamas.) The straight neckline was soon replaced by the V-shaped or California top. Combinations were made of silk crepe de chine, silk satin, or rayon knit and ranged from tailored and austere to ultra feminine.

## Corselette

The figure-hugging bias-cut garments of the 1930s looked best on the slender figure. Those with full figures would require the assistance of firm corsetry.

The corselette, also known as an "all-in-one" or "long-line" was the foundation of choice for most stout women. An inner belt propped up the abdomen, while the outer layer prevented unsightly bulges and created a smooth line from bust to thigh. All this was achieved through heavy canvas, Para rubber, steel boning, hooks and eyes, and tight lacing. These torture chambers were given tricky names like Y.B.Stout and Dia-trim. "You're 3 to 6 inches slimmer the minute you put on this marvelous reducing garment," touted the National Bellas Hess advertisement. Each corselette contained four metal/rubber hose garters suspended from adjustable elastic supporters. As the decade progressed, lace-up corsets were worn mainly by elderly women, while younger women preferred the newer, more comfortable Lastex foundations.

## Girdle and Pantie-Girdle

Girdles and pantie-girdles made of two-way stretch Lastex were the last word in comfort and control from the early 1930s

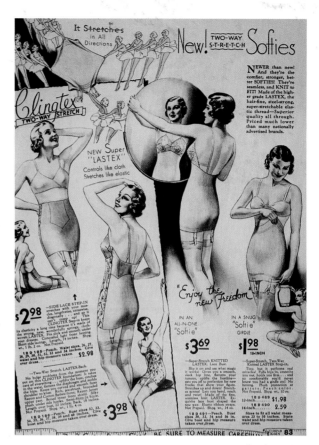

Sears, Roebuck and Co. catalog page (1933-34) advertising girdles and long-line corsets made of the new two-way s-t-r-e-t-c-h fabric called Lastex. "Stretches with your muscles lengthwise, crosswise, diagonally, and so it can't creep up. It takes care of everything... uplifts the bust, cinches in the waist, flattens the diaphragm, and molds the hips."

on. The "roll-on," which consisted of a seamless tube of circular-knit Lastex, let you "bend, reach, twist, and sit without riding up." Since earlier corsets and girdles were difficult to launder, they were worn over other undergarments which absorbed perspiration and body oils. Lastex girdles, on the other hand, were easy to wash and could therefore be worn next to the skin. By 1935, many girdles featured the new Talon slide fastener (zipper). Each girdle contained four metal hose garters suspended from adjustable elastic supporters.

## Vest

The vest was a simple tubular undergarment for the upper torso. It had a straight drawstring top (often with a picot edge) and ribbon straps. It was generally hip or thigh length and was worn tucked into knickers or panties. Glove silk or rayon knit were the common fabrics used to make this tailored garment.

## Union Suit

Also known as "long johns," these tailored all-in-one garments were worn in cool weather by both sexes and all ages. They were made with a round or scooped neckline; built-up shoulders or straps; long, short, or no sleeves; and long or short legs. Union suits were produced in form-fitting ribbed knit cotton, rayon, wool, or combinations of these fibers and often featured picot edging. With the advent of central heating, long knitted union suits were not the necessity they once had been.

## Slip

Early slips (a carry-over from the 1920s) were tubular and cut on the straight of the fabric with a straight neckline. The bias-cut figure hugging dresses of the 1930s, however, required bias-cut slips with no extraneous fabric. Full-length evening slips were often cut with a deep V at the back in keeping with low-backed evening gowns of the early '30s. Day slips followed the prevailing dress lengths, mid-calf or longer through 1937, just below the knee from 1938-40. The V-shaped "California top" soon replaced the straight top and an arched or inverted V-shaped seam was placed just under the bust. A "shadow-proof" double-front panel was added, particularly to summer slips, so that the outline of women's thighs and crotch were not visible through sheer dresses. Slips of the late '30s contained a slight flair at the hem to enhance the fashionable fuller skirts introduced at this time. This flair was often achieved by the use of a pleated or gathered flounce attached to the bottom of the slip. Adjustable straps became commonplace by the late 1930s.

Slips were made of silk satin, silk crepe de chine, and rayon. White cotton broadcloth and nainsook were also available. Early slips were made in pastel colors such as flesh, tea rose, Nile green, light blue, and buttercup. Black, navy, and burgundy were added to this spectrum later in the decade.

## Petticoat

To enhance the fuller skirts produced towards the end of the decade, the 1939 Sears catalog featured a flared petticoat or half slip. It was made of taffeta and was touted to produce "just the right polite rustle," known as *frou-frou* to the French. It was composed of flared gores with a full pleated flounce at the hem.

## Dress Shields

Crescent-shaped dress shields made of gum rubber covered with cotton nainsook were pinned to the inside of a dress, blouse, or sweater at the armseye to protect the garment from perspiration stains.

## Garter Belt

Garter belts were designed to support stockings and were worn by those slender women who did not need the intense constraints of a corset or girdle. They were made of *coutil*, poplin, or rayon striped or figured cotton with elastic sides. Each garter belt contained four metal hose garters suspended from adjustable elastic supporters.

## Hose

Sheer silk chiffon stockings were the most coveted and also the most expensive stockings on the market. Rayon was the inexpensive substitute for silk and consequently the everyday hose for most women during the depression. Ribbed cotton *lisle* and wool were used for sport and for added warmth in winter.

In 1938, the du Pont Company introduced the first lightweight, completely synthetic fiber which it called "nylon." It was ideal for hosiery as it was strong, elastic, mildew and moth resistant, and when hung up wet, needed very little ironing. Nylon was less absorbent than other textiles and therefore dried quickly. Women were just beginning to appreciate the advantages of nylon when it was taken off the market to make parachutes during the Second World War.

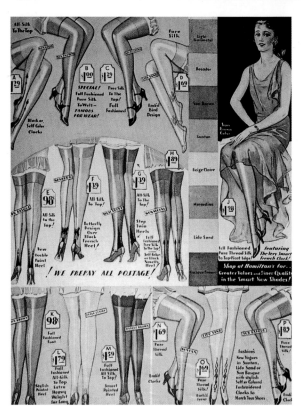

*Hamilton Garment Co.* advertisement (1930) for fancy silk hose with decorative heels and embroidered clocks.

Stockings of the early 1930s featured "clocks," a fashion first worn by men during the 16th century. It consisted of an embroidered arrow motif over the ankles which resembled the hand of a clock. Another decorative but short-lived feature of the early 1930s was the dark reinforced sole and heel which was visible above the back of the shoe. It often took the shape of a pointed dagger, steps, double steps, double arrows, minarets, or butterflies. The desirable "full-fashion marks" or "fashioning marks" were small dots in the knit along the seam created by increasing or decreasing stitches.

Knee-length stockings, with Lastex bands at the top, were available circa 1935. They were an ideal alternative under the longer skirts and wide-leg pants of the period.

Hosiery was produced in various flesh tones including beige, taupe, suntan, sable, blush, nude, onion skin, champagne, and a medium gray called "gunmetal."

# SLEEPWEAR

## Nightgowns

Nightgowns of the early 1930s were loose, shapeless, dartless tubes, a carry-over from the 1920s. Cotton nightgowns with square, V, or U-shaped necklines were hand embroidered in the Philippines and Puerto Rico. The waistline became a bit more defined on some nightgowns by the use of vertical pin tucks and/or a half girdle (sash) attached at the side seams and tied at the back.

Nightgowns of the mid-to-late 1930s featured high waists and were cut on the bias for a more figure-hugging fit. They became more elaborate, utilizing many of the same clothing details found on dresses of the period. These details included a small collar and a false placket with non-functioning buttons stitched down the center of the bodice. Cape, cap, and ruffled sleeves were also common.

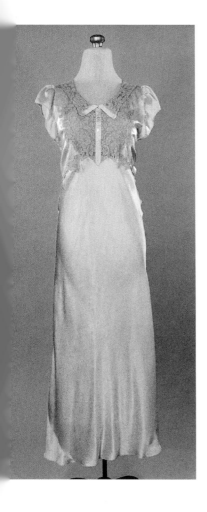

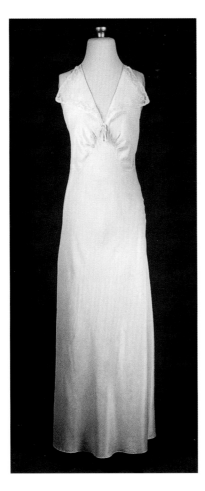

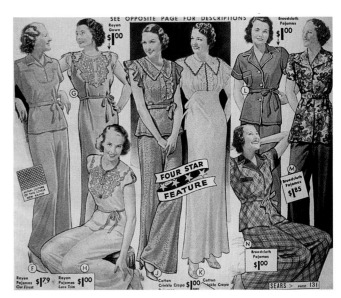

**Above:** Catalog page from Sears, Roebuck and Co. (1937) featuring nightgowns and pajamas. *(F,G,H)* Rayon. *(J,K)* Cotton crinkle crepe. *(L,M,N)* Man-tailored pajamas of cotton broadcloth. Note: sashes.

**Left:** Peach silk-satin nightgown featuring a lace collar and bodice with false placket, ruffled-wing sleeve, and bias-cut skirt. *Courtesy of Mary Anne Faust (Yesterday's Delights).* $50-$75.

**Far Left:** Peach silk sleeveless nightgown, empire waist, *rever* collar trimmed with lace. *Courtesy of Virginia B. Squair.* $40-$60.

By 1938-39, summer nighties resembled evening gowns. Their sleeveless V-neck tops were gathered into a high empire waistline. Winter gowns contained shoulder yokes and long sleeves. Some contained matching hip-length jackets or boleros.

Nightgowns were made of cotton batiste, silk crepe, rayon crepe, cotton crinkle crepe, and nainsook for summer and flannel for winter. Printed fabrics were frequently used for sleepwear as they were cheaper to produce than embroidery. Tea rose, light blue, Nile green, and yellow were the most common colors.

## Sleeping Pajamas

The word pajama stems from the Hindi word *"paejama,"* which means leg clothing. Early 1930s pajamas consisted of a loose tubular tunic with a *rever* or shawl collar and a girdled waist, worn over wide-leg pants. Popular colors for pajamas during the early 1930s were coral, honey dew, and Nile green. Stripes, plaids, florals, and abstracts were the common prints.

Pajamas of the mid-to-late 1930s contained a hip-length overblouse with either a full or a half girdle attached at the sides and tied in the back. Clothing details, similar to those found on nightgowns and dresses, were added to bodices. These details included Peter Pan or pointed collars, false placket fronts with decorative buttons, and cape, cap, baby doll, or ruffled wing sleeves. Some featured a bib front which created the look of a demure blouse.

When Claudette Colbert donned Clark Gable's pajamas in the movie *It Happened One Night,* it triggered a trend for man-tailored pajamas for women. They featured a hip-length button-front tailored shirt with a notched collar, contrasting piping, and a girdled waist.

In the late 1930s, shoulder yokes were added, creating the look of a loose-fitting smock. Puffed sleeves often created a square-shouldered

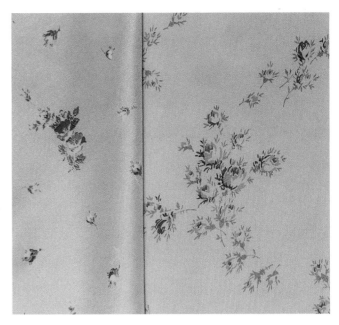

Silk fabric with miniature floral patterns used for lingerie during the 1930s. *Courtesy of Mary Anne Faust (Yesterday's Delights).*

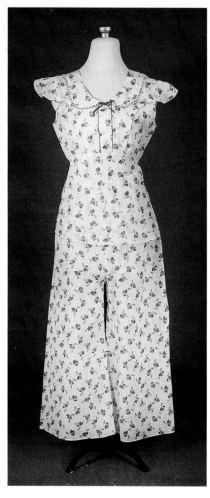

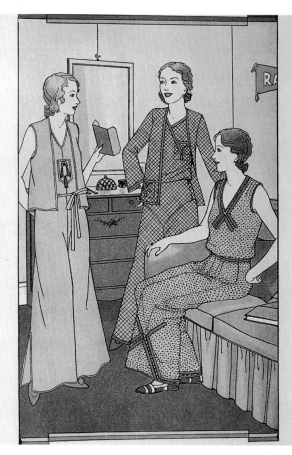

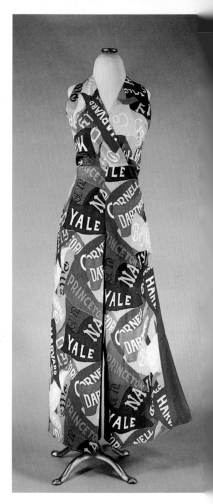

Floral-print cotton-batiste pajamas, Peter-Pan collar, false placket, ruffled sleeve, wide-leg pants, half sash ties in back, c. 1936-37. *Courtesy of Mary Anne Faust (Yesterday's Delights).* $60-$75.

Butterick pattern ad (1931) for wide-leg lounging pajamas and matching jackets. Suggested fabrics: gingham, dimity, or percale with contrasting bias binding.

One-piece cotton lounging pajamas in typical '30s novelty print featuring a collage of college-pennants. Wide legs were created by use of long red pointed *godets* on either side. $100-$125.

effect which continued into the 1940s. Wide-leg pants were typically used with pajama styles throughout the 1930s. Ski-style pajamas were an exception to the rule, however, featuring a rib-knit style neck and cuffs at the wrists and ankles.

Cotton batiste, rayon crepe, and cotton crinkle crepe (which needed no ironing) were used for summer, while cotton flannel and corduroy were used for winter. Pajamas were embellished with tucks, lace, piping, hem-stitching, embroidery, and ruffles. Florals were the most prevalent prints.

# LOUNGE WEAR

## Lounging Pajamas

Colorful lounging pajamas were introduced in the late 1920s and were worn for relaxing or informal entertaining in the home or at the beach. (For examples of beach pajamas see Sportswear, Chapter 6). While pajamas of the 1920s featured loose, hip-length "out-blouses," early 1930s styles called for "tuck-in" tops. These tops were usually sleeveless with a V or U-shaped neckline and flowing wide-leg pants. The tops often contained appliqués, some with wide sweeping lines resembling comet trails.

By 1934, lounging pajamas began to assume many of the clothing details used for dresses of the period. Man-tailored shirt-waist tops with notched collars were popular along with the classic middy blouse. Others had *rever* collars or cowl necklines. Russian-style hip-length tops contained a stand-up band collar, an off center closing, and a girdled waist. Practical three-piece ensembles contained a top, pants, and a tunic-length long-sleeved jacket or a short bolero with puffed sleeves.

Wide-leg pants creating the effect of a long skirt were used for pajamas throughout the 1930s. To increase the width at the hem, the sides of the legs were frequently cut away on either side from hip to hem, to allow for the insertion of long bias-cut triangular or arch-shaped *godets* in a contrasting color or print. Another decorative option was a contrasting band of fabric (from two to eighteen inches deep) stitched to the bottom of the pajama legs.

One-piece pajamas (resembling contemporary jumpsuits) often had a high arched or inverted V-shaped seam just under the bust. Some were made like bib overalls, while others featured a halter top. A belt or girdle was tied around the waist, or attached at the sides and tied at the back. Long bias-cut *godets* were also employed on the legs of one-piece pajamas for increased flare.

Lounging pajamas were made of cotton voile, cotton broadcloth, rayon knit, cotton crinkle crepe, and corduroy. They were made of solid or printed fabrics in florals, polka-dots, checks, and plaids. The collar, waist yoke, pockets, appliqués, and piping were often made of a color which contrasted with the rest of the garment. A print and a coordinating solid color, or twin prints were often used in the same garment.

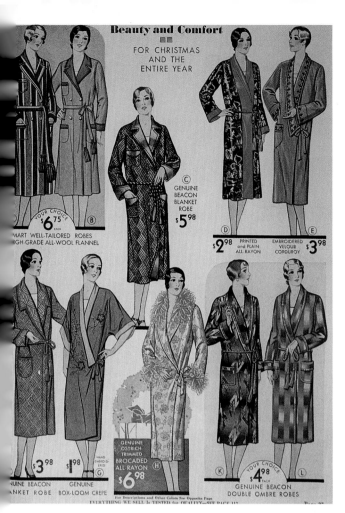

The Bellas Hess catalog (1930-31) offered these robes made from a variety of fabrics. (A,B) Wool felt. (D) Rayon. (E) Corduroy. (C,F,K,L) Beacon *ombré* blanket robes. (G) Crepe kimono. (H) Rayon-brocade *négligée*.

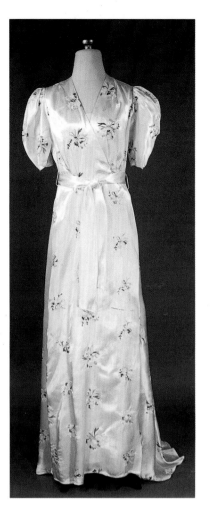

Surplice-style ivory rayon-satin robe, puffed sleeves and sash. Multicolored machine-embroidered flowers. $50-$75.

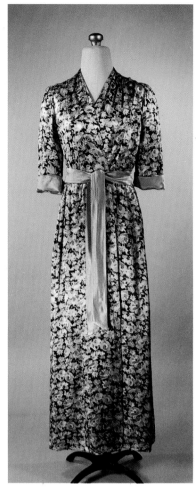

Surplice-style floral-print satin robe with peach satin cuffs and sash, hand made in 1938. *Courtesy of Marie Kozar.* $30-$40.

## Robes

*Bathrobes.* The majority of 1930s bathrobes had a surplice-style closing and a girdled waist. Many spring and summer robes of the early 1930s, were based on the Oriental kimono and were created from Oriental floral print fabric. The tuxedo collar and the bands at the cuffs and hem were often made of a solid contrasting color. Some models featured ruffles in place of the bands which created a feminine touch. Striped cotton-crepe robes with a tuxedo collar or pointed *rever* collar offered a more tailored look.

Soft fluffy Beacon robes were made of cotton blanket-cloth in solids or prints resembling flowers, leaves, dots, or abstract patterns. The shawl or notched collar, the cuffs, and the pockets were often made of a coordinating color, then edged with lustrous rayon cord. Blanket robes were girdled with rayon cord ending in tassels.

Bathrobes in the late 1930s had a more structured, fitted appearance. Sleeves, both short and long, were cut fuller at the top and were pleated into the armseye to create a puff which extended above the shoulders. Puffed sleeves formed a much broader shoulder line which remained in style throughout the Second World War. The tuxedo and *rever* collars were joined by the convertible collar, which resembled a notched collar when open and a short pointed collar when buttoned to the neck. The flared sweeping skirts were

**Right:** Sears, Roebuck and Co. catalog page (1939) advertising house coats with pleat-top sleeves and flared skirts. (A,B) Chenille. (C) Quilted rayon taffeta. (D) Spun rayon. (E) Rayon taffeta, zipper front. (F) Rayon taffeta, trapunto on sleeves. (G) Gypsy-style, rayon crepe, lime green top with bishop sleeves.

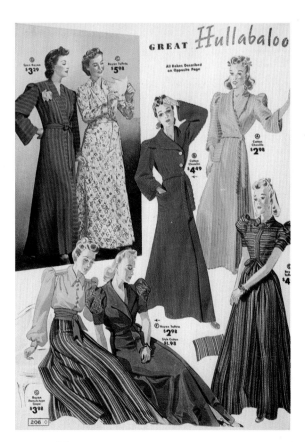

GREAT *Hullabaloo*

All Robes Described on Opposite Page

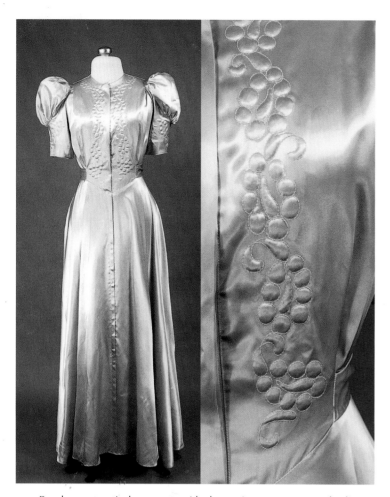

Peach rayon-satin housecoat with decorative trapunto over bodice and puffed sleeves, c. 1938-1939. $75-$85.

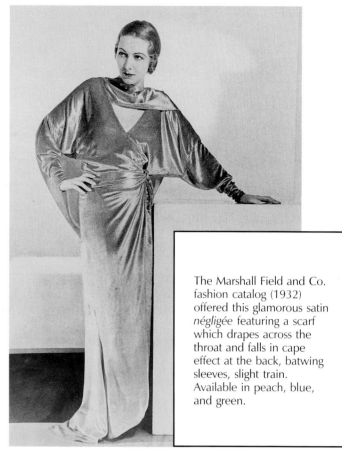

The Marshall Field and Co. fashion catalog (1932) offered this glamorous satin *négligée* featuring a scarf which drapes across the throat and falls in cape effect at the back, batwing sleeves, slight train. Available in peach, blue, and green.

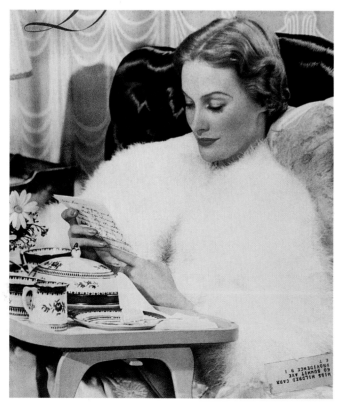

*Delineator* (2/37) image featuring a woman wearing a white marabou-feather bed jacket from Saks-Fifth Avenue. Note: short hair parted in the center.

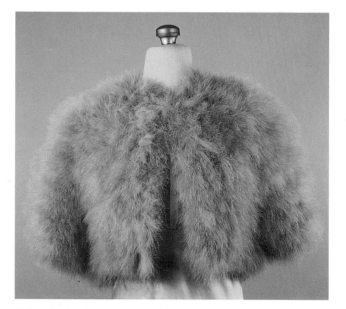

Taffeta bed jacket covered with pink marabou feathers. *Courtesy of Mary Anne Faust (Yesterday's Delights).* $125-$150.

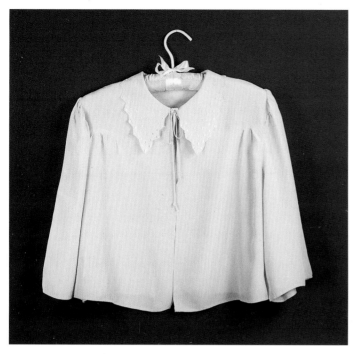

Peach rayon bed jacket with embroidered scalloped collar. $25-$35.

made from wide gores which were now cut on the straight of the fabric. Designers also began to utilize the new slide fastener (zipper) which was placed down the center front.

Common fabrics for summer robes were silk satin, rayon satin, cotton crepe, seersucker, organdy, and rayon containing alternating dull and shiny satin stripes. Winter robes were made of cotton blanket cloth, all-wool flannel, wool challis, velvety corduroy, quilted rayon taffeta, rayon moiré taffeta, terrycloth, rayon brocade, and chenille. Popular colors were royal blue, maroon, navy, brown, rose, burgundy, scarlet, and American Beauty (another name for Schiaparelli's "shocking pink").

*Négligées.* These long, loose, luxurious robes were worn in the privacy of the home or the boudoir. *Négligées* of the 1930s were usually made of satin or silk velvet trimmed with ostrich or marabou feathers. Hollywood seductress, Jean Harlow, was frequently photographed in sensual satin négliées and boudoir slippers.

## Bed Jackets

For the convalescent or for those who like to read or have breakfast in bed, a short bed jacket could be worn over the nightgown. It was generally made of silk crepe de chine, silk satin, lace, or rayon knit and decorated with embroidery, hemstitching, shirring, quilting, or lace. Pastels such as peach, tea rose, flesh, and pale blue were the most prevalent colors. The most unusual bed jackets of the decade, however, were made of fluffy marabou feathers. This style often doubled as an evening jacket.

## Slippers

*Felt Slippers.* Felt bedroom slippers were a carry-over from the 1920s. Some contained a moccasin-style U-shaped seam over the vamp, while others were plain. Some had ribbon laced through slits around the neck, and others had a turnover collar which was pinked at the edge or covered in a coordinating plaid fabric or soft fur. They were occasionally edged with two-toned rayon cord and accented on the vamp with a puffy pompon or ribbon rosette. These slippers were made in solid colors or mottled heather felt and had soft flat soles and heels. A similar slipper was made of quilted satin.

*Sheepskin Slippers.* Winter slippers were made of tan sheep's skin with the fleece on the inside creating a soft, warm lining. The tops were turned down to form a fuzzy collar. These slippers had wide round toes and flat soles.

*Backless Scuffs.* Scuff-style slippers contained fronts but no backs and a flat sole with no heels. This style often featured fur cuffs over the instep.

*D'Orsay Slippers.* Tailored d'Orsay-style boudoir slippers contained closed heels and toes with broad V-shaped open sides. They featured 1 3/4-inch Cuban or 1 1/2-inch military heels. They were commonly made of leather, corduroy, rayon crepe, satin, velveteen, or jacquard and occasionally featured fur or marabou cuffs over the instep for a glamorous look.

*Bridge slippers.* The Sears, Roebuck and Co. catalog described bridge slippers as "ideal for house wear yet a little more dressy than boudoir slippers." They were cut away at the sides in a gentle shallow curve and often featured bows over the vamps.

*Mules (Slingbacks).* "Mules" or backless slippers now featured new adjustable backstraps. These slippers were still referred to as mules in 1930s catalogs, however, as the term "slingbacks" had apparently not yet been coined. They were commonly made of kid, velveteen, or rayon satin and trimmed with appliqués, marabou feathers, gathered trim, or matching bows.

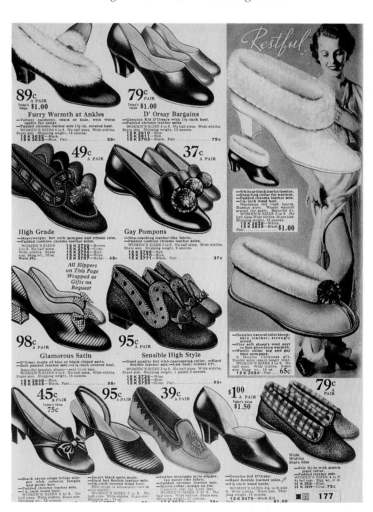

Sears, Roebuck and Co. catalog page (1935-36) displaying a variety of slipper styles including two *d'Orsay*, four felt, one bridge slipper, one slingback, two pajama bootees (boot), one lambskin slipper.

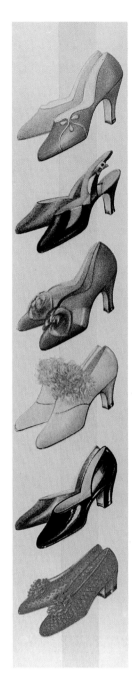

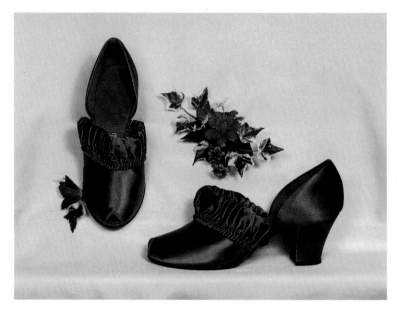

Above: Wine satin *d'Orsay* boudoir slippers, open sides and toes, Cuban heels, and gathered satin trim. Marked: Daniel Green Comfy. $75-$85.

Left: Daniel Green advertisement (3/31) for boudoir slippers. *(1,5) d'Orsay* slippers - peach crepe, black patent. *(2)* Sling-backs - black satin. *(3)* Bridge slippers - lavender with bows. *(4)* Pajama boots - pale green crepe and marabou. *(6)* Flat slipper - orange quilted satin with pompon.

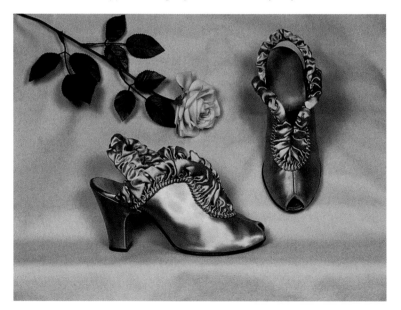

Blue satin boudoir slippers, gathered satin trim and back straps, open toes. Labeled *"frou-frou"* style in Daniel Green ad, 12/39. $80-$90.

**Pajama Boots.** Referred to as "bootees" in National Bellas Hess Co. catalogs, pajama boots covered the entire foot, ending just under the ankle. They were made of silk crepe or quilted satin and trimmed with marabou, rabbit fur, or lambs wool.

The most common colors for slippers were black, red, and blue. Slippers were often two-toned using the common combinations of red and black or blue and black. As the decade progressed, these colors were joined by Copenhagen blue (medium blue-gray) and burgundy.

# Chapter 3

# Day Wear

## DRESSES

After the waistline dropped to the hips in 1922, the natural waist remained invisible for nearly eight years. In his 1929 collection, French designer Jean Patou returned the waistline to its natural position. In the same collection he lowered the hemline for day dresses from the knee to just below the calf. Ironically the short, economical styles of the 1920s ended at a time when many women had little money to replace an outdated wardrobe. Some women of modest means were forced to sew an extra band of fabric to the hems of their short, outmoded dresses. Circa 1937, hemlines rose again to the knee where they remained throughout the Second World War.

The ideal woman was no longer a youthful "five foot two" with no trace of bust or hips. The consummate 1930s beauty was tall, slender, and mature with small rounded breasts and gently curving hips. This change was reflected in 1930s dress bodices which evolved from the flat two-dimensional quality of the 1920s to the full three-dimensional gathered bodices of the 1940s. Fashions gradually changed from the soft feminine styles of the early '30s, with their bias-cut undulating ruffles, to the masculine broad-shouldered styles of the late '30s and early '40s.

Many women took up sewing, crocheting, or knitting to provide clothing for themselves and their families. Companies such as McCall's and Butterick provided home seamstresses with patterns and easy to follow instructions for a wide variety of styles. Thread and yarn manufacturers offered instruction booklets for crocheting and tatting a variety of dainty collars, jabots, and *gilets* (dickeys).

### Madeleine Vionnet and the Bias Cut

Madeleine Vionnet was one of the most influential designers of the 20th century. In 1927, she developed the "bias cut" which revolutionized the principles of dressmaking and dominated fashion design for the next ten years. In the past, dress patterns had been placed on the fabric so that the lengthwise direction of the pattern (perpendicular to the waist) ran parallel to the warp threads and the selvage. Fabric cut "on the straight" is more rigid, with little or no "give" or stretch. With the bias cut, however, the pattern was rotated slightly so that the lengthwise direction was placed on the diagonal or at a 45 degree angle to the selvage. In the U.K. this was called cutting "on the cross."

Cutting on the bias created a natural elasticity in the fabric which Vionnet used to her advantage. This elasticity made fabric easier to drape and mold to the figure. Dresses cut on the bias clung subtly to the torso and hips, which gave them shape,

then fell in graceful fluted folds to the hem. This technique helped to soften the severe rectangular silhouette during the late 1920s, and created a more feminine look which continued into the 1930s. Because of the elasticity which the bias cut provided, Vionnet's dresses could be slipped over the head without the need for fastenings.

Vionnet had a great appreciation for the natural curves of the female figure. She believed in molding her garments to the natural figure, rather than forcing the figure to conform to her garments, as other designers had done in the past. She disap-

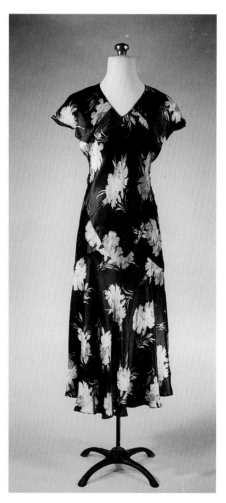

Bias-cut black-satin floral-print dress with cape sleeves, c. 1932. *Courtesy of Cedar Crest Alumnae Museum, Gift of Ellie Laubner.* $65-$85.

proved of corsets and forbid her models to wear them. As you might imagine, bias-cut garments were comfortable to wear, however, they required a well-proportioned figure to look their best.

Vionnet's genius lay in the unique cut of her garments. When other designers visualized a dress, they saw a front and a back fastened together by side seams. Vionnet saw a cylinder. She draped and cut the fabric "in the round" on a half-size articulated mannequin which she placed on a revolving piano stool. By rotating the mannequin she could created pattern pieces which wrapped around the figure. For example, the front of a dress might extend into a portion the back. These pieces were then enlarged to form human-size patterns.

Seams cut and stitched on the straight were often too rigid and unyielding for bias-cut garments. Therefore, diagonal or curved seams were frequently used for better elasticity. Vionnet often took this concept a step further by using supple fagoted seams, a construction technique which also served as a decoration. Narrow rolled hems or picot edging were often used in lieu of the conventional bulky hem.

Vionnet was also known for her complex construction details which fulfilled the need for decoration as well. She often arranged pin tucks so that they outlined various shapes, i.e., triangles, diamonds, or lozenges. By positioning the shapes in rows of graduated sizes she was able to shape the fabric to the contours of the body. Shaping could also be achieved by varying the size of the tucks. Since these delicate details would have gone unnoticed on dark or printed fabrics, Vionnet often chose solid colors in delicate pale tints such as banana, flesh, cactus, beige, mauve, lavender, pink, and peach for this intricate work. As you might imagine, the complex construction of Vionnet's creations made them very difficult to duplicate.

## Fabrics

The soft supple fabrics commonly used for bias-cut garments were crepe de chine, satin, georgette, silk velvet, lamé, lace, mousseline de soie, charmeuse, rayon, and printed sheers like georgette and chiffon. Although cutting garments on the bias did not necessarily require more fabric, it did require wider widths to prevent an overabundance of piecing seams. It is felt that through Vionnet's urging, the French textile industry began to produce fabrics in wider widths.

The flagging economy triggered a sharp decline in the use of costly silks and an increase in inexpensive fabrics which were once considered too inferior for fashionable clothing. As a practical alternative to silk, Chanel promoted the use of cottons such as piqué, muslin, lawn, eyelet, lace, and voile for day and evening wear. Organdy, dotted Swiss, and other stiffer fabrics were ideal for crisp stand-out ruffles or large puffy sleeves. White organdy was often used for "ingénue" dresses, as it created an air of youth and purity.

The depression also created a demand for less costly synthetic fabrics. Rayon, the inexpensive substitute for silk, became the predominate fiber for clothing worn by middle class Americans. Schiaparelli was always eager to try new technology and enjoyed being the first to introduce a novel new product. She experimented with a textured rayon fabric called "tree bark crepe" and a transparent cellophane-like material called "Rhodophane," which she used for scarves, evening bags, shoes, and see-through capes.

**Prints.** Prints were very common for day wear and increased in popularity as the decade unfolded. As a result of the faltering economy, the costly embroidery of the flamboyant 1920s was, for the most part, replaced by less expensive printed fabrics. Prints became important to the busy housewife as they were less likely to show soil or stains than solid colors and were, therefore, easier to maintain. Mini-floral prints were especially popular along with geometric shapes, stripes, and plaids. Polka dots were very popular and psychologically uplifting during the depression as they were associated with balloons, bubbles, clowns, and lighthearted merriment.

"Twin prints" consisting of positive and negative patterns were also popular. Fabric with white dots on a navy background could be used for the dress, while contrasting navy dots on a white ground were used for the collar and cuffs.

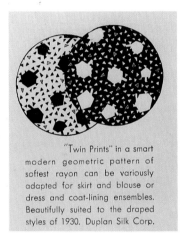

"Twin Prints" in a smart modern geometric pattern of softest rayon can be variously adapted for skirt and blouse or dress and coat-lining ensembles. Beautifully suited to the draped styles of 1930. Duplan Silk Corp.

*Delineator* illustration (4/30) of "Twin" or "positive and negative" prints.

Many clever novelty prints chronicled the events and the cultural history of this period. One such colorful print featured men and women drinking alcoholic beverages surrounded by the names of mixed drinks and the number 33 (a reference to the repeal of prohibition in 1933). The Chicago World's Fair (1933) and the New York World's Fair (1939) were the inspiration for many colorful prints featuring fair logos and modern pavilions. Collage prints were very popular and featured such subjects as the names of fashion magazines, newspapers, nightclubs, radio stations, song titles, and colleges.

Prints with romantic cupids and bleeding hearts were inspired by the abdication of Edward VIII of England and his subsequent marriage to Wallis Simpson. To commemorate the coronation of George VI in 1937, manufacturers printed fabrics featuring royal motifs such as English lions, Tudor roses, Scottish thistles, Prince of Wales plumes, the Union Jack, the coronation coach, and of course royal crowns. Prints were also created to commemorate the maiden voyage of the luxury liner the Queen Mary in 1936.

In 1935, Schiaparelli commissioned Culcombet, the prestigious French textile manufacturer, to print fabric featuring a collage of newspaper clippings about herself in different languages.

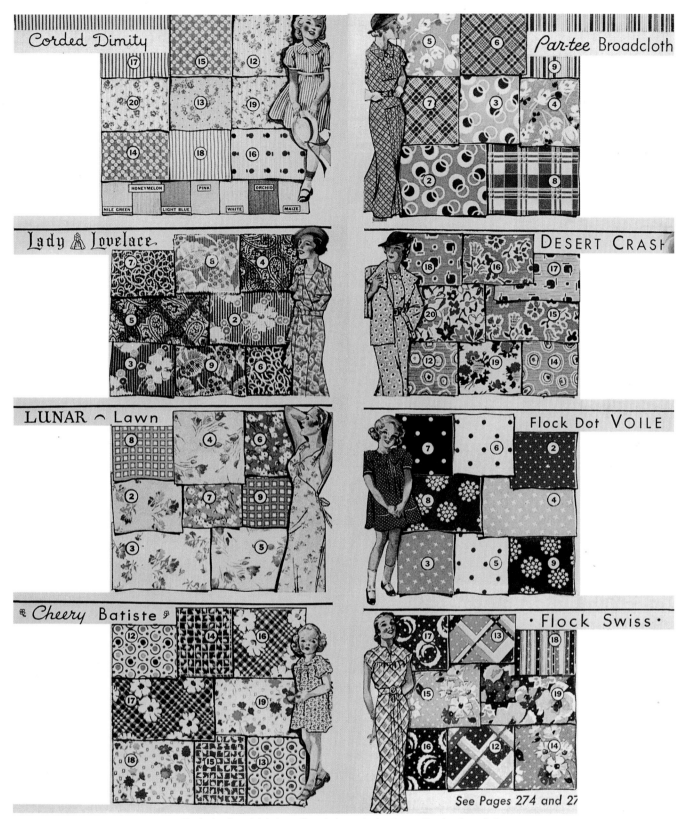

Corded Dimity

Par-tee Broadcloth

Lady Lovelace

DESERT CRASH

LUNAR ~ Lawn

Flock Dot VOILE

Cheery Batiste

Flock Swiss

See Pages 274 and 27

Typical printed fabrics offered through the Sears, Roebuck and Co.
catalog (1936) including dimity, lace, lawn, batiste, broadcloth,
crash, voile, and dotted Swiss. Note: bubble prints - upper right.

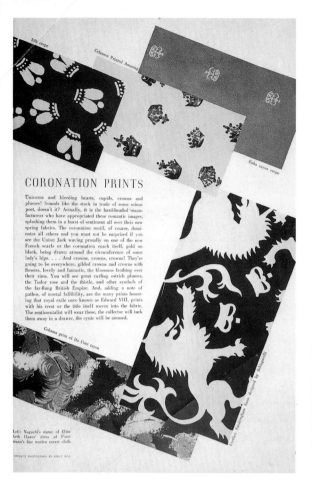

*Harper's Bazaar* (2/37) featured these printed fabrics created to commemorate the abdication of Edward VIII and the coronation of George VI of England. They include crowns and plumes, plus an English lion print designed by Schiaparelli.

Black and white silk print composed of film strips forming Elsa Schiaparelli's initials "E.S." from 1936. *Courtesy of the Allentown Art Museum. Gift of Kate Fowler Merle-Smith, 1978.26.351.*

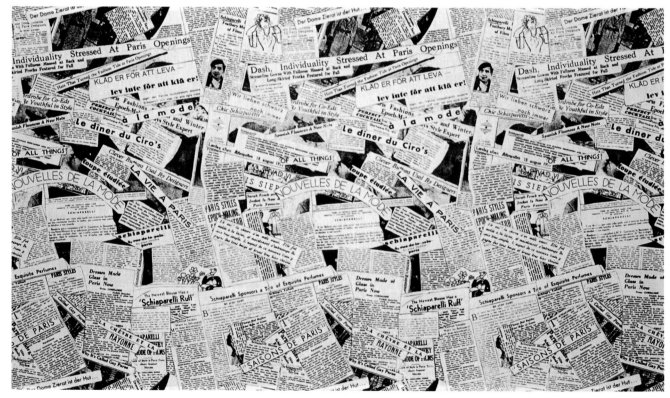

Cotton chintz fabric by Culcombet for Schiaparelli featuring a collage of newspaper articles about her in different languages, 1935. *Courtesy of the Allentown Art Museum. Gift of Kate Fowler Merle-Smith, 1978.26.352.*

She used this fabric to create unusual sportswear and handbags. Schiaparelli also commissioned a print called *Subways of Paris* in 1936. This print contained multicolored linear squiggles, representing the various train routes on a Paris subway map, interspersed with drawings of various Parisian tourist attractions. In 1938, she created what is known as her "tear dress" using *trompe-l'oeil* (trick of the eye) fabric inspired by Salvador Dali. It featured rips and tears which appeared three dimensional, yet were just printed on the fabric. (For additional prints see the World's Fair scarf in Sportswear, Chapter 6 and the college pennant scarf in Hair and Headgear, Chapter 8.)

***Colors.*** Still popular during the first half of the decade were the dynamic color combinations typical of Art Deco which included black and white, black and red, and black and green. The early 1930s also saw a continuation of the three popular medium-density colors of the 1920s. They were soon replaced, however, by deeper more intense shades of the same colors. Sunset orange became rust, Nile green intensified to forest green, and sunny yellow turned to gold or butterscotch. These colors were joined by *vieux* (old) rose, wine or burgundy, purple, plum, lime green, teal, and skipper blue (royal) during the second half of the decade. Schiaparelli's contribution to this range of fashionable colors was her famous "shocking pink," a vibrant pink with a hint of blue. Sears, Roebuck and Co. adopted a similar color and called it "American beauty."

The well-dressed woman made a concerted effort to color coordinate her ensembles. Fashion magazines and mail-order catalogs pictured matching ensembles consisting of a hat, bag, shoes, and gloves all of the same color to complement a solid-color frock or to match one of the colors found in a print dress. Pattern magazines suggested coordinating the solid color of the collar, cuffs, and belt with the print of the bodice and skirt. The fabric of a jabot might be repeated in the trim of a hat, or the color of a scarf might match that of the gloves.

## Afternoon Dresses

# 1930-1931

The hemline for afternoon dresses of the early '30s fell just below the calf. These dresses were characterized by soft supple fabrics, romantic colors, and a multitude of undulating ruffles.

V and U-shaped necklines were popular along with numerous collar styles, the most common of which was the feminine "cape" collar. The bias cut caused this collar to fall in soft fluted folds, in much the same way as a bias-cut skirt. It covered the upper arms in summertime, taking the place of short sleeves. This style was often accented at the neck with an artificial flower, a brooch, or a dress clip. The front of the cape collar could be extended to form panels which were tied in a square knot or a bow over the bodice. An ultra-feminine look was achieved when scallops or soft ruffles were added to the collar's edge. The cape collar was occasionally placed over long fitted sleeves in winter.

The popular *Pierrot* collar was named after the French pantomime comedian whose clown suit contained a wide round ruffled collar. (*Pierrot* was the French counterpart to the character Pedrolino from the famous *Commedia dell'Arte* or Italian Renaissance comedy.) The *Pierrot* collar, worn by women of the 1930s, was usually made of gathered or finely-pleated fabric or lace.

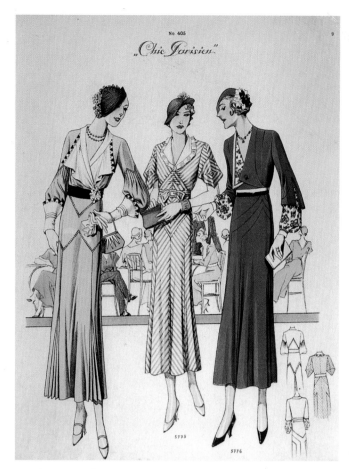

French pattern illustrations (1932) of bias-cut afternoon dresses. *Left:* Draped-*jabot* collar, bishop sleeves, wide-*gauntlet* cuffs, skirt has zigzag seams. *Center:* Striped fabric reveals intricate bias-cut marquetry, *rever* collar. *Right:* Asymmetrical *rever* collar, bishop under sleeve. Note: low head-hugging hats and *pochettes*, 1932.

The soft classically-draped "cowl" neckline was the contribution of Madeleine Vionnet. For this style, the supple bias-cut fullness of the bodice was draped in graceful U-shaped folds over the bust. To encourage this draping, a small nickel-sized metal weight was often suspended on a cord from the edge of the neck fabric on the inside of the bodice. (See photograph in Evening Wear, Chapter 4.) The cowl neckline was also created by the use of shirring at the shoulders.

The "jabot" collar consisted of wide pointed *revers* (lapels) made of soft supple fabric which were allowed to drape in soft folds over the bodice. The "shawl" collar was also popular. The lower ends were often extended to form a large floppy bow at the base.

"Jabots" were created in various ways and were made from self fabric or lace. A square of fabric could be attached by one point to the center of the neckline and allowed to cascade down the bodice. A semi-circle of fabric could become a jabot by attaching the midpoint of its straight edge to the center of the neckline. A narrow rectangular strip of fabric could also be attached vertically to the bodice by stitching along one lengthwise edge. The opposite edge was then allowed to fall into undulating serpentine folds. A soft, floppy, self-fabric or contrasting bow was often attached at the center of the neckline or collar; or a vertical row of butterfly bows might be fastened down the center of the bodice.

The important sleeve styles for this period were the fitted, the cape, the bell, and the bishop sleeve. The bishop sleeve was a long, full, set-in sleeve which was gathered into a short cuff at

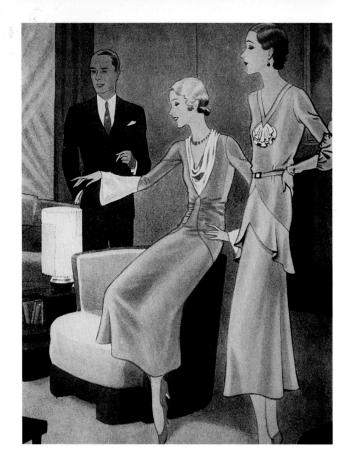

*McCall's* advertisement (12/30) featuring a bias-cut afternoon dresses. *Left:* Cowl neck, shirred waist, bell sleeves. *Right:* Jabot at V-neck, bias-cut flounce at diagonal hip seam.

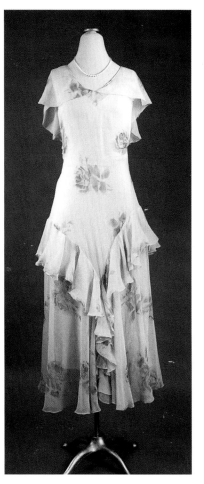

Romantic bias-cut floral-print chiffon dress with cape collar and bias-cut flounce at diagonal hip seam. 1930-31. $80-$120.

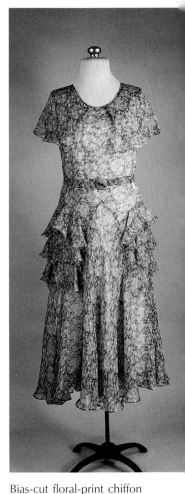

Bias-cut floral-print chiffon dress with cape collar, belt at natural waist, flounces over the hips, 1930-32. $75-$110.

Original French fashion illustration, from the *Atelier* (studio) Bachroitz, which appeared in *Chic Parisian*, c. 1931-32. Brown bias-cut velvet, *gauntlet*-style cuffs, flounces over hips, fox-fur scarf, swagger-brim hat, and *pochette*.

the wrist or a longer 12-inch cuff extending from the wrist to the elbow. This longer cuff was often decorated with a row of closely spaced buttons. Interest was beginning to focus on the area around the wrist. The "jabot" sleeve was unique to the '30s and consisted of a fitted sleeve with a jabot-like ruffle attached at the wrist. High-fashion *"gauntlet"* sleeves featured stiff exaggerated cuffs which flared out from the wrist like Cavaliers' *gauntlets* (gloves).

Dresses from 1930 and 1931 not only had a seam and/or a belt which gave new definition to the natural waist, they usually retained a seam or some form of detail at the hip as well (a last vestige of the 1920s dropped waist). This may have been the fashion industry's way of providing a gradual transition to the higher natural waistline of the '30s. This hip seam joined the upper portion of the skirt to the bias-cut lower portion which fell in soft undulating folds to the hem. This hip seam could be horizontal, diagonal, zigzag, asymmetrical, stepped, curved, or an up-turned or down-turned point. A bias-cut flounce was often inserted into this seam. It usually encircled the body, however, short flounces were sometimes created to rest solely over the hips.

The December 1930 issue of McCall's magazine featured "tunic frocks," which were basically dresses with knee-length overskirts. The hem of these tunics could be horizontal, diagonal, scalloped, or asymmetrical. Tunic dresses would remain in style throughout the decade.

Fabric was often shaped to the waist by creating blocks of shirring at the center front, center back, or sides. Another alternative was a narrow vertical strip of shirring from the center of the neckline to the center of the hips. A two-inch strip of self fabric was often attached over this shirring so that the gathers seemed to radiate from it.

A long arched or triangular-shaped portion of the skirt was frequently cut away from hip to hem on either side to allow for the insertion of *godets*. *Godets* were often wider than the section which they replaced, thus producing a soft flare at the sides of the skirt. (This popular technique was also used in the design of evening gowns, wedding dresses, and even lounging pajamas.) *Godets* were usually the same length as the skirt. Longer *godets* were used, however, to create the fashionable uneven hem—a sophisticated style used by Augustabernard in the late '20s. Handkerchief hems, a carry-over from the two previous decades, remained fashionable for the first few years of the decade.

A hip-yoke effect was often created by shirring along the side seams from the waist to the hips. This produced horizontal gathers over the hip area. A hip yoke was also created by stitching together multiple horizontal strips of fabric.

## 1932-1936

The overall look of this period was more tailored than the preceding years. Emphasis was now placed solely above the waist; while the long slender skirts remained relatively unadorned. Bodices were decked with numerous forms of structural and decorative details.

The cowl neck remained popular as well as the chelsea, Peter Pan, *Pierrot*, and jabot collars. Jabots of all kinds were extremely popular. They were joined by ascots, artificial flowers, and butterfly bows in contrasting colors. Bows tended to grow in size as the years progressed. Enormous butterfly bows, unique to the mid-1930s, covered the bodice with tips extending to the outer reaches of the shoulders, often dwarfing the wearer. *Faux* bows were created when a rectangular piece of fabric was pushed into and out of two vertical slashes in the bodice. Square scarves were folded diagonally and tied at the neck, or draped asymmetrically over one shoulder. They were also placed around the neck with the ends pushed through two horizontal slashes, similar to the *faux* bow.

Tunic tops, basque bodices, and tops with peplums were very popular and featured a belt over the natural waist. Shoulder yokes and saddle shoulders (the yoke and sleeve in one), with their horizontal seams, helped to created the illusion of breadth. The fullness of the bodice was often gathered into the shoulder yoke, creating a peasant look. The yoke was frequently made in a different color, print, or texture to contrast with the rest of the dress.

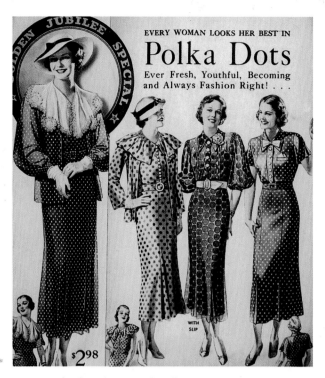

Sears, Roebuck and Co. catalog illustration (1936): bias-cut polka-dot day dresses. *(1)* Navy and white flocked-dot voile, lace-trimmed linen collar, matching jacket, bishop sleeves. *(2)* Brown dots on rose or turquoise crepe, *Pierrot* collar, matching jacket. *(3)* Navy on white chiffon, full three-quarter sleeves. *(4)* White dots on brown or navy crepe.

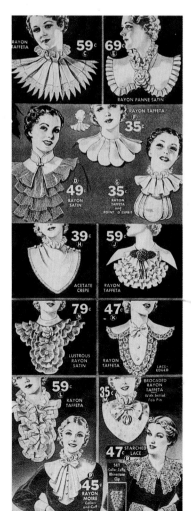

This Sears, Roebuck and Co. illustration (1936-37) offers a selection of dickeys, collars, and *jabots* made of organdy, lawn, crepe, rayon taffeta, satin, *moiré*, and lace.

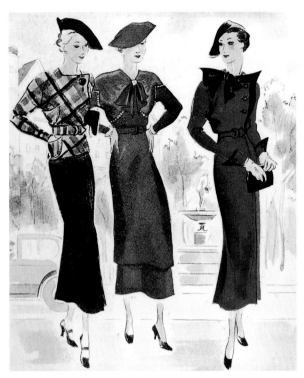

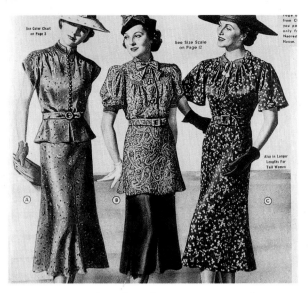

Berth Robert advertisement (1934) for semi-made afternoon dresses. *Left:* Heather-plaid basque top with belt, asymmetrical closing. *Center:* Tunic dress, fagoted seams, satin *jabot*, rhinestone dress clip. *Right:* Red wool dress, black velvet bow and trim on asymmetrical closing and *gauntlet* cuffs.

Montgomery Ward catalog advertisement (1937) for afternoon dresses. *Left:* Two-piece rayon print containing royal crowns (in commemoration of coronation), shirred shoulders, closely spaces buttons, peplum, and self belt. *Center:* Paisley tunic top with puffed sleeves, musical-note buttons, self-fabric belt. *Right:* Drawstring neckline, short bell sleeves.

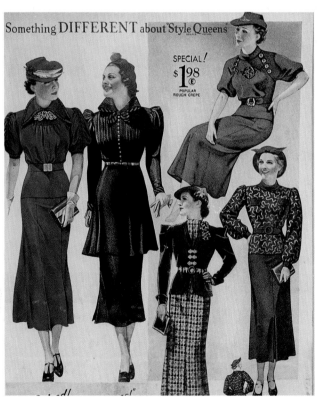

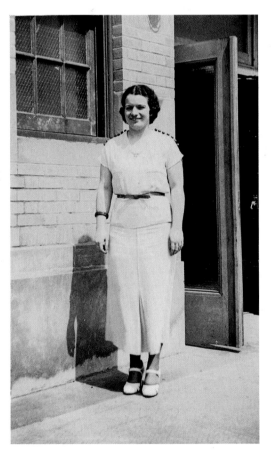

Illustrated on this Sears, Roebuck and Co. catalog page (1936-37) are: *(1)* Red crepe, belted basque top, shirred bodice and sleeves. *(2)* Black crepe tunic top, tucked bodice, gather-top sleeves. *(3)* Green belted basque top, rolled collar, buttons along raglan seam, embroidered medallion. *(4)* Brown velveteen basque jacket, tuck-top sleeves, plaid scarf, belt, and skirt. *(5)* Wine basque top, embroidered vermicelli pattern. Note: three peak-style hats.

Author's Aunt Eleanore wearing a belted basque-style blouse with Bakelite buttons at the shoulders and a contrasting belt. Note: hair with central part, Bakelite bangle, 7/36. *Courtesy of Eleanore Miller.*

Cape, cap, and puffed sleeves were all popular for summer dresses. Layers of ruffles were often attached to the armseye, adding breadth to the shoulders.

The full bishop sleeve, containing either short or long cuffs, remained in style. The diagonally seamed "raglan" and wedge-shaped "batwing" sleeves were also stylish. The fitted sleeve was worn alone or in conjunction with a dwarf cape or capelet.

The "Juliet" sleeve, named for Shakespeare's heroine, featured a fitted sleeve surmounted at the top by a small puffed sleeve. The revival of this style was inspired by the costume worn by actress Norma Shearer in the movie version of *Romeo and Juliet* in 1930.

Long, slender bias-cut skirts often rose above the natural waist to the bust, where they ended in an arched, pointed, or scalloped seam. In addition, a self belt was often worn over the natural waist, accented by a buckle, belt slide (buckle without a hasp), or clasp. Pointed or arched *godets* were still inserted into the sides of skirts, creating a slight flare.

Four, five, or six gored skirts were also stylish. A central box pleat, one or two inverted pleats, or clusters of knife pleats were all very common. Short pleats emanating from the knees were often employed for additional freedom of movement. Bias-cut skirts were often made of stripes which converged in an up-turned or down-turned V at the center seam.

Dresses were often made with matching jackets. These jackets were straight or fitted, single or double breasted, and hip or 3/4 length. They could be collarless or feature a notched or a wide pointed *rever* collar. Fitted jackets were often made with a belt over the natural waist. Boleros, favored by Schiaparelli, were either waist-length or rib-length jackets with straight or curved front edges.

Common dress fabrics were velvet, wool, satin, jersey, linen, semi-sheer crepe, dotted Swiss, organdy, chiffon, silk *matelassé* (a luxurious fabric with a raised pattern made on a jacquard loom).

Dark colored dresses with a white collar and cuffs were popular, thus mirroring the dark shirts and light ties worn by men at this time. Two contrasting colors or textures were often used in the same dress, such as wool and satin, or wool and velvet. Print dresses often had a solid collar, yoke, and cuffs.

## 1937-1939

The styles for 1937 through 1939 were decidedly masculine, a look which would prevail through the Second World War. The fluttering ruffles of the early '30s were replaced by gathers, shirring, and smocking. Gathers served a dual purpose. They were important to the structural design of a garment as they helped to shape the fabric to the figure, particularly around the bust. They also provided the garment with a form of decorative detailing. Gathers appeared in endless varieties and combinations and could be found at the neckline, shoulders, shoulder yoke, waist, waist yoke, top of the sleeve, and down the outside of the sleeve. Whole yokes and even pockets were often shirred or smocked as a form of decoration. For one very common style, the fullness of the bodice was gathered into both the shoulder yoke at the top and the waist yoke at the bottom, creating ripples of fabric over the bust. This style was used in conjunction with a narrow V-shaped neck opening. When gathers were used on printed fabric, the result could be quite busy.

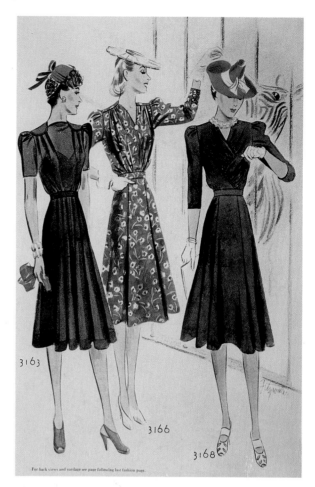

Featured in this *McCall's* advertisement (4/39) are afternoon dresses with gathered bodices and short full skirts. Note: orange hat with snood.

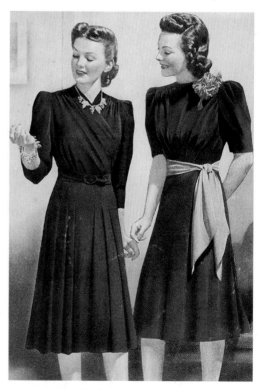

Shown in this Sears, Roebuck and Co. catalog illustration (1939) are solid-color rayon-crepe knee-length "background" dresses (good for displaying jewelry, scarves, or flowers.) *Left:* Gathered and draped surplice bodice, pleated skirt, self belt. *Right:* Gathered bodice and sleeves, pink flower and sash. Note: charm bracelet and necklace.

35

Princess-style dresses, which contained two long continuous seams from shoulder to hem, made an appearance during this period. Also in demand were two-piece dresses consisting of a straight skirt and either a knee-length tunic, a hip-length basque bodice, or a peplumed top. Many dresses with short bolero jackets were worn with a colorful, gypsy-style sash in either solid or printed fabric.

Broad shoulders became very common during the late 1930s. They were created by the use of small shoulder pads or wide puffed sleeves which were gathered or pleated into the armseye. The "cap" sleeve was also establishing itself as an important style to watch.

New A-line style gored skirts, featuring shorter knee-length hemlines, were illustrated in fashion magazines in 1937 and in mail-order catalogs by 1938. Some skirts still arched or peaked above the belt, giving the illusion of a waist yoke. Belts were now *de rigueur* with buckles made of bakelite, metal, or wood. (See examples of belt buckles, slides, and clasps in Accessories and Related Items, Chapter 12.)

Common fabrics were rayon crepe, taffeta, dotted Swiss, organdy, cotton piqué, eyelet, flock-dot cotton voile, and cotton crinkle crepe.

Ornamentation took the form of machine-made peasant embroidery, trapunto, and "spaghetti cord" bows. (See full explanation of trapunto in Lingerie, Chapter 2.) Braid was also stitched to garments forming decorative designs called *passementerie*.

## Town and Country Dresses

Town and country dresses were worn for business and shopping in the city or for spectator sports and picnics in the country. These tailored dresses were devoid of the soft feminine ruffles and frilly jabots so prevalent in afternoon frocks.

Typical of this look was the classic shirtwaist dress which enjoyed immediate and continued success throughout the decade. Bodices were often decorated with pin tucks and patch pockets. Common collars were the Bermuda, Peter Pan, shawl, and chelsea. The *rever* and the more masculine notched collars were often accented with parallel rows of topstitching called "railroad" stitching. Many of these styles featured a contrasting ribbon bow at the base of the collar. Collarless V-shaped necklines were also prevalent. Shirtwaist dresses were available in sleeveless or short-sleeved models in summer and long fitted sleeves, often styled with French cuffs (for cuff links), in winter.

The tailored "jacket frock" (also known as a "jacket dress," a "suit dress," or a "two-piece" dress) was also popular. The accompanying jacket took on a variety of forms. The straight, hip-length boxy jackets of the early '30s were generally beltless, while the newer fitted hip-length jackets were often belted over the natural waist. Notched and *rever* collars were commonly used on these jackets. Bolero jackets gained favor during the second half of the decade and were often paired with dresses featuring colorful waist sashes.

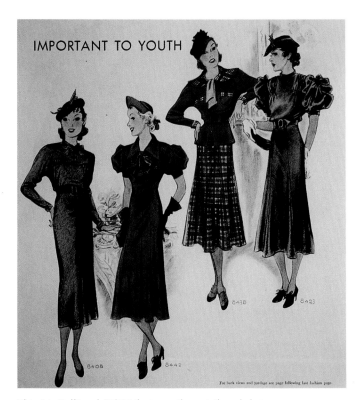

Displayed in this *McCall's* advertisement (1935) are tailored shirtwaist dresses. Note: scarf treatment, row of buttons.

This *McCall's* ad (9/35) features three tailored dresses.
*(1)* Shirtwaist with saddle shoulder, gathered bodice.
*(2)* Princess-style, puffed sleeves. *(3)* Belted jacket with peplum.
*(4)* Butterfly sleeves.

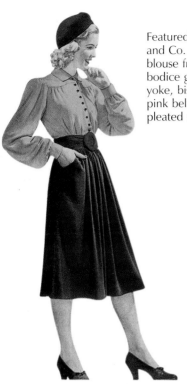

Featured in this Sears, Roebuck and Co. catalog ad (1939) is a blouse frock with lime-green bodice gathered to shoulder yoke, bishop sleeves, shocking pink belt, and skipper blue pleated skirt. Note: turban.

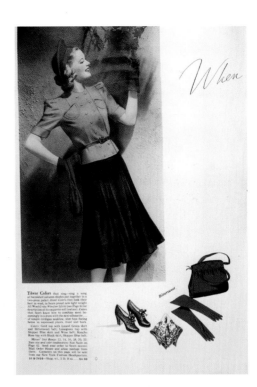

This Sears, Roebuck and Co. ad (1939-40) offers a coordinated ensemble in popular colors of late '30s. Gold square-shoulder basque-style jacket, forest-green pleated skirt and oxford shoes, rust hat, belt, gloves, and purse.

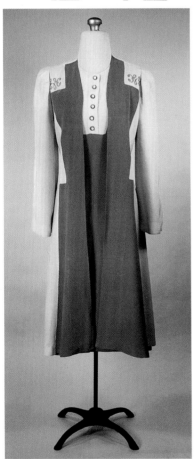

Cream and rust rayon-crepe dress and unlined coat, slightly padded shoulders and rust embroidery. *Courtesy of Pam Coghlan (Odds and Ads).* $100-$130.

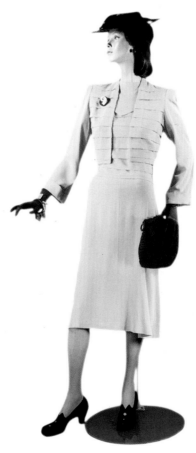

Rose-crepe suit dress, padded shoulders, horizontal tucks on bodice and jacket. $100-$125.

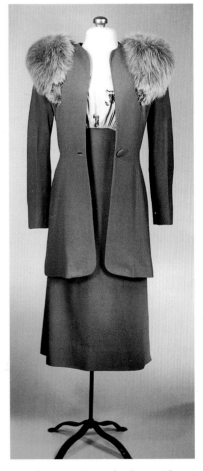

Suit dress. Empire-style dress with beige and brown print bodice, rust wool skirt. Matching jacket with fox fur trim, padded shoulders, late '30s. Label: Eisenberg Original, *Courtesy of Cedar Crest Alumnae Museum.* $250-$300.

The "blouse frock," which resembled a blouse and skirt of two different fabrics, was actually a dress. This style was often designed in twin prints or in a print with a coordinating solid.

The "little black dress" with a white collar and cuffs, introduced by Chanel in the 1920s, was still *de rigueur* in every stylish wardrobe. Collars and cuffs were often made of white cotton piqué, linen, or crepe and were either buttoned or basted onto a dress for easy laundering.

Town and Country styles were usually made of more durable, less fancy fabrics such as tweed, herringbone, tartan, challis, wool crepe, wool jersey, corduroy, and flannel for winter; seersucker, batiste, rayon, cotton mesh, cotton piqué, linen, silk crepe, silk shantung, and silk pongee for summer. Stripes, plaids, and polka dots were the most common prints.

**Housedresses and Aprons**

Hoover wraparound apron dresses, called "Hooverettes," were very popular, as they adjusted to any figure with a button or ties at the side. They had a reversible front so that when one side was soiled, the wearer could have a clean front again by simply reversing the sides. (Left over right, then became right over left.) Feminine versions featured a lace or ruffle trimmed shawl collar, while the more tailored versions had notched collars.

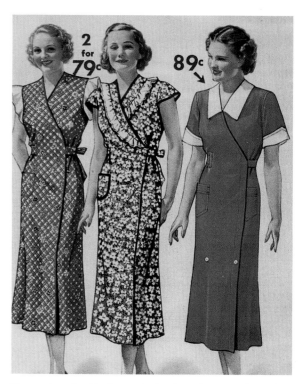

Shown here in this Sears, Roebuck and Co. catalog ad are cotton surplice-style wraparound Hooverette housedresses with reversible fronts.

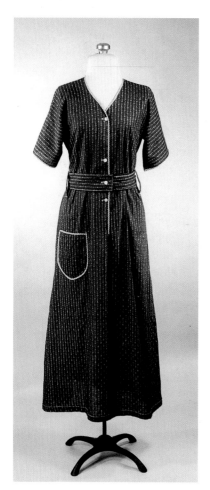

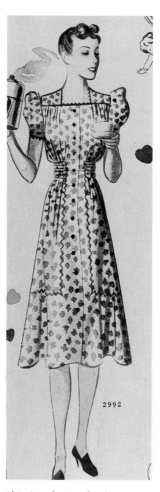

Cotton roller-print housedress, striped bias binding along the front opening and the pocket. *Courtesy of Judy Carpenter*. $25-$45.

This Simplicity ad (2/39) features a cotton print housedress with gathered bodice and puffed sleeves.

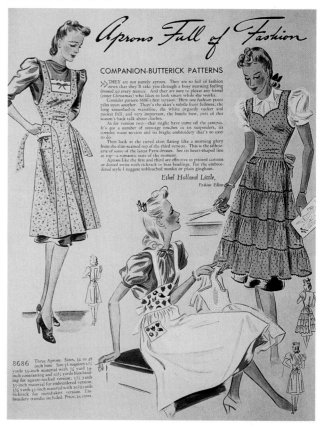

Butterick ad (12/39) for cotton aprons. *Left:* white organdy tucker and pocket frill. *Center:* suspenders and corselette waist. *Right:* sweetheart neckline, tiered skirt.

Other housedress styles included the princess and the shirt-waist, which were either double or single breasted. The V-neckline or the Peter Pan collar were commonly used with these styles. Pin tucks, rickrack, and bias binding highlighted the bodice, while practical patch pockets accented the skirt. Common fabrics for these utility frocks were cotton broadcloth, percale, gingham, and poplin. The collar and cuffs were often made of white cotton to contrast with the solid or mini-print fabric of the dress.

**Maternity Dresses**

Maternity dresses appearing in mail-order catalogs of the '30s were touted as "keeping your secret for months" and "cleverly concealing so your friends will never know."

Three basic maternity styles emerged during the 1930s. The first was a wraparound dress (similar to the Hooverette) with a side tie and "generous overlap" which could be "easily adjusted to every figure change." The second style consisted of a full hip-length smock with deep pleats in front and back. This smock was worn with a wraparound "bodice-top skirt" to match. The third style was a loose-fitting sack dress with fullness gathered into the shoulder yoke. It could be adjusted to the figure through the use of a self sash tied at the waist.

Common fabrics used for maternity dresses were cotton lace, cotton voile, eyelet batiste, printed dimity, cotton muslin, cotton broadcloth, and rayon crepe.

The full swagger-style coat was popular for those mothers-to-be who were pregnant over the winter months. (See an example of the swagger coat in Outerwear, Chapter 7.)

# SUITS

Fashion magazines promoted suits as ideal travel ware. The June 1938 issue of *McCall's* recommended, "The costume that one travels in should look well with one's luggage. Suitcases and printed dresses, for instance, just do not go together. But suits and bags complement each other extravagantly. Also, a suit is thoroughly in the picture whether you go by train, car, bus, boat, or airplane." (1938:107)

Beginning in the early '30s, suits took on a broader, more masculine look through the use of shoulder pads. Lapels also became wider as the decade progressed.

## 1930 - 1931

For the first two years of the decade, suits remained remarkably similar to those of the late '20s. Long, straight, hip-length jackets had fitted sleeves; however, short capes were occasionally attached at the shoulders.

Suits were made of textured fabrics such as nubby English tweed, Scottish tartan, checks, herringbone, bouclé, flannel, and wool jersey. Both single and double-breasted styles were popular. Shawl and notched collars were common, as were collars without *revers* (lapels) and *revers* without collars.

## 1932 - 1936

Hip-length, basque-style jackets were produced in either single or double-breasted styles. A belt was usually worn over

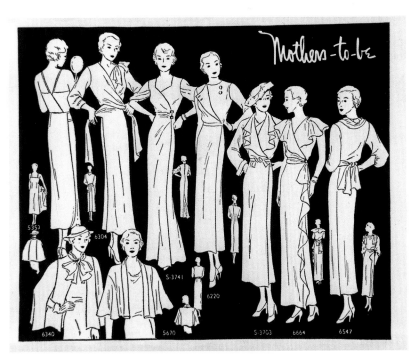

*Vogue Pattern Book* ad (11/34) for mother-to-be expandable wrap fashions: (5353) slip, (6304) dress, (3741) evening gown, (6220) dress, (3703) coat with jabot collar, (6664) afternoon dress with cape collar, (6547) dress, (6340) cape, (5670) capes.

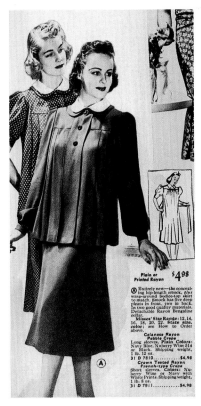

Sears, Roebuck and Co. catalog ad (1939-40) offering a rayon maternity outfit. Hip-length smock with five deep pleats, wrap-around skirt.

the jacket at the natural waist. Short fitted jackets with nipped-in waists were also popular. They featured square or cut-away corners and notched collars and were worn with or without a belt.

Man-tailored suits with classic blazer-style jackets were also offered. They included hip-length, single-breasted jackets with notched collars and double-breasted jackets with peaked lapels. The single-breasted versions were either fastened with two or three buttons or featured an edge-to-edge closing fastened by one single "link button" (similar to a cuff link). These jackets were often made with an "action" back featuring an inverted-pleat and a stitched-to-the-waist half belt similar to men's suit jackets of the 1930s.

Full three-quarter or thigh-length "swagger" jackets were another alternative. They featured an unfitted front and a full swinging back suspended from a shoulder yoke. Roomy patch pockets created a smock-effect.

The "tunic" suit, introduced circa 1936, had a knee-length jacket with a belt at the waist. This style was mainly worn in winter and was often trimmed with fur along the edge of the collar and hem.

Sleeves on suit jackets varied. Straight fitted sleeves and pleat-top sleeves were used throughout the decade. Pouch-style sleeves with fullness over the elbow were used from the middle '30s through the end of the decade. Loose-fitting raglan sleeves which widened toward the wrist were generally used for swagger jackets. The long, slender suit skirts ended below the calf.

Gilbert Adrian, head designer at MGM studios, created suit jackets with broad masculine shoulders and fitted waists for the assertive roles played by Joan Crawford. This look called "hard chic" became her trademark and set an international trend which continued through the war years.

In 1936, Schiaparelli designed her famous "desk" suit based on a drawing by Salvador Dali. The pocket flaps were embroidered to resemble drawers with metal rings as drawer pulls.

# 1937-1939

Fitted basque and tunic-style jackets remained in style through the end of the decade. Short jackets with tiny peplums were also popular. The swagger jacket was now produced with a long tuxedo collar. Short A-line suit skirts ended just below the knee.

Tailored suits with classic single or double-breasted blazer-style jackets were offered with matching reefer-style topcoats. These practical three-piece "wardrobe" suits became universally popular during the Second World War as they were warm, durable, and could be mixed and matched, creating several practical ensembles.

The use of nubby tweeds and tartans was inspired by the movie *Mary of Scotland* in 1936, staring Katharine Hepburn and Fredric March. Tweeds were produced in solids, checks, and plaids. Those with white silk nubs were called "snowflake" tweeds, while "monotone" tweed contained various tints, shades, or tones of the same hue.

Winter suits were made of pebbly crepe, gabardine, and flannel in wool or camel's hair. Spring and summer suits were made of cotton gabardine, cotton twill, and cotton piqué and were often unlined.

***Gilet***. Also known as a plastron, vestee, *blousette*, or dickey, the *gilet* could be worn as an alternative to a blouse. It consisted of a front and a back panel fastened at the shoulders, with an attached collar or jabot. When tucked into the V-neckline of a suit jacket, it gave the appearance of a blouse. Cotton, linen, silk crepe, silk-foulard, satin, and satin jacquard were favorite fabrics for blouses and *gilets*. (For examples of blouses see Sportswear, Chapter 6.)

## Fasteners

***Buttons.*** The period from 1934 to 1940 was the heyday for unusual buttons. Bright whimsical buttons were ideally suited to the 1930s, as they were an inexpensive antidote to the doldrums of the depression. For many women, the failed economy meant making do with last year's frocks. What better way

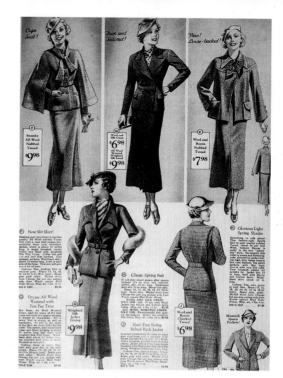

Montgomery Ward (1935) offered these wool suits with long straight skirts. *(F)* Tweed, belted jacket, cape effect over fitted sleeves. *(H)* Fitted double-breasted jacket. *(K)* Swagger jacket, shoulder yoke, bell sleeves. *(G)* Railroad-stitched collar, spirals of fox fur. *(J)* Man-tailored pleated action back, half belt, notched collar.

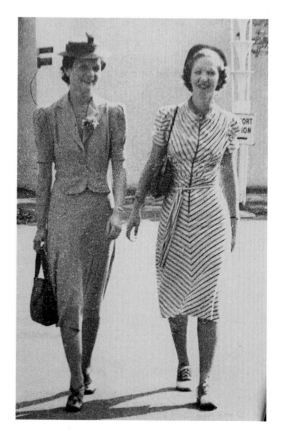

Author's mother Elizabeth and friend Ethel at the World's Fair, June 1939. *Left:* Saucer hat, blue suit, short jacket with slight peplum, puffed sleeves. (My mother wore this as her wedding suit when she married my father, April 8, 1939.) *Right:* Dress with converging diagonal stripes, saddle shoes. *Courtesy of Ethel Hoyt.*

to liven up an old dress (or a new dress for that matter) then by adding a few cheerful buttons—perhaps ones that looked like flowers, animals, fish, or even insects. Wealthy women enjoyed these creative buttons as well, as they were considered quite chic and great conversation pieces. (For further information and examples of unique '30s buttons, see Accessories and Related Items, Chapter 12.)

**Belts and Belt Buckles.** When the waist returned to its natural position in the early 1930s, it signaled the return of the belt. Belts were often fastened with unique buckles, belt slides (buckles without hasps), and clasps made of a variety of materials. (For further information on belts, buckles, slides, and clasps see Accessories and Related Items, Chapter 12.)

Unfortunately, when 1930s dresses are found today, the belts are often missing. Many 1930s dresses have an empire waist and appear not to need a belt. However, if you examine the side seams you will probably find chain stitched or self-fabric belt loops. Soft silk ribbon sashes in complementary colors appeared in many fashion illustrations of the 1930s and would be an acceptable substitute for a missing self belt.

**Hooks and Eyes.** When a side placket was required, it was fastened with snaps, or hooks and eyes.

**Zippers.** Automatic metal "slide fasteners," were introduced for luggage, handbags, boots, and girls' leggings circa 1927. Schiaparelli pioneered the use of zippers by incorporating them in her garments beginning in 1930. Circa 1934, manufacturers were beginning to use zippers for women's jackets, men's trousers, and bathing suits. Zippers were not in general use for women's dresses, however, until the late '30s. (These are factors to consider when dating vintage garments.) Zippers not only made dressing quicker and easier, they provided a smoother, neater finish to a garment. They were also less expensive and less time consuming to stitch into garments than hooks, eyes, snaps, or buttons. Unfortunately, people were just beginning to appreciate the many benefits of zippers when the government removed them from the market to conserve on metal for the war effort.

Daytime styles fell into two basic categories. First were fancy "afternoon dresses" designed for luncheons, card parties, matinees, races, and afternoon tea. Second were "town and country" styles which included tailored dresses worn for spectator sports, travel, business, shopping, or a day in the country.

# ADDITIONAL DESIGNERS

**Edward Molyneux.** Designer Edward Molyneux won a sketching contest sponsored by the designer Lucile and worked for her in London until the First World War. He served as a captain in the British Army where he sustained multiple injuries including the loss of one eye. He opened a salon in Paris in 1919 and produced designs for tailored suits, pleated skirts, and matching ensembles in the classic understated colors of grey, navy and beige. His reserved designs were the antithesis of the flamboyant fashions produced by Schiaparelli.

**Maggie Rouff.** The Maison Drécoll, where her parents worked as directors, was the launching pad for designer Maggie Rouff. She opened her own house in 1929 and is known for her day wear, sportswear, and lingerie. She often created garments made of various types of fabric all in the same color. Monograms, fichus collars (scarf-like), and the color blue-purple were all common among her designs.

# CARE OF GARMENTS

Caution should be taken when washing printed fabrics from the 1930s. They are not all colorfast and darker colors may bleed into lighter ones. It is best to test a small corner before plunging the entire garment into the wash tub.

# Chapter 4

# Evening Wear

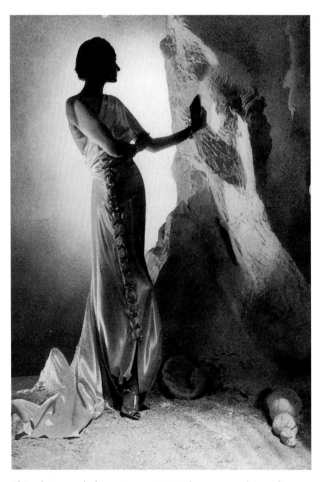

This photograph from *Vogue* (1936) features a white rayon-satin evening gown by Vionnet. The fabric is draped over one shoulder, a row of rhinestone bows accent the skirt. (The deep shadows and surrealistic backdrop were typical of fashion photography of the 1930s.)

## EVENING GOWNS

The stock market crash of 1929 brought an abrupt end to the wild-spirited parties and reckless spending of the flamboyant twenties. Gone were the costly beading and sashaying fringe characteristic of 1920s evening wear. Designers now relied less on applied ornamentation and more on sophisticated cut and fluid lines to produce some of the most stunning evening wear of the twentieth century.

From 1925 to 1928, hemlines for evening dresses ended just below the knee. In 1928 and 1929, French designer, Louiseboulanger, lowered the hems of her gowns to the floor in back, creating bi-level skirts. In his 1929 collection, Jean Patou lowered the entire hemline to the instep, where it remained throughout the decade. This signaled the return of long, elegant evening wear.

Evening fashions were evolving from the soft, feminine styles of the late '20s and early '30s, to the masculine, broad-shoulder designs of the late '30s and early '40s.

It was a general rule of thumb that the more bare the shoulders and arms, the more formal the gown. Gowns for white-tie occasions were sleeveless and often exposed the shoulders and back as well. (Occasionally, the most formal of gowns featured a semi-circular train, a last vestige of Victorian/Edwardian fashion.) Gowns for cocktails, dinner, and less-than-white tie occasions had covered shoulders and often some form of sleeve.

### Madeleine Vionnet and the Bias Cut

In 1927, the influential French designer, Madeleine Vionnet, developed the bias cut, a technique which would dominated the fashion scene through 1937. This novel technique for placing pattern pieces on the fabric revolutionized the fashion industry. The bias cut created a natural elasticity in the fabric which was instrumental in shaping the fabric to the body. Vionnet had a great appreciation for the natural, fluid lines of the feminine figure. She was responsible for the clinging, supremely-sensual evening gowns commonly associated with the 1930s. (For further information on Vionnet and the bias cut see Day Wear, Chapter 3.)

### 1930-1931

The soft, classically-draped "cowl" neckline was another of Vionnet's contributions to fashion. For this style, the bias-cut fullness over the bodice was draped in graceful U-shaped folds. To encourage this draping, a small nickel-sized metal weight was often suspended by a cord from the edge of the neckline, on the inside of the bodice. The cowl neckline could also be created by the

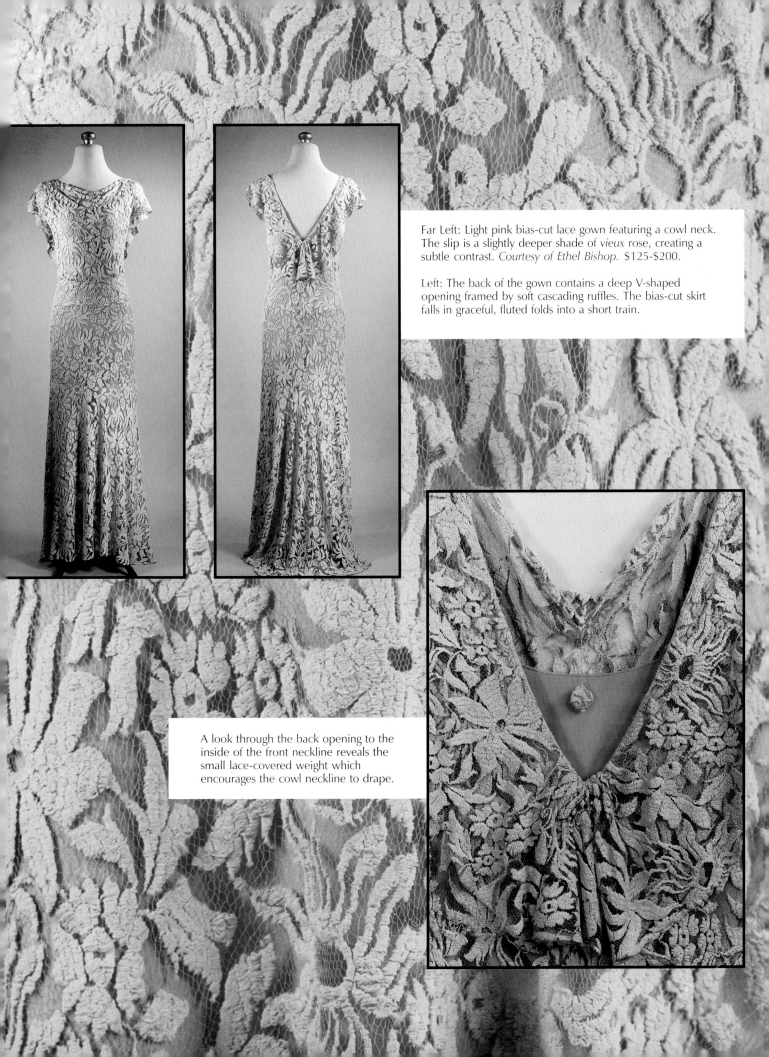

Far Left: Light pink bias-cut lace gown featuring a cowl neck. The slip is a slightly deeper shade of *vieux* rose, creating a subtle contrast. *Courtesy of Ethel Bishop.* $125-$200.

Left: The back of the gown contains a deep V-shaped opening framed by soft cascading ruffles. The bias-cut skirt falls in graceful, fluted folds into a short train.

A look through the back opening to the inside of the front neckline reveals the small lace-covered weight which encourages the cowl neckline to drape.

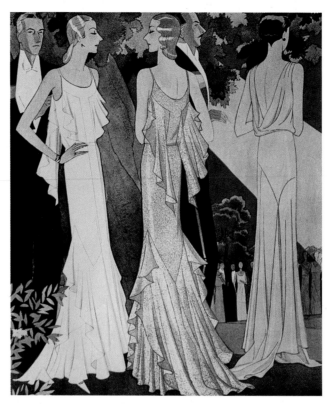

This colorful *McCall's* illustration (7/30) features formal bias-cut evening gowns. *Left and Center:* Fluttering-chiffon flounces cut at oblique angles cascade from bodice and skirt. *Right:* Deep gracefully-draped cowl neckline doubles as a hood (also known as a "cowl hood," derived from a monks habit).

use of shirring along the ridge of the shoulders. Upon occasion, a deep cowl neckline could be found at the back of an evening gown.

The '30s woman no longer flung her legs in every direction on the dance floor. Instead, she danced sedately "cheek to cheek" with her partner. While assuming this position, the backs of gowns were plainly visible. A perfect reason to continue the fashion for plunging V and U-shaped backlines, a sensual look introduced in the late '20s. Many gowns were completely backless with either vertical, crisscrossed, or converging V-shaped straps. The straight camisole-style bodice with spaghetti straps was also popular.

The soft cape collar fell in flutes folds over the arms, serving as short sleeves. In some cases this collar was removable, turning a cocktail ensemble into an evening gown. A ruffle was often added to the edge of this collar for an ultra-feminine look.

The sides of the skirt were often cut away from hip to hem for the insertion of long, arch-shaped or pointed *godets*. These *godets* were wider than the sections which they replaced, and the added fullness gently flared in soft undulating ripples at the sides. An ultra-feminine look was created when a three or four-inch wide flounce was inserted into this *godet* seam. The soft, supple fabric of the flounces cascaded down the skirt in graceful serpentine folds.

Gleaming satin, lustrous silk velvet, and supple crepe were the three most popular fabrics used for evening gowns during the early '30s. Satin was most common in black or white; however, other colors were also used. Silk velvet appeared in the deep rich shades of sapphire, garnet, purple, burgundy, pumpkin, rust, bronze, forest green, and black. Other fabrics common to this period were chiffon, mousseline de soie, georgette, net, lace, organdy, charmeuse, and gold and silver lamé. Furs such as fox,

ermine, sable, and mink were used to trim the collars, cuffs, and borders of winter evening gowns and wraps.

The flagging economy also touched off a trend for cotton, which was once considered too common for fashionable evening wear. As a practical alternative to expensive silks, Chanel used such fabrics as lawn, organdy, piqué, chintz, eyelet, tulle, and lace for her evening collection in 1930.

Organdy, dotted Swiss, voile, taffeta, moiré, and other stiffer fabrics were ideal when crisp stand-out ruffles or large puffy sleeves were desired. Affordably priced rayon remained a practical alternative for the modest budget. Prevalent colors for these fabrics were peach, white, pale pink, pale green, powder blue, dusty rose, geranium red, and beige. Strong contrasting color combinations such as black and white were very fashionable. To this spectrum of color Schiaparelli added her vivid "shocking pink" which became one of her well-recognized trademarks. Printed fabrics including florals, polka dots, plaids, checks, and stripes continued to grow in popularity.

### 1932 - 1936

During the first half of the decade, evening wear fell into two dissimilar categories. On the one hand was the "*ingénue* look" characterized by soft, romantic gowns with rippling flounces of fluffy chiffon or billowing sleeves of crisp organdy. On the other hand was the "seductress look" exemplified by Jean Harlow, sex symbol of the 1930s. Her slinky bias-cut satin gowns clung to the fluid lines of her body, creating a sleek, sensual elegance which many women tried to emulate.

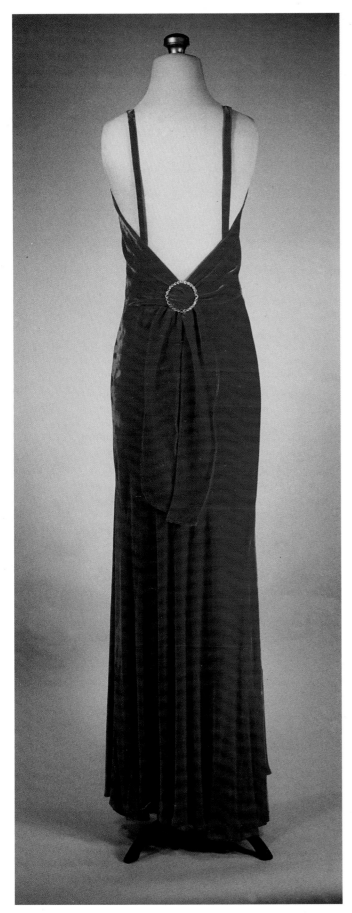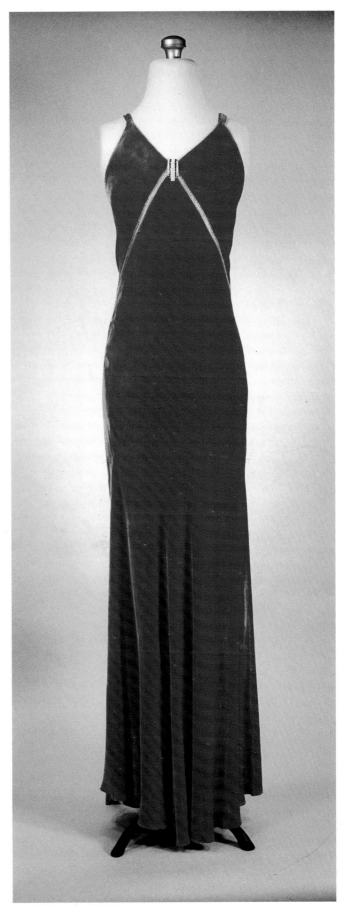

Orange bias-cut silk velvet gown with diagonal fagoted seams. Low-cut back contains spaghetti straps and sash which is fastened with rhinestone belt slide. (Worn by pianist to concert performance.) *Courtesy of Mary Anne Faust (Yesterday's Delights.)* $80-$125.

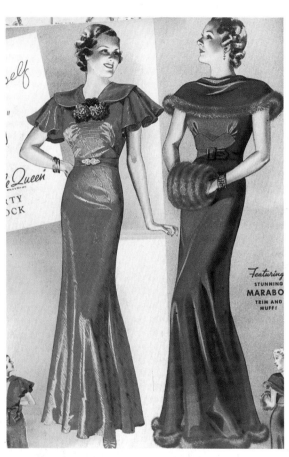

Sears, Roebuck and Co. evening gown illustrations (1936-37). *Left:* Red rayon-*moiré* gown, round collar, cape sleeves, blue silk flowers, self belt with mirror-image clasp. *Right:* Royal-blue crepe empire-style gown, self belt. Cape collar, muff, and hem trimmed with marabou feathers.

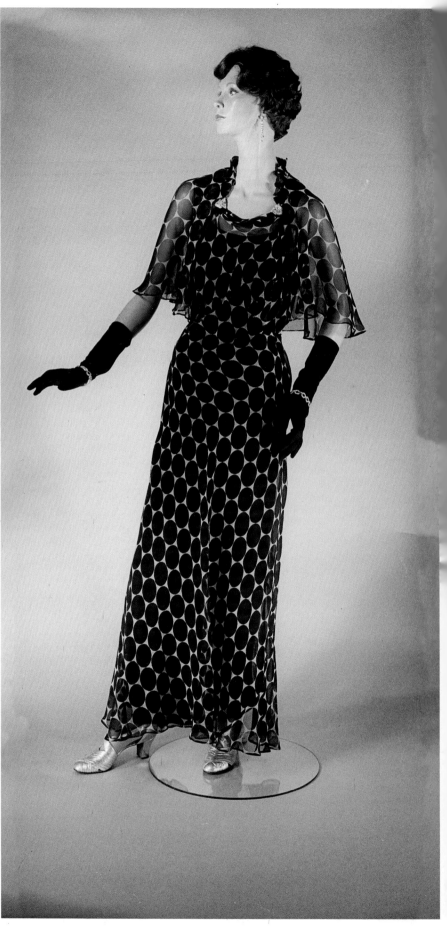

Black and white polka-dot chiffon evening gown, cape sleeves, rhinestone dress clips. *Courtesy of Cedar Crest Alumnae Museum, gift of Ellie Laubner.* $150-$200.

# Ingénue-Style Gowns

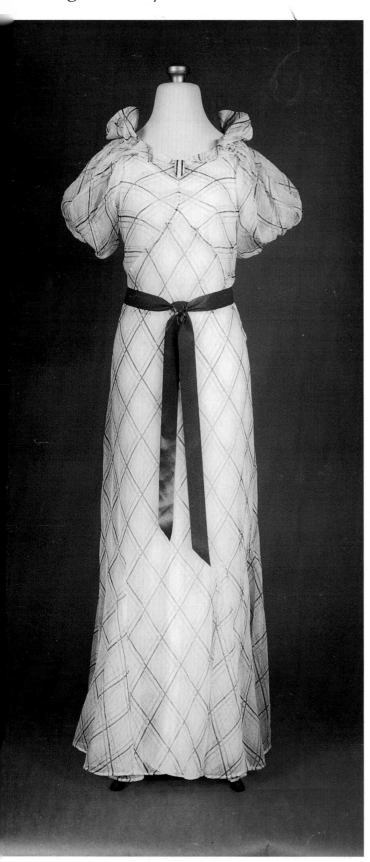

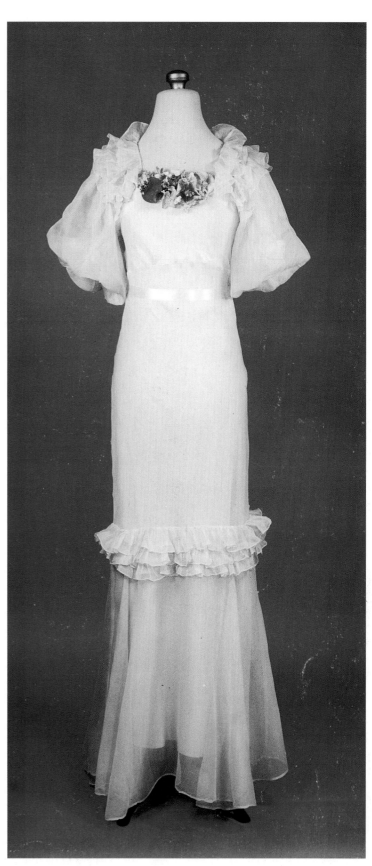

The bias cut is plainly visible on this green, blue, and white plaid organdy gown with empire waist, ruffled collar, and puffed sleeves. (Belt missing.) $60-$90.

Bias-cut peach chiffon gown with three rows of ruffles over the shoulder and around the knees, empire waist, puffed sleeves, cluster of multicolored silk flowers. $75-$110.

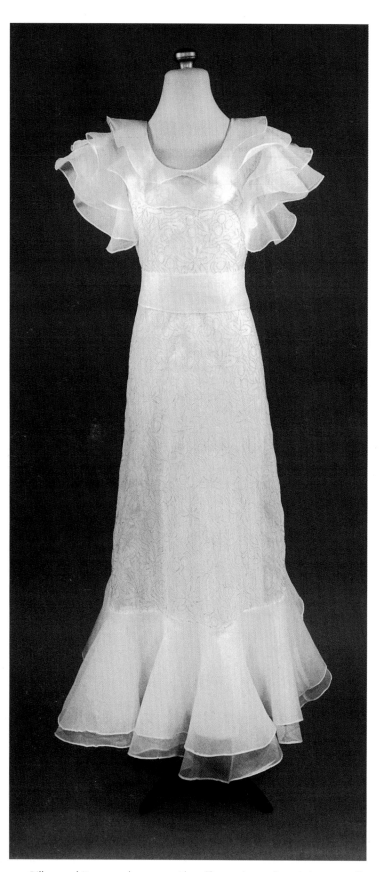

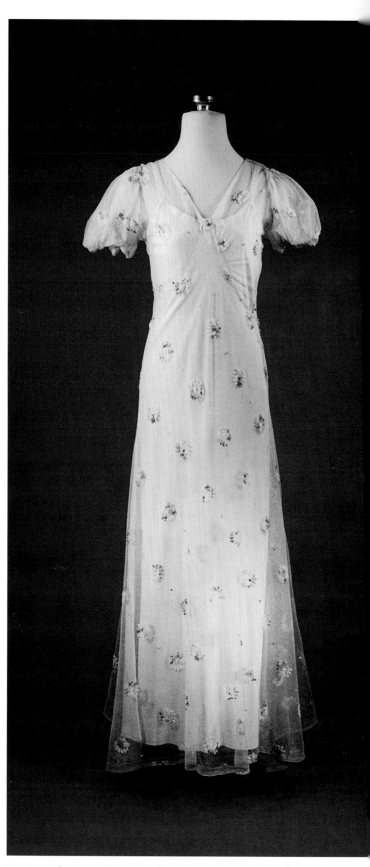

Billowy white organdy gown with ruffles at the neck and sleeves, self sash, bias-cut flounce at the hem. This gown is similar to the Letty Lynton dress. *Courtesy of Rose Jamieson.* $75-$100.

Empire-style gown of peach-tulle with small embroidered flowers, puffed sleeves, peach slip. *Courtesy of Cedar Crest Alumnae Museum, gift of Ellie Laubner.* $60-$80.

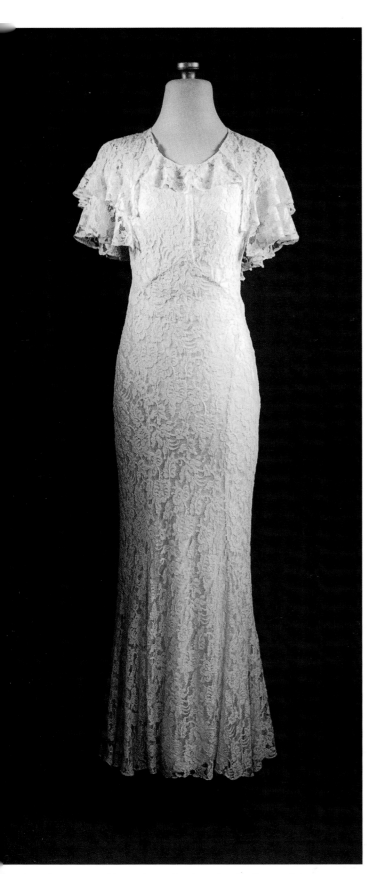

Ivory lace gown with empire waist, sleeveless bodice, and short detachable cape with two layers of ruffles. $75-$100.

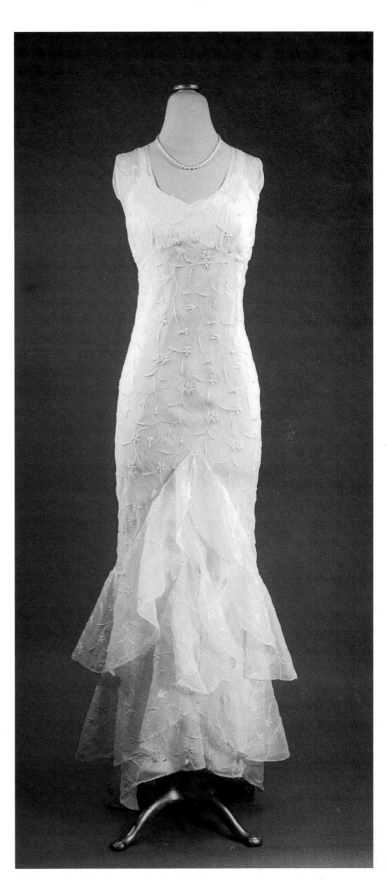

White embroidered-organdy sheath gown, empire waist, double-flounced skirt. $125-$175.

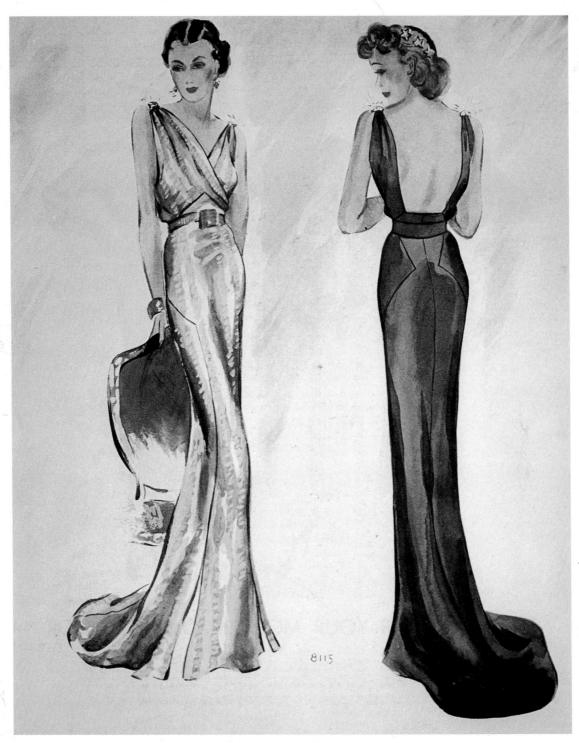

McCall's fashion illustration (12/35) features a bias-cut satin gown by Agnès-Drecoll. *Front*: Surplice-style bodice with V-shaped neckline. *Back*: low-cut square opening. Note: Juliet cap, dress clips and matching belt buckle.

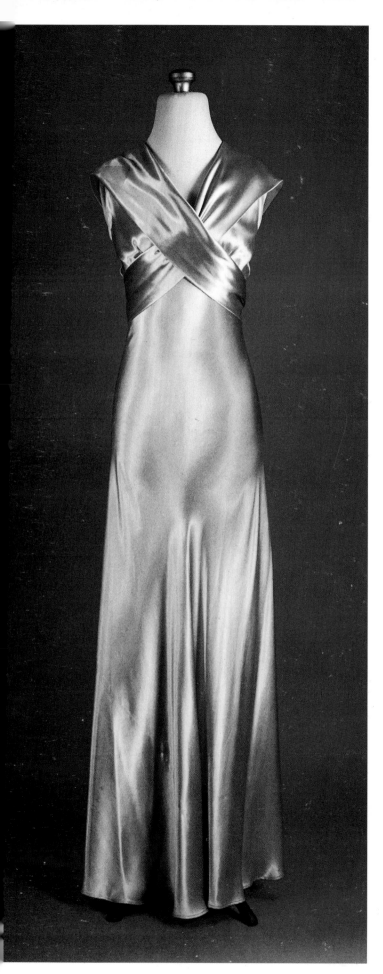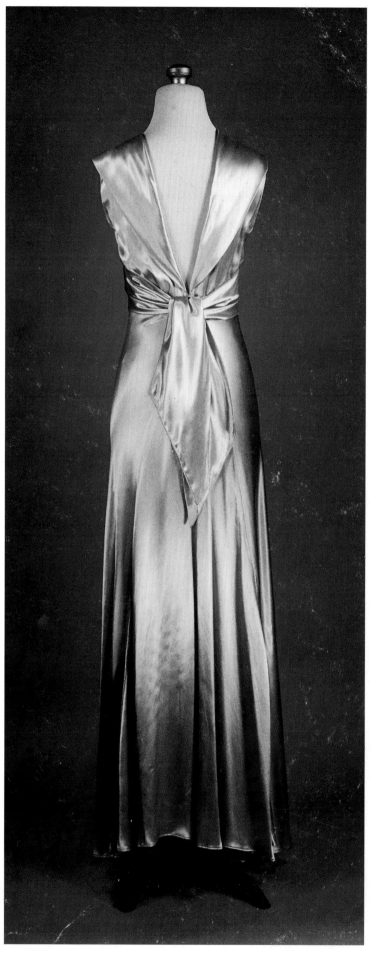

Lustrous gold-satin bias-cut gown, two wide panels start at the waist in back.
They frame the deep V-shaped opening, then pass over the shoulders, crisscross
the bust, and finally tie at the waist in back. $150-$175.

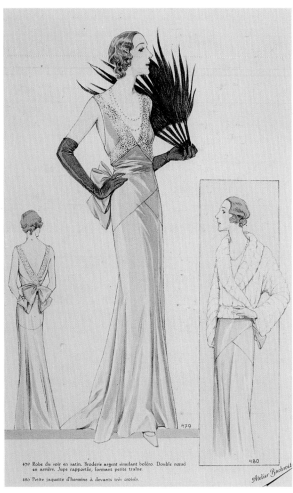

479 Robe du soir en satin. Broderie argent simulant boléro. Double nœud
en arrière. Jupe rapportée, formant petite traîne.

480 Petite jaquette d'hermine à devants très croisés.

Atelier Bachroitz

Original French fashion illustration (c. 1931-32) from the
*Atelier* (studio) Bachroitz. Pale-green satin evening gown
featuring silver embroidery. Open back accented with
embroidered straps in "V" formation, large butterfly bow,
and petit train.

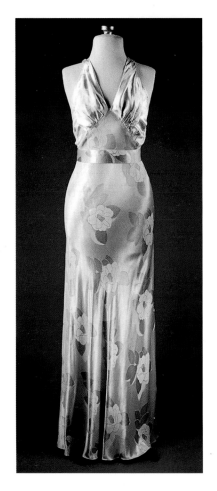

Off-white satin floral-print halter-
style gown with empire waist and
self belt, 1935. *Courtesy of Cedar
Crest Alumnae Museum, gift of
Constance Parkes Washburne.*
$150-$175.

This *McCall's* illustration (12/35) features a bias-
cut gown by Lelong. *Front:* princess-style, V-
neck. *Back:* crisscross straps, slightly train. Note:
dress clips at the shoulders and at center back.

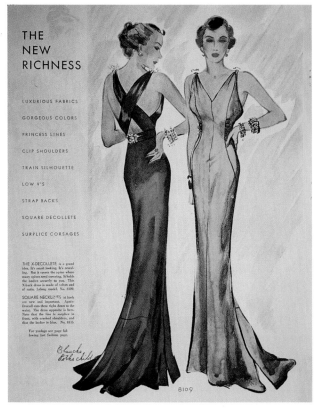

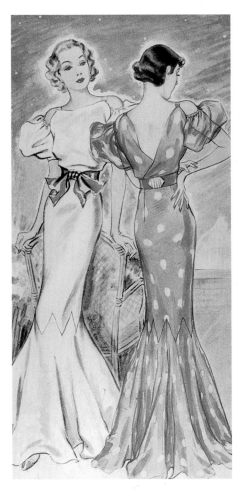

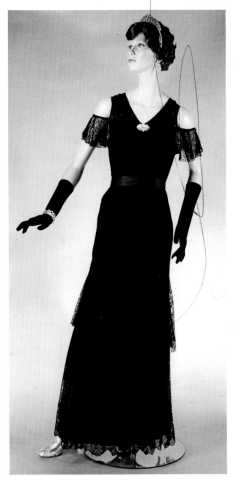

*McCall's* illustration (8/34) for an organdy cold-shoulder gown, *faux* puffed sleeve, exposed shoulders, ribbon sash, flared fishtail skirt.

Black-lace cold-shoulder gown, black-lace flounce encircles the bodice and arms leaving the shoulder exposed, layered skirt. $150-$200.

The popular "cross-over" sash-style bodice started with two four-foot-long strips of four-inch-wide self fabric attached at the base of the deep V-shaped opening at the back. These strips ran up either side of the V-shaped back opening, then over the shoulders to crisscross between the breasts in front. From there they ran under the breasts and around to tie at the waist in back.

"Cold shoulder" gowns, which revealed the curve of the shoulders, were a product of the years 1932 through 1934. This style began with a sleeveless gown featuring either built-up shoulders or narrow straps. A four or five-inch-wide flounce of fabric or lace was wrapped horizontally around the upper arms (and occasionally the bodice as well), giving the impression of detached sleeves. When this flounce was gathered across the top and bottom, it resembled a detached puffed sleeve.

The classic Victorian "bertha" collar made a reappearance during the 1930s. It consisted of a five to six-inch flounce or gathered ruffle which hung in graceful folds from a wide neckline. Unlike the 19th-century bertha collar, however, this flounce often cascaded from the edges of a plunging V-shaped "backline" as well.

Another of Vionnet's creative contributions was the "halter" neckline. For this style, the bodice fabric was drawn up into a narrow band on either side which then passed over the shoulders and buttoned or tied behind the neck. This left the back, shoulders, and arms exposed. A variation of the halter style featured one or two vertical strips of fabric connecting the halter with the top of the skirt in back. When made of black crepe with a large white-piqué notched collar, the gown took on a very tailored look. The halter was often used in conjunction with a high pointed or arched empire-style skirt which ended just under the bust. Unlike the empire-style dresses of the early 19th century, the skirt was fitted at the natural waist. The halter became a popular style, not only for evening gowns, but for nightgowns, sundresses, playsuits, and swimsuits.

"Wing" sleeves consisted of a single or double layer of gathered ruffles attached to the upper portion of the armseye (armhole). Fabrics such as organdy, dotted Swiss, voile, taffeta, and moiré were often used to create the desired stiffness.

The popular "Letty Lynton" dress was named for the style worn by Joan Crawford in the 1932 movie *Letty Lynton*. Created by Hollywood designer Gilbert Adrian, this crisp white or-

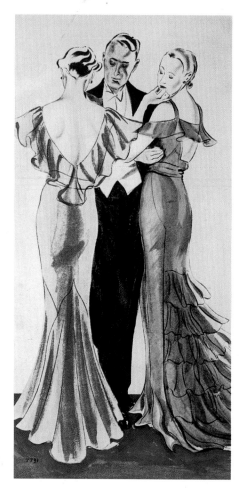

*McCall's* evening gown illustrations: *Left:* A cascading ruffle frames the deep-V neckline and covers the shoulders with softness, graceful fishtail skirt. *Right:* Cold-shoulder gown. Flounce encircles the bodice and arms, series of flounces simulate a mini bustle with train.

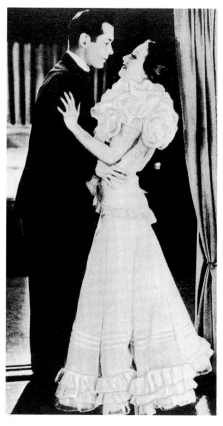

The Letty Lynton dress (1932) designed by Gilbert Adrian for Joan Crawford in the movie "Letty Lynton."

gandy dress featured multiple rows of narrow ruffles over the sleeves, the peplum, and around the hem. This style was widely copied and R.H. Macy in New York alone sold half a million copies.

The bishop and cape sleeves remained in style for dinner gowns. The unique "draped sling" sleeve began as a square kimono sleeve which was gathered along the ridge of the shoulder. Short puffed sleeves were also gaining in popularity.

Tunic-style gowns were offered during the mid-thirties and featured a knee-length over skirt attached to the waist of the evening gown. Skirts were generally bias cut, molding themselves to the hips and thighs, then falling in gentle fluted folds to the hem. The "fishtail" skirt, which fanned out from the knees to the hem, was created by the addition of wide bias-cut *godets*.

Common fabrics used during this period were chiffon, organdy, crepe, lace, tulle, and transparent velvet. Changeable and checkered taffeta, embossed figured satin, floral prints on black backgrounds, and polka dots were all prevalent. The most popular colors were black and white followed by strawberry, turquoise, mauve, gray, burgundy, and blue. Printed fabrics were extremely popular.

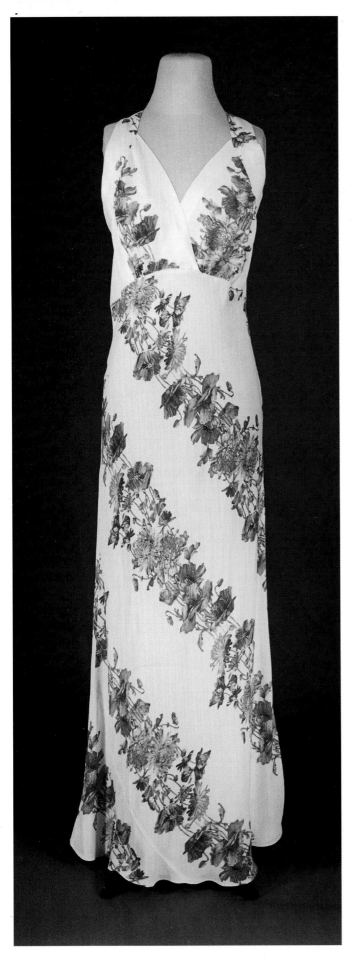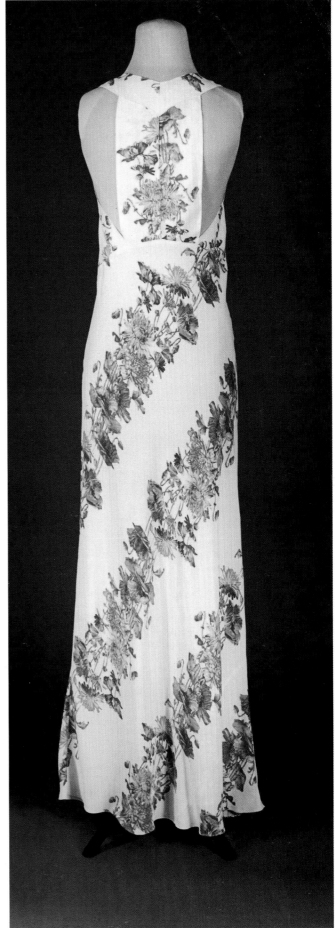

This bias-cut floral-striped rayon gown features a variation of the halter. Back view reveals two vertical panels connecting the halter to the top of the skirt. *Courtesy of Mary Anne Faust (Yesterday's Delights).* $75-$110.

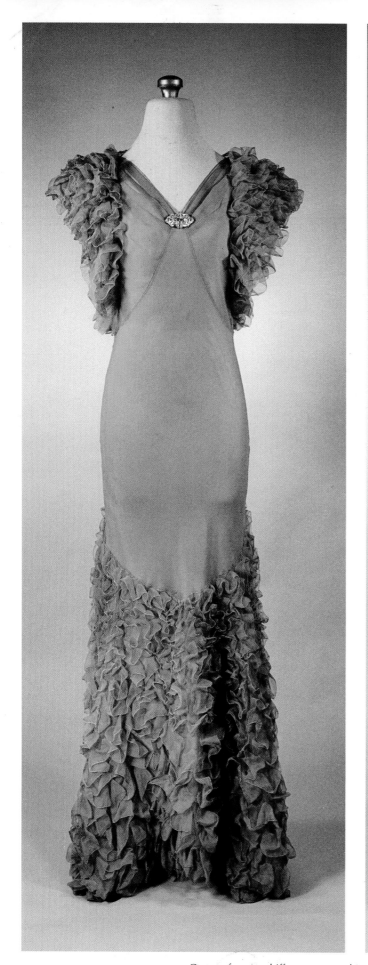
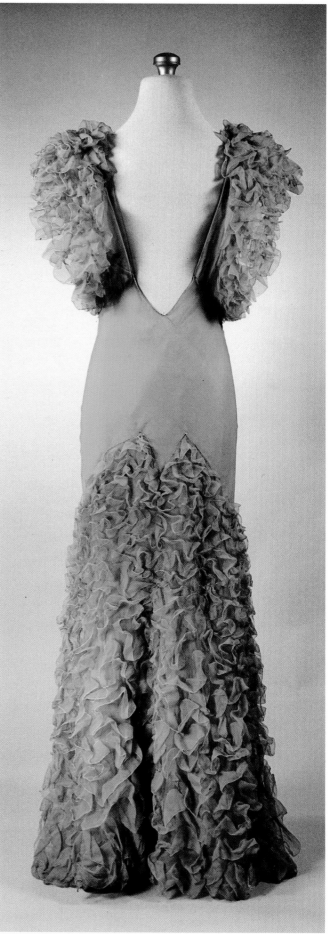

Gown of green chiffon over matching slip, multiple rows of ruffles
enhance broad-wing sleeves and skirt. Note: similarity to Letty
Lynton dress. Label: NRA, 1933-34. $175-$200.

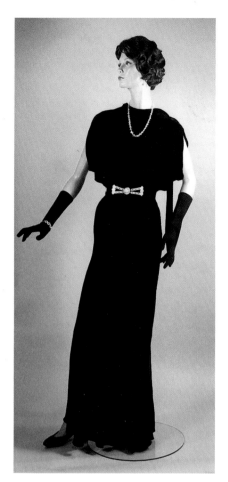
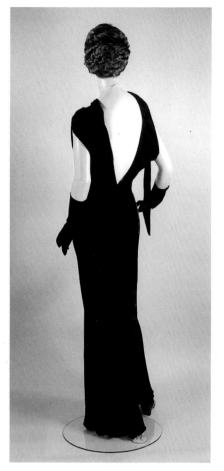
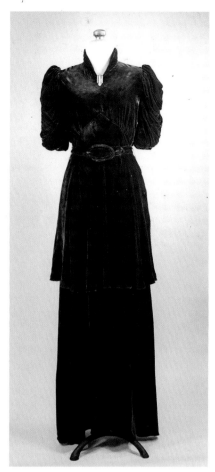

Black bias-cut silk-velvet gown, "draped-sling" sleeves. The rolled collar in front extends to form two narrow "flying panels" on either side of the deep V-shaped opening in back, self belt with rhinestone clasp. $125-$150.

Blue silk-velvet tunic dress with stand up collar, puffed sleeves, and self belt. $100-$150.

## 1937-1939

Practical diner/dance ensembles were offered which could easily pass from one activity to the another. Removing the short cape, bolero, swagger jacket, or over-blouse revealed the sleeveless (often backless) evening gown beneath.

Gathers became the most common detail used on evening gowns of the period. They were instrumental in shaping garments to the contours of the bust, the shoulders, the waist, and the arms. They were also used in the creation of puffed sleeves.

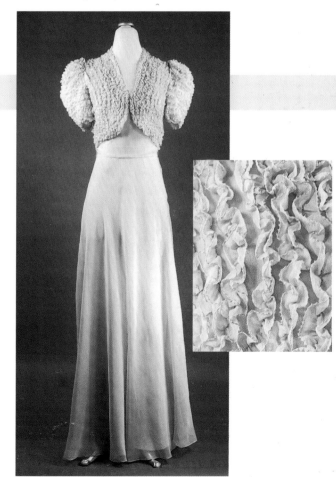

Bias-cut chiffon gown with gathered heart-shaped bodice worn over matching slip. Short bolero jacket covered with multiple rows of gathered ruching. c. 1935. *Courtesy of Ethel Bishop.* $100-$150.

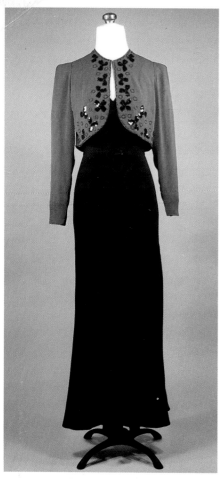

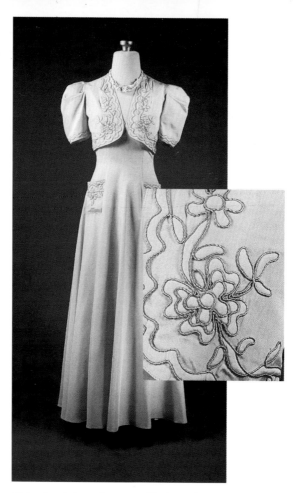

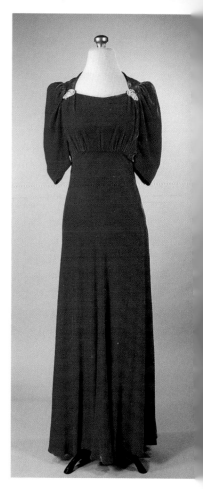

Black crepe gown with heart-shaped bodice and shoulder straps. Red silk-crepe long-sleeve bolero jacket accented with black sequins and bugle beads. *Courtesy of Kemerer Museum, gift of Mrs. Edmund Martin.* $200-$225.

Pink-taffeta halter-style gown with elevated waist and full gored skirt. Bolero jacket and patch pockets decorated with trapunto outlined in *passementerie* (cord), c. 1938-39. $125-$150.

Bias-cut burnt-orange silk-velvet dinner dress with empire waist, slightly puffed sleeves, and rhinestone dress clips. $120-$150.

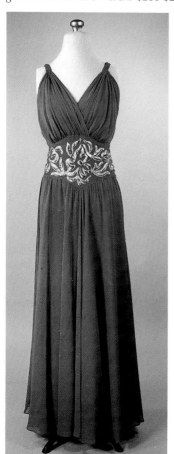

Sheer rust crepe evening gown with heart-shaped gathered bodice, waist yoke accented with padded gold *lamé* appliqué work, c. 1938-39. *Courtesy of Sue Steiner.* $125-$175.

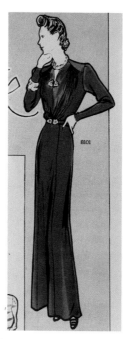

*La Press* advertisment (1/21/39) for a blue-velour dinner dress, V-neckline, bodice gathered into shoulder yoke and waist, rhinestone dress clips and matching belt clasp.

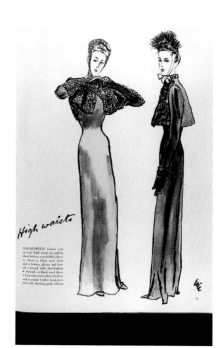

These black-wool jacket dresses by Schiaperelli appeared in *Vogue* (12/37). *Left:* Bolero, gloves, and bonnet covered with shoe buttons. *Right:* Embroidered bolero, feathered bonnet.

A decorative form of quilting known as "trapunto" was used on clothing and accessories during the late 1930s and 1940s. Unlike conventional quilting, which is often used for warmth, trapunto was created primarily for ornamentation. It gave dimension to the design which was most effective on solid-color fabric. (For more information and examples of trapunto see Chapters 2, 7, and 9.)

Sleeveless gowns with V-shaped necklines were still very much in style. The V-neck could be created by various means. One was the surplice-style bodice featuring two overlapping triangles which were formed into the shoulder straps at the top and gathered into the waist seam or waist yoke at the bottom. (Waist yokes were usually triangular or diamond-shaped.) A similar effect was created by using the same gathering technique on two triangles placed side by side.

The heart-shaped and straight-camisole bodices contained thin spaghetti straps fastened on either side of the bust or converging at the center front, forming a large V. For a feminine touch, the neckline was trimmed with pleated or gathered ruffles of fabric or lace. These two bodice shapes were also used for strapless gowns, a style pioneered by debutante Brenda Frazier. (See photo of Brenda Frazier in a strapless gown in Historical Overview, Chapter 1.) These gowns often featured a wide sash or cummerbund at the waist. Although introduced in the late '30s, strapless gowns did not become common place until after World War II.

The "sweetheart" neckline was introduced in the late '30s. It was similar to a square neck, however, the base line featured two arches—one over each breast—which resembled the top of a heart. This neckline was often used in conjunction with large puffed sleeves.

In the mid-to-late 1930s, gowns with fuller, more voluminous skirts were introduced, a reflection of the trend towards Victorian-revival fashions. They were called "Winterhalter" gowns after the renowned mid-19th century painter. He is known for his paintings of the Empress Eugénie of France wearing *bouffant* hoop skirts.

The fullness of 1930s skirts was achieved by the use of three different techniques. The first involved the use of numerous wedge-shaped gores which widened towards the hem. Taffeta shot with metal, organza, moiré, and satin were popular fabrics for this style of skirt. The second technique featured three to eight gathered flounces stitched in horizontal layers, each overlapping the top of the flounce below it. The illusion of breadth was further emphasized when the layers were made of horizontal stripes. The third technique involved three or four graduated tiers, each wider then the one above. Each tier was gathered slightly at the top, then stitched to the bottom of the tier above it. This style was often made of sheer fabrics such as tulle, chiffon, or lace over a taffeta underskirt.

There was also a growing trend toward more tailored two-piece evening ensembles. A long gored skirt of silk jersey, crêpe, satin, or taffeta might be paired with a silk-foulard basque-style jacket or a gold-lamé over blouse with a belted waist and bishop sleeves. A print blouse with a coordinating cummerbund or a sleeveless evening sweater were other alternatives.

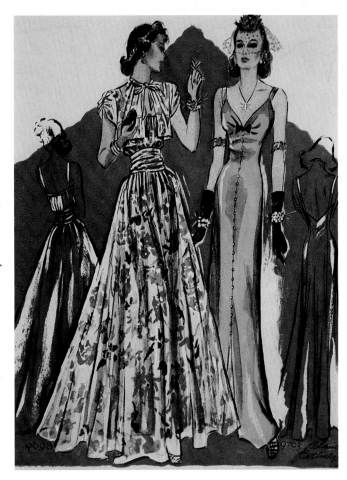

Summer gown from *McCall's* (1938): *Left:* Evening gown features bolero jacket with short gathered sleeves, cummerbund, and full Winterhalter skirt. *Right:* Sheath gown with heart-shaped neckline and row of buttons. Note: evening headpiece.

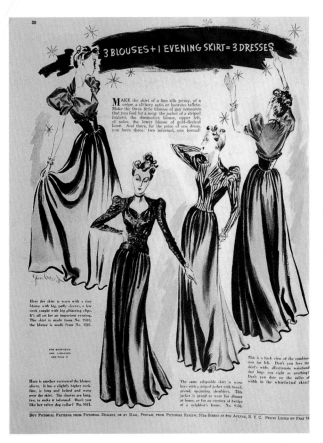

This *Pictorial Review* advertisement (2/39) features three evening ensembles using one basic skirt. (1 & 4) Blouse - puffed sleeves, sweetheart neckline, corselette. (2) Basque top - sweetheart neckline and belt. (3) Fitted jacket - puffed sleeves.

# DINNER SUITS

The "dinner suit" made an appearance towards the end of the decade. It consisted of a bolero or short peplum jacket with broad shoulders and a long matching skirt. Crepe, wool, velvet, and bouclé were the common fabrics. (See bridal attendant's evening suit in Bridal Wear, Chapter 5.)

Beautifully embroidered evening jackets, became one of Schiaparelli's trademarks. She commissioned the most prestigious embroidery firm, the Maison Lesage, to design exquisite embroideries which are now considered works of art. Prancing ponies, acrobats, and performing elephants graced boleros for her "Circus" collection in 1938. Astrological signs and heavenly bodies were embroidered on a midnight blue evening jacket for her "Astrology" collection that same year.

## Ornamentation

Dress clips were the most popular form of jewelry produced during the 1930s. They were produced in white gold or platinum with pavé-set diamonds, rubies, sapphires, and emeralds for the well-to-do. For the more modest budget there was a silver set with marcasites or rhodium-plated base metal with pavé-set rhinestones. These pieces looked particularly striking against the deep, rich colors of silk velvet.

Sold singly or in pairs, dress clips were often clipped to the center of sweetheart or V-shaped necklines or at the corners of the square, sweetheart, or boat necklines. Clips could add interest to the shoulders or accent a deep back opening. They could even add style to an evening bag or hat. (For further information and examples of dress clips and double-clip brooches see Jewelry, Chapter 11.)

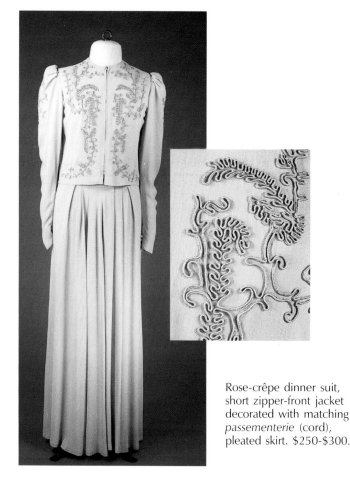

Rose-crêpe dinner suit, short zipper-front jacket decorated with matching *passementerie* (cord), pleated skirt. $250-$300.

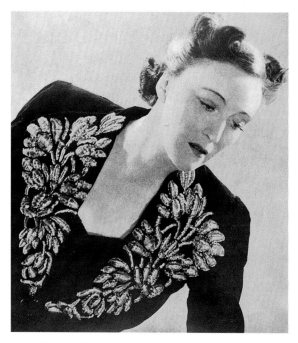

This Schiaparelli dinner suit appeared in *Harper's Bazaar* (1/38). The plum-velvet jacket was lavishly embroidered in iridescent purple and silver threads. The slender skirt was slit to the knee. Note: up-swept hair.

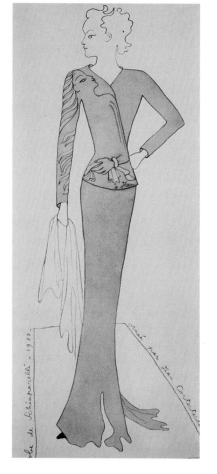

*Harper's Bazaar* (3/37) published this illustration of Schiaparelli's gray-linen dinner suit. Surrealist artist Jean Cocteau designed the silhouette which was embroidered on the jacket in gold sequins and bugle beads.

### Fasteners

***Buckles, Clasps, and Belt Slides***. Evening gowns often contained self belts accented with glittering Art Deco style mirror-image clasps, buckles, clasps, or belt slides (buckles without hasps) decorated with pavé-set gemstones or paste. Three-piece sets including two clips and a matching belt clasp were also offered. In lieu of a belt, a wide silk or rayon satin ribbon was often used for evening gowns.

***Hooks and Eyes.*** Evening gowns requiring side plackets were fastened with hooks and eyes and/or snaps. Back openings were often fastened with closely-spaced covered buttons and *rouleaux* loops, a loop created from a narrow tunnel of the dress fabric with or without a cord for filler. (For an example see Bridal Wear, Chapter 5.)

***Zippers.*** By the end of the decade metal "slide fasteners" (zippers) were beginning to appear in women's dresses. Just as women were beginning to appreciate the benefits of this revolutionary new fastener, however, the government restricted the use of metal for the duration of the war.

# ADDITIONAL DESIGNERS

***Mme. Grès (Alix)***. French *couturiere*, Mme. Grès, opened her own *couture* house in Paris in 1923. Like Vionnet, she had an appreciation for the well-formed feminine figure. She designed her garments by draping, pinning, and basting the fabric directly on a live model. Her special talents lay in her ability to manipulate the fabric into meticulous pleats and undulating folds. Seldom influenced by contemporary fashion trends, her gowns exhibited an understated simplicity and timeless elegance reminiscent of the ancient Greeks. Her favorite fabrics were silk and wool jersey, silk crepe, chiffon, and mousseline de soie. Her design house was closed by the Germans in 1942.

***Mainbocher.*** American-born designer, Main Rousseau Bocher, attended the Chicago Academy of Fine Arts and studied in London, Munich, and Paris. He worked as fashion editor, then editor-in-chief of French Vogue from 1923 to 1929. In 1930, he combined his first and last names and became the first American designer to open a salon in Paris, attracting many wealthy American clients. Mainbocher was famous for his bias-cut evening dresses and dinner suits. He received international acclaim when Wallis Simpson called upon him to design the blue crepe wedding dress she wore for her marriage to the Duke of Windsor. Mainbocher's designs were always tasteful and refined with a certain understated elegance which appealed to the mature woman. He closed his *maison de couture* at the outbreak of World War II, and opened a salon in New York.

# CARE OF EVENING GOWNS

When stored on a hanger for many years, bias-cut garments tend to stretch. (They often look as though they had been worn by a seven-foot-tall toothpick.) The shape of the garment can also become distorted. This may be avoided by storing bias-cut garments flat in boxes. Clothing should not touch ordinary paper, cardboard, or wood as they contain acids which may burn fabrics. For this reason, it is best to store garments in acid-free boxes lined with acid-free tissue paper. Another alternative is to wrap the garment in unbleached muslin.

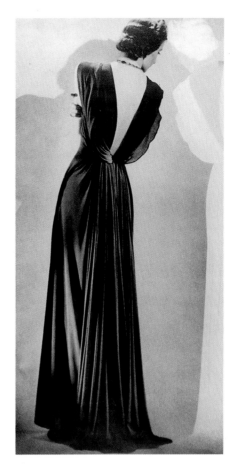

This elegant evening gown, pictured in *Harper's Bazaar* (1/38), was designed by Mme. Grès. It featured a low neckline and her trademark — classically draped pleats.

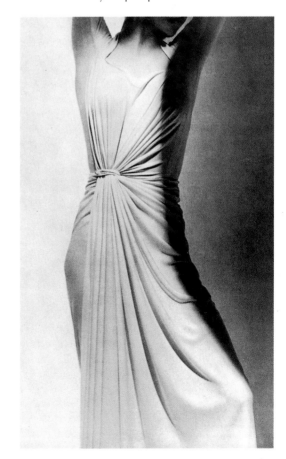

This photograph published in *Harper's Bazaar* (3/15/38) illustrates Mme. Grès unique talent for draping which sets her creations apart from the ordinary. Note: sweetheart neckline.

# Chapter 5

# Bridal Wear

## WEDDING GOWNS

For many brides who were married during the depression, a formal wedding was out of the question. It was not unusual for couples to wed in the home of the bride's parents with a few relatives and friends looking on. The bride wore her best dress and carried a bouquet of flowers picked fresh from the garden.

For the handy bride, McCall's pattern magazine offered a practical sleeveless gown which could be worn with the matching jacket for the marriage ceremony and without the jacket as an evening gown. Some resourceful brides dyed their wedding dresses after the wedding in an effort to maximize their use.

For those brides fortunate enough to have a church wedding, a gown was carefully chosen. Many wedding gowns were patterned after evening gowns of the period and featured the same details and elements of design. The halter-style gown, however, with its open back and shoulders was considered inappropriate for church weddings. White, the symbol of virginity, was still the traditional color for brides.

Unlike the short, tubular wedding dresses of the preceding decade, 1930s bridal gowns were long, sophisticated, and bias cut for a smooth, body-hugging fit. Arch-shaped *godets* were often inserted in the sides of the skirt for a soft flare. Bridal gowns contained little or no applied ornamentation. Curved or diagonal seam lines, gathers, and an occasional belt or artificial flower were the only forms of decoration. They were fastened down the back with 15 to 30 closely-spaced self-covered buttons and self *rouleaux* loops (a loop created from a narrow tube of the dress fabric with or without a cord for filler). Many gowns ended in a semi-circular train.

As with evening gowns of the '30s, the most popular fabric was lustrous silk satin. Lace, velvet, organdy, silk crepe, chiffon, and mousseline de soie were other commonly used fabrics.

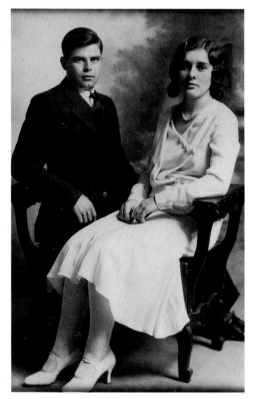

This bride wears a champaign-colored dress and ankle-strap shoes, 1932. After the wedding she dyed her dress to maximize its use. *Courtesy of Erma Updegrove.*

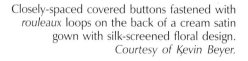

Closely-spaced covered buttons fastened with *rouleaux* loops on the back of a cream satin gown with silk-screened floral design. *Courtesy of Kevin Beyer.*

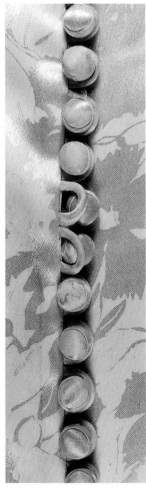

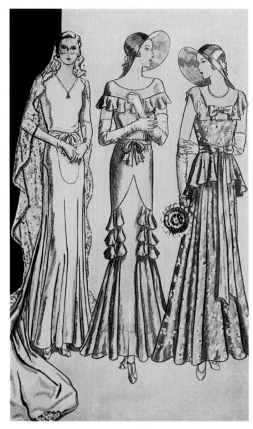

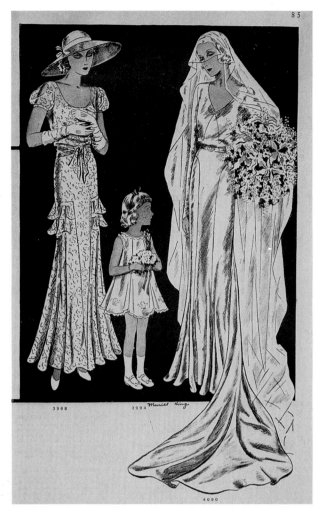

*Delineator* bridal-wear patterns (3/31). *Bride* - White satin bias-cut gown, fitted sleeves, girdled waist, long arched *godets* at sides of skirt, train, and long lace veil. *Maid of Honor* - Bias-cut chiffon, scoop neck, girdled waist, horizontal flounces around bodice and at knees, skirt flares below knees. *Bridesmaid* - Bias-cut printed georgette with scoop neck, ruffled peplum, flared skirt, velvet ribbon bows. Note: garden party hats and long white gloves.

Bridal wear patterns from *Delineator* (9/32). *Bridesmaid* - Blue bias-cut lace gown with scooped neck, puffed sleeves, self sash, and two flounces below each hip, wide-brimmed garden party hat with down-turned brim. *Flower girl* - Blue sleeveless chemise-style dress with lace trim. *Bride* - Bias-cut satin gown with a V-neck, large pointed collar, self belt, gored skirt with a train.

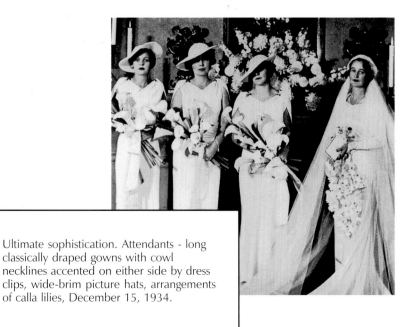

Ultimate sophistication. Attendants - long classically draped gowns with cowl necklines accented on either side by dress clips, wide-brim picture hats, arrangements of calla lilies, December 15, 1934.

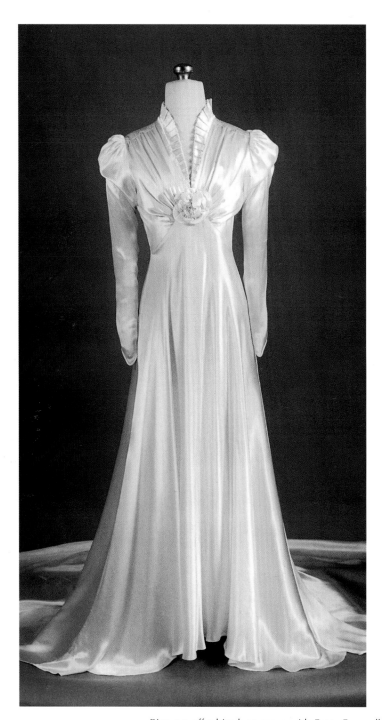
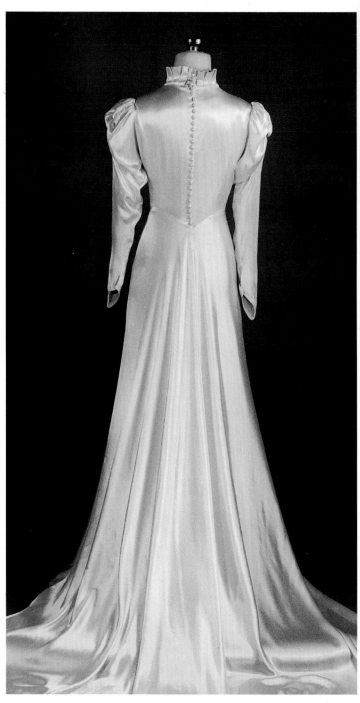

Bias-cut off-white lace gown with Peter Pan collar and semicircular train, sleeves have a slight fullness at the top, then taper to a snug fit from elbow to wrist. Back reveals a row of closely-spaced covered buttons with *rouleaux* loops and a lace half belt. $200-$300.

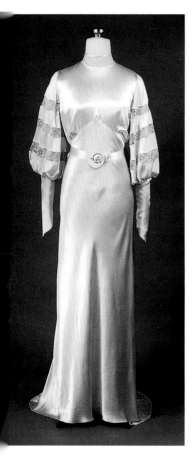

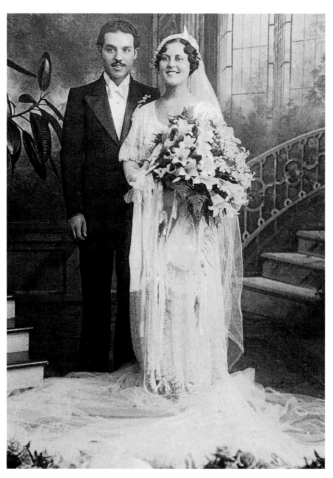

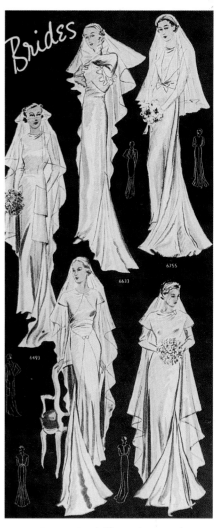

Bias-cut crepe-back satin gown, high band collar and bishop sleeves accented with rows of Chantilly lace, self belt, skirt slightly trained. c. 1932-34. *Courtesy of Kevin Beyer.* $200-$250.

White lace gown featuring bishop sleeves with wide cuffs, small head-hugging lace cap accented with pearls, "star-cut" crystal pendant, bouquet of white lilies, c. 1932-34. *Courtesy of Rose Jamieson*.

*Vogue Pattern Book* illustrations (10/34) featuring five wedding gowns. *From top right (6755)* - Pointed *revers* with fitted sleeves. *(6633)* - Empire waist with standing collar and ruffles fastened at the armseyes. *(6493)* - Cowl neck with layered flounces over the hips. *(S-3619)* Diagonal seaming, short sleeves with long fitted under sleeves. *(S-3691)* - Simple lines with short sleeves over long fitted sleeves.

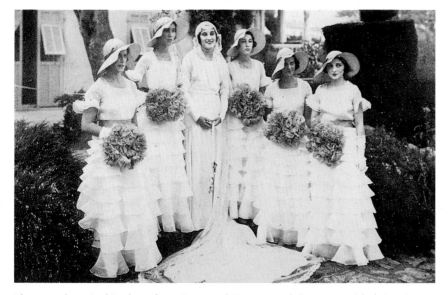

The attendants in this photo from *Town and Country* (10/1/31) wear wide-brim picture hats and pale organdy gowns with multiple horizontal flounces.

65

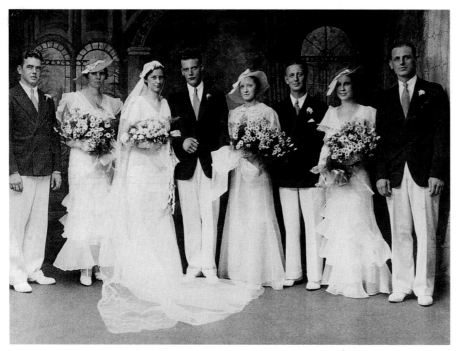

*Bridesmaids* - White organdy gowns with double-cape sleeves, flounced skirts, wide-brimmed transparent-horsehair picture hats with yellow satin ribbons, bouquets of daisies. *Maid of Honor* - yellow hat. 1934. (See bridal gown in accompanying photo.) *Courtesy of Samuel and Margaret Haldeman.*

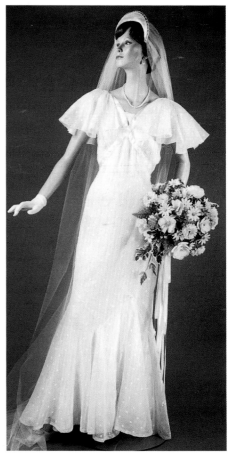

White organdy gown with embroidered coin dots, cape sleeves, skirt flared below the knees, 1934. *Courtesy of Samuel and Margaret Haldeman.* $200-$250.

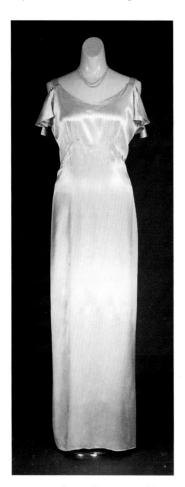

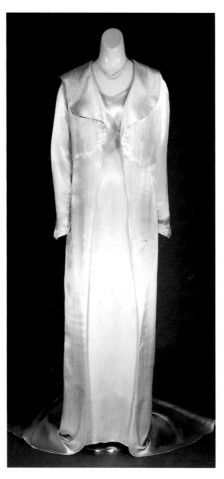

Lustrous white silk-satin wedding gown with scooped neck, empire waist, and *jabot*-like ruffles under the arms. Matching silk satin coat features wide shawl collar, long pointed sleeves, and ends in a train, 6/11/35. *Courtesy of Elizabeth Irons.* $250-$300.

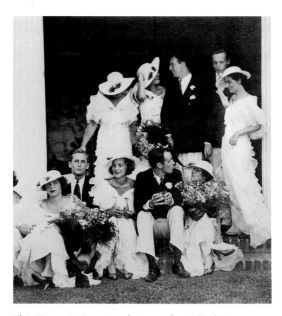

This *Town & Country* photograph (12/15/34) displays the last word in femininity! These romantic organdy gowns have wide décolleté necklines and heaps of frothy ruffles over the upper arms and the sides of the skirts. The picture hats are the icing on the cake.

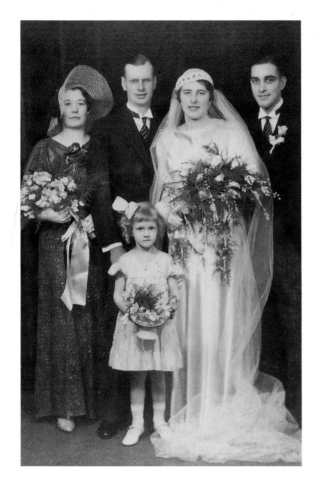

*Bride* - white satin gown with a cowl neck, bishop sleeves, white satin snug-fitting cap with lattice-style trim. *Bridesmaid* - blue lace gown, horse-hair hat with wide asymmetrical brim. *Flower girl* - white dress. *Men* - black morning coats and gray striped trousers, 1935. *Courtesy of Margaret Place.*

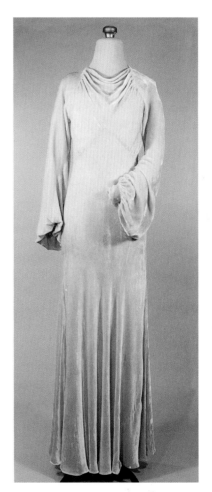

Gown of ivory bias-cut silk-velvet, cowl neckline, bishop sleeves, 1935. (Similar to illustration at left.) *Mary Anne Faust (Yesterday's Delights).* $150-$200.

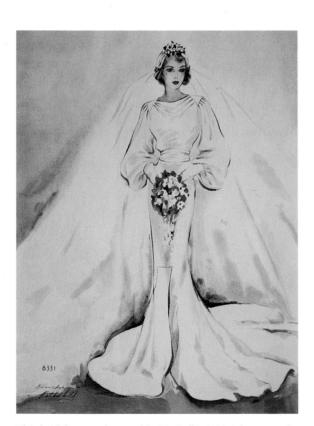

This bridal gown, featured in *McCall's* (1935) has a cowl neckline and full bishop sleeves. The sweeping train features a slit at the center front, allowing a glimpse of the wedding slippers as bride walks.

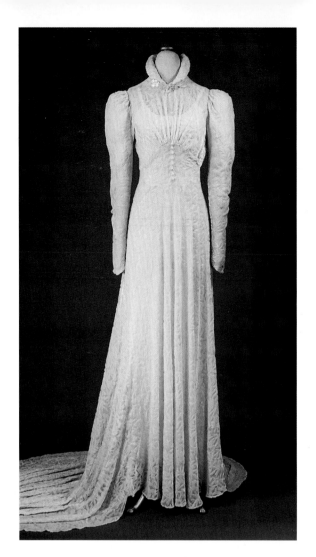

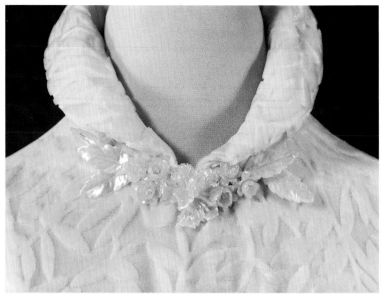

Gown of ivory silk velvet with "burnt-out" foliate motif, leg-o-mutton sleeves, cluster of wax flowers at base of curled Peter-Pan collar. Bodice gathered at empire waist, skirt accented by row of covered buttons. *Courtesy of Kevin Beyer.* $300-$350.

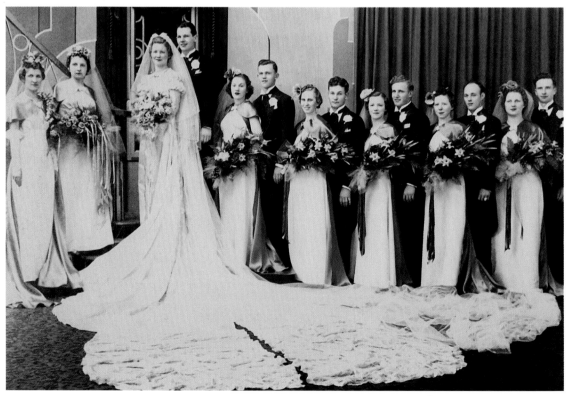

*Bride* - gown with Juliet sleeves and a voluminous train and veil. *Attendants* - gowns with gathered bodices, short sleeves, and long gloves, small round satin capes in a contrasting color. *Men* - cutaways with wing collar shirts and cravats. Note: Art Deco background.

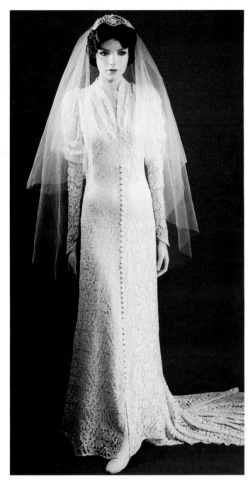

Bias-cut off-white lace gown contains a gathered bodice, sleeves full to the elbow, then fitted to wrist, vertical row of covered buttons on skirt. Worn with white crocheted Juliet cap and veil. *Courtesy of Joan York.* $200-$250.

Brides generally wore long-sleeved gowns while their attendants often wore short. There were three main sleeve styles used for wedding gowns. The decade began with the straight fitted sleeve, a carry-over from the 1920s. A puffy fullness began to form at the top of the sleeve, eventually culminating in a full-blown Juliet sleeve towards the end of the decade. This sleeve was influenced by the costumes worn by Norma Shearer in the film version of *Romeo and Juliet* in 1936. The full bishop sleeve was another favorite, beginning in the early 1930s and overlapping the other two styles. It had either a short cuff at the wrist or a longer 12-inch cuff which extended from the wrist to the elbow. This longer cuff was often decorated with a row of closely spaced covered buttons.

A variety of necklines were used including the square, the scoop, and V-neck. The soft, classically-draped cowl was another option. The Peter Pan, ruffled *Pierrot*, and high-band collars were all common during this period. A high, inverted V or U-shaped waist seam was common with a belt at the natural waist.

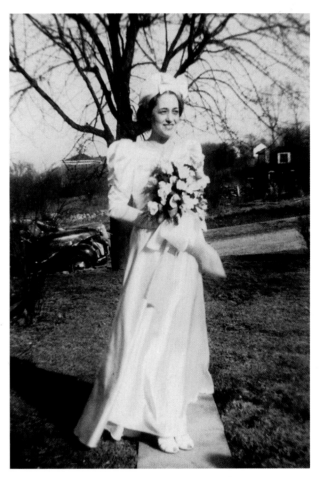

Ivory satin gown with a sweetheart neckline and gather leg-o-mutton sleeves, matching hat has an up-turned brim with asymmetrical self bow, 2/18/39. *Courtesy of Adeline Laudenslager.*

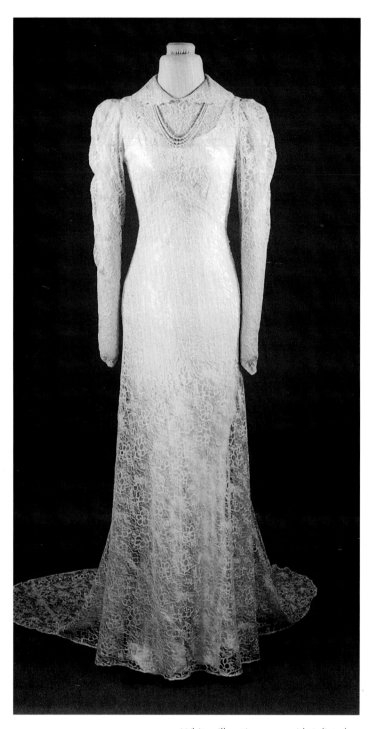
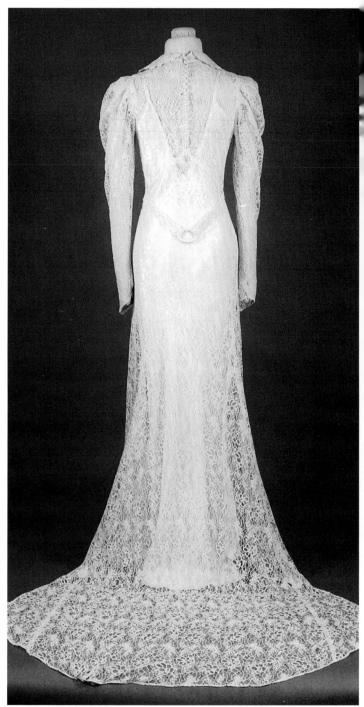

White silk-satin gown with Juliet sleeves, gathered bodice, V-neck accented with pleated trim and a *chou* (rosette), full skirt with semicircular train, back fastened with 25 covered buttons and *rouleaux* loops. $300-$350.

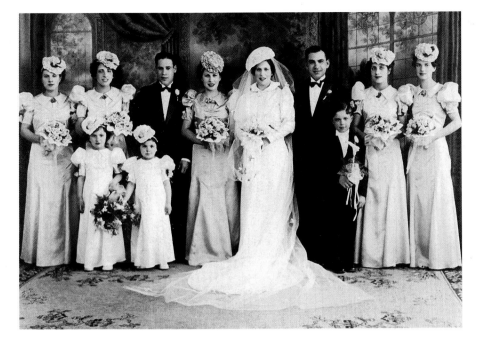

*Bride* - Gown with Peter Pan collar and long sleeves. *Bridesmaids* - pastel taffeta gowns with puffed sleeves, small pointed collars, and vertical gathers down the center of bodices, each carries a nosegay. *Flower girls* - mini versions of the bridesmaid's gowns. All wear tilting doll hats with concentric rows of ruffles, c. 1938-39.

One of the most famous wedding dresses of the decade was designed by Mainbocher for the marriage of Wallis Simpson to Edward VIII on June 3, 1937. Since this was Mrs. Simpson's third marriage, white (signifying virginity) was out of the question. She wore instead a long slender medium blue-gray silk crepe dress with a matching long-sleeved jacket, on the order of a dinner suit. The fabric of the jacket bodice was gathered into the neckline above and into the two arched panels at the waist below. A vertical row of closely-spaced self-covered buttons was the only decoration. She wore a small blue straw hat decorated with blue and pink *coq* (rooster) feathers designed by French milliner, Caroline Reboux. (For a wedding photo of the Duke and Duchess see Historical Background, Chapter 1.) In the spring of 1937, the Duchess purchased numerous outfits for her trousseau from the houses of Mainbocher, Paquin, and Molyneux. Also included were fashions chosen from Schiaparelli's Music Collection.

## ATTENDANTS' GOWNS

Attendants' gowns were usually floor length with short puffed or cape-style sleeves and occasionally a Peter Pan collar. During the early years, attendants' gowns were soft and feminine with rippling ruffles on the bodice and skirt, which echoed evening gowns of the period. Gowns of the later 1930s were a bit more tailored. Organdy, georgette, lace, and chiffon were commonly used in summer, while satin, crepe, lace, and velvet were used in winter.

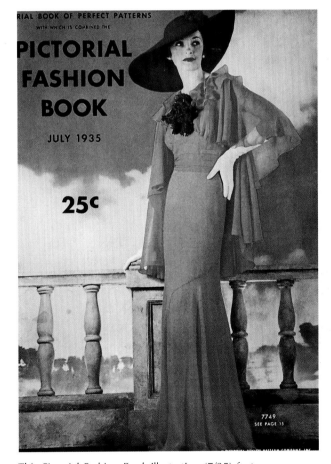

This *Pictorial Fashion Book* illustration (7/35) features an ensemble suitable for a summer garden wedding. Salmon silk-chiffon bias-cut gown, bi-layer bias-cut cape with ruffled neckline, deep-blue wide-brimmed hat by Lilly Daché, elbow-length gloves by Aris.

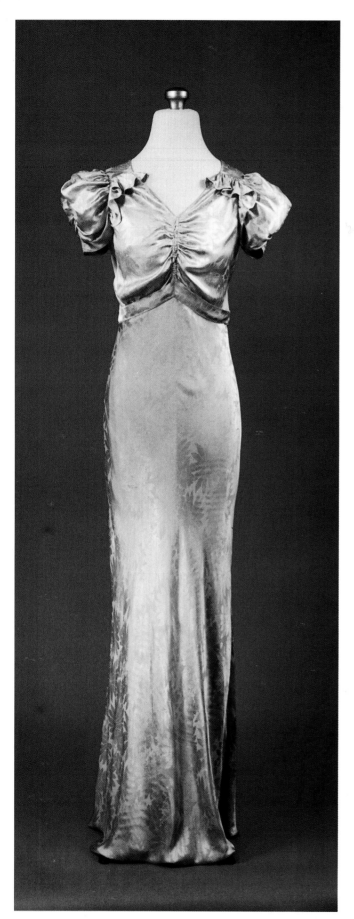

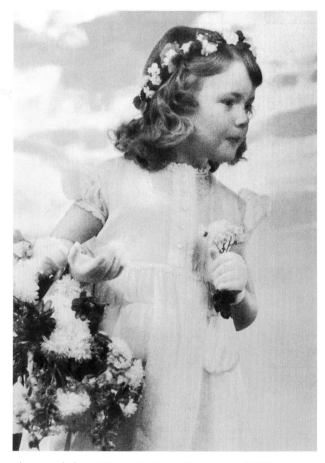

Photograph from *Woman's Home Companion* (6/37) shows a flower girl wearing a white dotted-Swiss dress with lace-trim, baby-doll sleeves, and a wreath of purple and white flowers.

Bridesmaid's gown. Gold satin with silk-screened all-over daisy pattern, puffed sleeves, bodice contains vertical gathers down the center, c. 1937-39. *Courtesy of Kevin Beyer.* $125-$150.

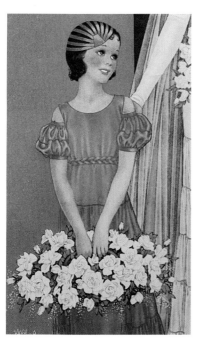

*Delineator* illustration (6/33) featuring a flower girl wearing a blue satin cold-shoulder gown with *faux* puffed sleeves, tiered skirt. Headpiece of blue satin ribbons which converge at the front and back.

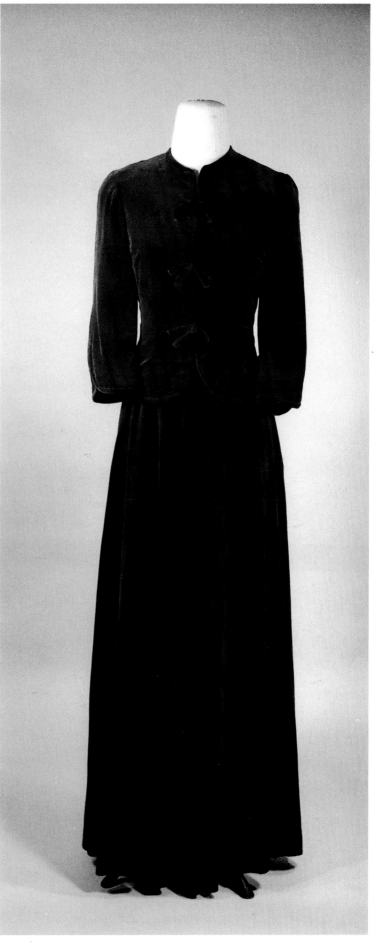

Bridesmaid's evening suit. Short purple velveteen jacket with cutaway corners, self-fabric bows along the zippered closure, padded shoulders, long gored skirt. c. 1938-39. *Courtesy of Mary Anne Faust (Yesterday's Delights).* $150-$175.

# BRIDAL HEADPIECES

***Small Head-Hugging Headpiece.*** During the early '30s, small head-hugging hats were popular. They were decorated with seed pearls and were worn tilted over the right eye.

***Halo-style Headpiece.*** During the first few years of the decade, brides continued to wear the halo-style headpiece of the late '20s. This consisted of a fan-shaped piece of gathered organdy or lace wired to spread in semi-circular fashion framing the face. This halo was attached to a close, head-encompassing cap.

The cap soon began to recede towards the back of the head, exposing more of the hair. Eventually all that remained was the halo itself, resembling an ancient Greek *stephane*. The halo was often made of white satin which was stiffened with buckram for body and decorated with seed pearls. Attached to the base of the halo was a U-shaped spring-tension wire band which gripped the sides of the head. A net veil was attached along the bottom edge of the halo.

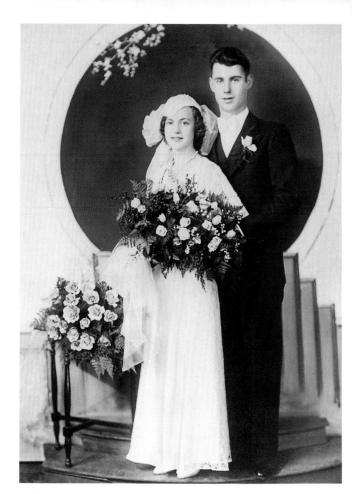

Bride wears close-fitting pointed hat accented with a large bow at the back.

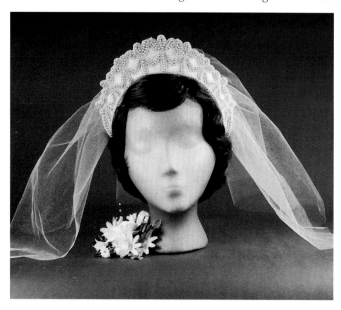

Satin halo-style headpiece decorated with pearls and seed beads. $50-$75.

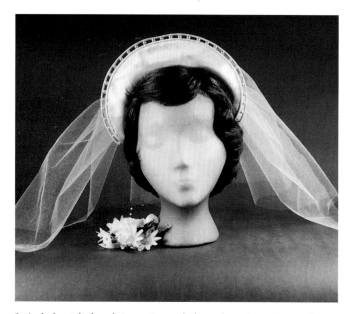

Satin halo-style headpiece trimmed along the edge with pearls. Label: Bonwit Teller & Co. $50-$75.

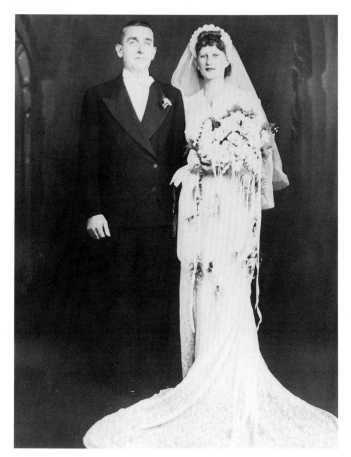

Scalloped halo-style headpiece.

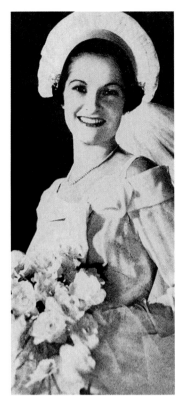

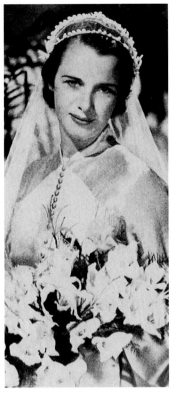

This *McCall's* advertisement (10/35) features a white cap with sheer halo and veil, cold-shoulder-style gown.

*Ladies' Home Journal* advertisement (11/35) featuring two bands of flower buds to hold this bridal veil in place.

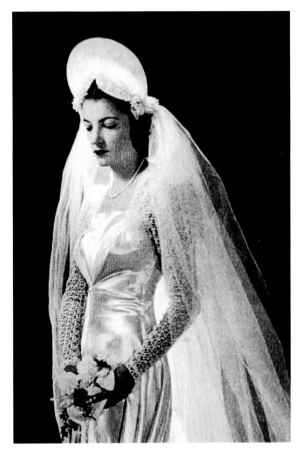

Circular halo attached to flower decked headpiece with floral clusters over each ear. White satin gown features long fitted lace sleeves. *Courtesy of Rose Jamieson.*

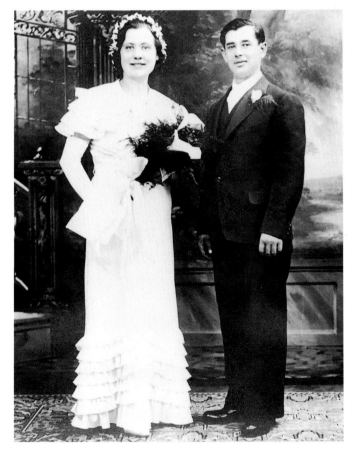

Bride wears a wreath of flowers over her hair, 5/3/34. *Courtesy of William W. Hoffman, M.D.*

**Floral Bands and Wreaths.** One or more bands of the traditional wax orange blossoms were worn over the top of the head, ear to ear. These were also available with silk, organdy, or muslin flowers. Similar to the floral bands was the wreath of artificial flowers which encircled the head. A veil, if desired, was attached at the back.

**Veils.** Some brides fastened the end of their veil snugly over the head, then decorated the edge with a band of flowers. Others preferred to lay a veil loosely over the top of the head so that seven or eight inches fell down over the face, veiling the eyes.

**Skull Cap.** The skull cap became a popular choice for brides during the second half of the decade. It consisted of a shallow dome-shaped crown which hugged the back of the head. It was often made of the same fabric as the gown and decorated with seed pearls or a cluster of flowers over each ear. More tailored versions were decorated with rows of piping.

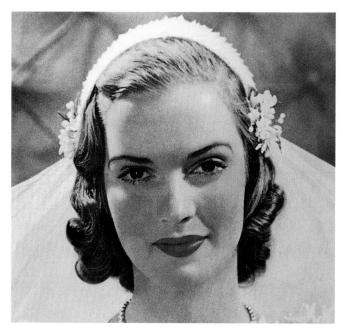

This *McCall's* cover photo (6/38) features a bride wearing a skullcap accented with clusters of wax orange blossoms over each ear.

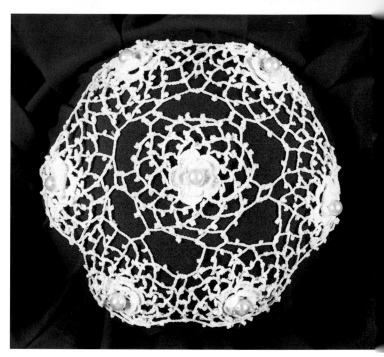

Top view - Crocheted Irish-lace Juliet cap containing three-dimensional flowers with pearl centers. *Courtesy of Joan York.* $90-$125.

*Juliet Cap.* Similar in shape to the skull cap, the Renaissance-style Juliet cap was made of delicate, crocheted mesh often accented with pearls.

# ATTENDANTS' HEADPIECES

*Picture Hats.* The most popular head covering for bridal attendants during the first half of the decade was the wide-brim "garden party" or "picture" hat. These romantic-style hats featured a shallow dome-shaped crown and a wide brim which was either turned down evenly all around or drooped in front and back. They were made of transparent horsehair, cellophane braid, or straw and decorated with ribbons and/or flowers.

*Doll Hats.* These zany little hats began with a round, slightly-domed felt form decorated with concentric rows of ruffles and/or flowers. They teetered precariously over one eye and were held in place by an elastic or back strap.

# ACCESSORIES

Brides often wore a short strand of pearls and matching pearl earrings. White silk or kid gloves, white satin shoes, and stockings completed the ensemble. Matching wedding and engagement rings were introduced during the 1920s. Smaller diamonds were often set in "illusion settings" at this time, to give them a larger appearance.

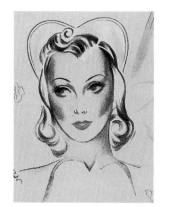

An illustration from *Pictorial Review* (5/38) featuring a heart-shaped headpiece used for brides as well as for bridesmaids into the 1940s. Bonwit Teller. Note: page-boy hair style.

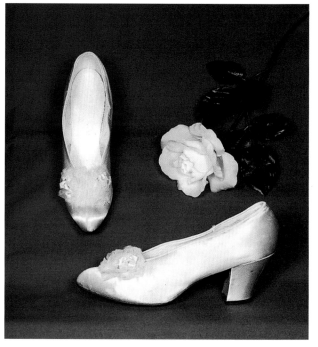

White satin wedding slippers with chiffon and satin ribbon puffs, Cuban heels. $85-$100.

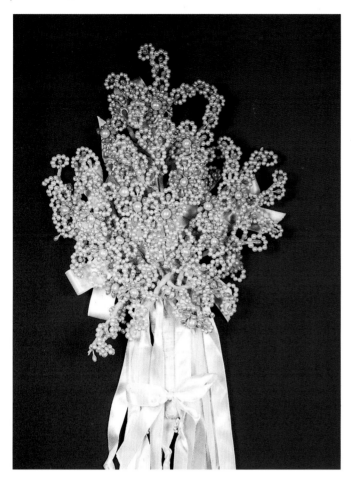

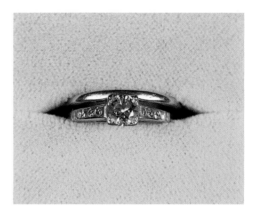

White-gold engagement ring featuring a diamond in an illusion setting flanked by eight smaller diamonds, plain wedding band, 1935. Both marked: W 18K. *Courtesy of Margaret Place.*

Unique bridal bouquet made entirely of pearls wired together to form flowers. *Courtesy of Mary Anne Faust (Yesterday's Delights).* $150-$200.

## BRIDAL BOUQUETS

Bridal bouquets were receding in size from the enormous bouquets carried by 1920s brides. Roses were the traditional favorite with sophisticated calla lilies a close second. Nosegays were popular for bridesmaids, while flower girls carried a basket of flowers or petals.

## BRIDAL WEAR FOR MEN

For information on men's morning suits (cutaways) worn for formal daytime weddings, refer to Men's Wear, Chapter 13.

# Chapter 6
# Sportswear

## CASUAL LEISURE-TIME CLOTHING

The active life style of American women created a demand for practical sports clothing. American sportswear companies produced Hollywood-inspired casual wear which was both comfortable and attractive.

Fashionable Europeans enjoyed vacationing in the Tyrol regions of Austria, Bavaria, and Germany. This heightened interest in the area inspired Tyrolean-style sportswear including ski outfits and accessories, *dirndl* skirts, shorts with embroidered braces (patterned after lederhosen), and masculine-style Tyrolean hats.

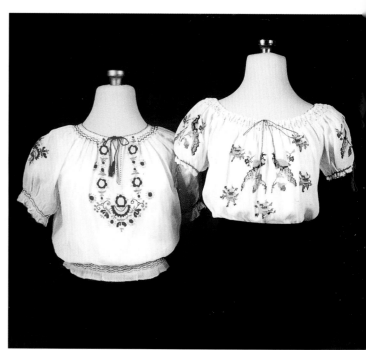

Smocked and embroidered peasant blouses. *Left:* White cotton, floral design in satin stitch. *Right:* Rayon crepe, peacocks and flowers in cross stitch. *Courtesy of Cedar Crest Alumnae Museum, Gift of Ellie Laubner.* $40-$60.

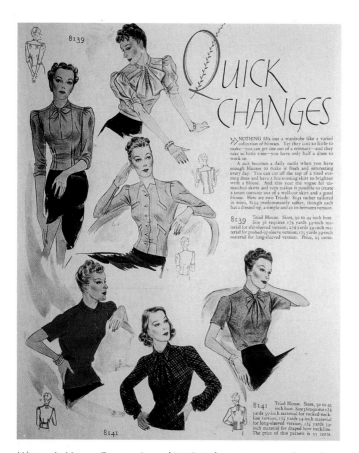

*Woman's Home Companion* ad (11/38) featuring a sampling of "tuck-in" and "out" blouses.

### Blouses

Very few blouses were offered in mail-order catalogs during the first few years of the decade. Most were straight, unfitted hip-length overblouses, usually with a V-shaped neckline, a carry-over from the 1920s. Blouses and skirts became more popular as the decade progressed, and were offered in both hip-length overblouse and "tuck-in" styles. Some versatile blouses could be worn "in" or "out." The overblouse became more fitted circa 1932 and was worn with a belt or a narrow self sash tied over the waist.

Common collar styles were the chelsea, stand-up ruffle, notched, *rever*, rolled, and cowl neckline. During the first half of the decade, blouses contained all manor of fussy details. Bodices were decorated with rippling jabots, ascots, middy ties, and floppy bows. Ruffles, ruching, or accordion-pleated trim were often stitched vertically along the center front opening. Unique to the '30s was the enormous butterfly bow which covered the bodice and extended to the outer reaches of the shoulders. Towards the end of the decade, blouses became more tailored with Peter Pan or notched collars, and rows of vertical tucks. Common sleeve styles were the short, puffed, and bishop sleeve. Peasant-style blouses smocked and embroidered with "gay" colored yarns were also popular.

Blouses were made of a wide range of fabrics, the most common of which was silk or rayon crepe. Also used was silk or rayon satin, rayon or cotton knit, cotton lace, broadcloth, cotton piqué, organdy, batiste, voile, lawn, moiré, and taffeta. They were generally made in solid colors, although stripes, and polka dots were also offered. Typical colors were white, beige, brown, red, navy, copen blue (medium blue), light blue, tea rose (light pink), and maize. After 1937, American beauty (shocking pink), wine, gold, lime green, dark green, and royal blue were added.

## Sweaters

Sweaters increased in popularity as the decade progressed. They were quite snug fitting and were referred to as "hug-me-tight" sweaters in one period catalog.

*Pullovers* were often knit in raised stripe, cable, diamond, or zigzag patterns. They were made with short or elbow-length puffed sleeves or full-length fitted sleeves. Sleeves usually ended

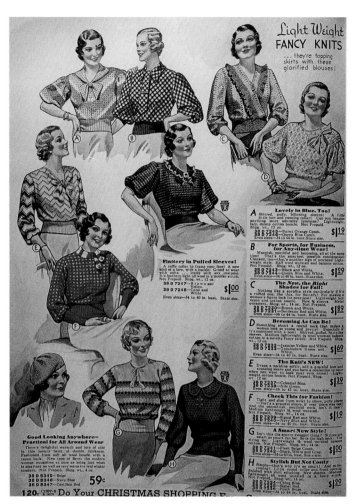

This Sears, Roebuck and Co. (1933-34) catalog page is devoted to patterned pull-over sweaters featuring a variety of neck lines and sleeves.

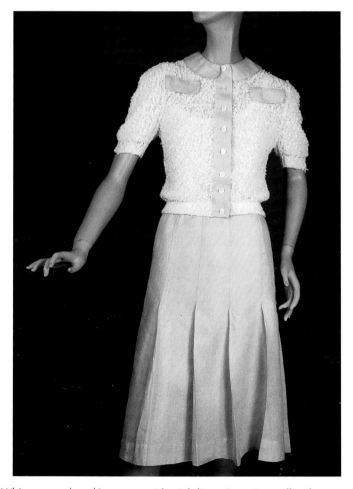

White cotton-*bouclé* sweater with pink linen Peter Pan collar, *faux*-pocket flaps, and center-front panel. Matching linen skirt contains top stitched knife pleats. *Courtesy of Ethel Bishop.* $75-$100.

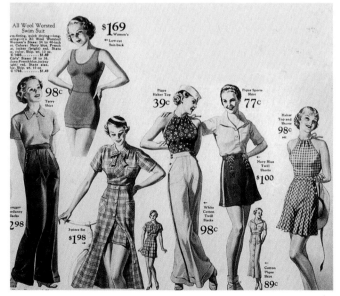

Montgomery Ward catalog illustrations (1935) of casual sportswear. *(1)* Zippered terry-cloth top, wide-leg corduroy pants. *(2)* Wool-knit swimsuit. *(3)* Cotton-plaid blouse, shorts, wrap skirt. *(4)* Piqué halter, wide-leg cotton-twill pants. *(5)* Cotton piqué sport shirt, twill shorts. *(6)* Cotton-check halter and shorts.

in a 2 to 2 1/2-inch rib-knit band (wider 4-inch bands were sometimes used on full sleeves). The waist was also banded, often with a wide 3 to 4-inch band which gave the sweater a slight, high-waisted appearance. Common necklines were the V, square, jewel, and crew neck. The middy and the Peter Pan collars were popular along with the surplice-style closing. Necklines were often accented with a self bow. Warm turtleneck sweaters were suggested for skiing, skating, and other outdoor sports. Sweaters were made of wool worsted, cotton, rayon, and various blends of these fibers. Novelty bouclé yarn was also popular.

**Cardigans** changed very little from the 1920s. They were still cut straight to the hips with a V-shaped neckline. Some were collarless, while others contained either a shawl, notched, or *rever* collar. "Sweater sets," introduced in the 1930s, consisted of a long-sleeve crew-neck cardigan over a short-sleeve crew-neck pullover.

## Skirts

When the hemline dropped below the calf in 1930-31, skirts became long and slender. They often contained inverted or knife pleats from the knees down, or a kick pleat in back for better mobility. Some skirts were accented with a row of decorative buttons down the center front or off to one side. Patch pockets were another decorative option.

In 1937, hemlines rose above the calf, where they remained until the end of the Second World War. Skirts became A-line in appearance which was achieved through the use of gores (8 to 12 per skirt). Pleated skirts were also popular, featuring accordion or stitched-down knife pleats. *Dirndl* skirts, which originated in the Tyrol region, consisted of several yards of fabric gathered to a narrow waistband. Wider "swing" skirts were popular with teenager girls, as they allowed for the freedom of movement needed for dancing to the "swing" music played by the big bands.

Skirts were generally tailored and were worn with or without a belt. They were made of cotton piqué, silk, gabardine twill, sharkskin, wool flannel, worsted, tartan, or tweed. Common colors were black, navy, brown, tan, and gray with white and pastels reserved for summer. Gathered *dirndl* skirts of the late '30s, usually contained horizontal stripes.

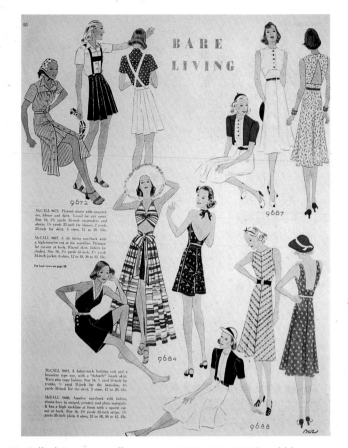

*McCall's* leisure wear illustrations (1938). *(9672)* Tailored blouse, pleated shorts with lederhosen-style suspenders, wrap skirt, babushka. *(9687)* Sun frock with back opening, bolero. *(9684)* Halter-top swimsuit, halter, wrap skirt, shorts. *(9688)* Sun frock, bolero.

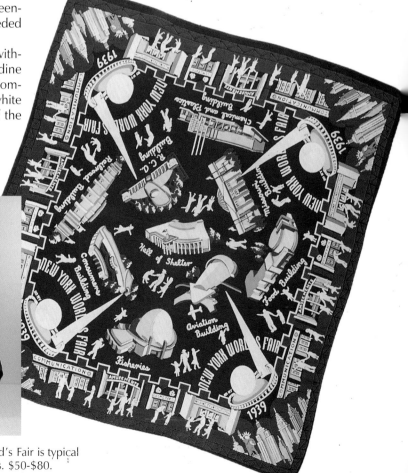

This silk souvenir scarf from the 1939 New York World's Fair is typical of the colorful novelty prints offered during the 1930s. $50-$80.

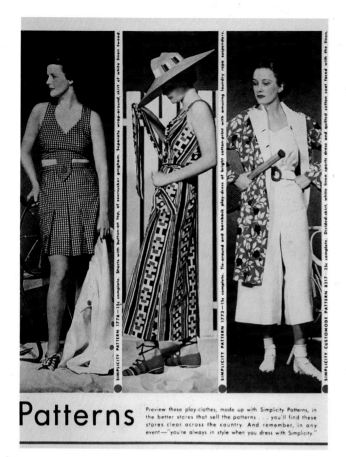

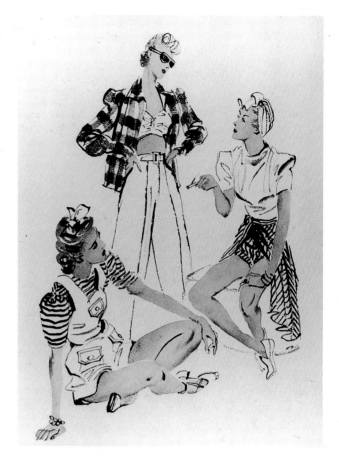

Play clothing by Simplicity Patterns (7/35). (1) Shorts with button-on top of seersucker gingham. Separate wrap-around skirt of white linen. (2) Wrap-around bareback sundress in geometric print worn with espadrilles and sun hat. (3) Quilted cotton jacket and white linen playsuit with divided skirt. 7/35.

*Vogue* sportswear illustrations (7/1/39). (1) White cotton piqué overalls. (2) Red and white silk plaid jacket, white sharkskin slacks and halter. (3) White jersey blouse, navy and white striped jersey bloomers and overskirt.

## Halters

The halter top often took the form of two side-by-side triangles (one over each breast) which were tied at the back of the neck and the middle of the back. Another resembled a sleeveless, backless shirtwaist dress with a notched collar, which passed around the back of the neck, forming a halter. While long halters were tucked into a pair of shorts or a skirt, short halters revealed a few inches of the midriff. It was usually necessary to go without a brassiére when wearing a halter. Halters were made of the same fabrics as playsuits which are described later in this chapter.

## Sundresses

Sundresses were an important part of a woman's summer wardrobe and there were many variations to choose from. Open-back dresses, a carry-over from the late '20s, were designed to show off the "sunburned back." Most were sleeveless and contained a deep square, V, or U-shaped opening at the back. Some had a bodice with straps which tied or buttoned over the shoulders.

The halter-style sundress appeared circa 1935. One version featured a sleeveless V-neck top which extended to tie at the back of the neck. Another resembled the shirtwaist-style halter described above. Sundresses were commonly made of cotton broadcloth, gingham, chintz, linen, cotton piqué in solids, mini prints, and polka dots. When bias-cut sundresses of the early '30s were made of striped fabric, the stripes often converged in the center front in an up-turned or down-turned V. "Railroad" stitching was a popular form of ornamentation for tailored dresses. It consisted of numerous parallel rows of closely-spaced top stitching.

## Pants

Trousers were a comfortable alternative to dresses and skirts for leisure wear. Their popularity increased during the 1930s, due in part to the indorsement of advocates like Greta Garbo and Katharine Hepburn. Slacks of the 1930s were inspired by the "gob" pants worn by sailors. They were extremely wide at the hem and were produced with or without cuffs. Many were accented with large buttons on either side of the drop-front closing. They were made of such fabrics as linen, denim, cotton twill, gabardine, duck, and wool jersey. Common colors were white, navy, brown, red, green, burgundy, and rust.

Cotton overalls for women were offered from the early '30s and would became the uniform for many women working in war plants during the Second World War.

## Culottes

Culottes were the combination of pants and a skirt. They had the advantage of separate legs for mobility, with the look of a skirt when the wearer was standing with legs together. Culottes were worn with a middy blouse or a tailored camp shirt. They were usually made of denim, linen, or cotton twill.

## Shorts

The *Delineator* for June 1933 reported, "The pajama isn't out...but it is suffering a slight eclipse due to the popularity of shorts. They are wearing shorts for beach games, for tennis, for hiking, and all such. Smartest in flannel or linen, worn with a mannish shirt..."

Wide-leg shorts of the 1930s often contained four to six pressed-down pleats, which created the look of a short skirt.

Some styles were fastened with a large button on either side of the drop-front closing, similar to sailor pants. Navy and white were the most popular colors. Shorts with braces (suspenders), patterned after lederhosen, were often pictured in fashion magazines of the 1930s, a reflection of our growing awareness of German nationalism.

## Playsuits

The one-piece playsuit, introduced circa 1935, was suitable for a variety of sports. The top could resemble a tailored shirtwaist or one of the many variations of the halter. The bottom was either shorts, culottes, or a short pleated skirt. For more versatility, playsuits were often made with matching or coordinating wraparound skirts, which could be either long or short. These gathered skirts could be buttoned down the front; however, it was fashionable to leave a few of the buttons open towards the bottom. Playsuits were made of cotton broadcloth, linen, seersucker, glazed chintz, cotton piqué (plain or printed), knits, and terry cloth. Popular colors for playsuits were white, blue, red, green, and yellow. The most common prints were mini florals, polka dots, geometrics, and nautical motifs.

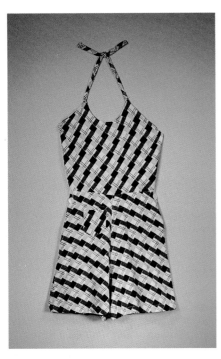

Halter-style cotton-piqué playsuit. *Courtesy of Cedar Crest College Alumnae Museum, gift of Ellie Laubner.* $40-$50.

## Babushkas (Head Scarves)

Head scarves were not new to sportswear. They were worn over the forehead as a part of the bathing costume during the teens and early twenties. Circa 1937, head scarves reappeared. This time, however, they were folded diagonally and tied under the chin in the manner of a Russian peasant's babushka. Head scarves remained in style through the 1950s and were particularly popular with younger women. Sewing magazines of the late 1930s encouraged women to make a babushka to match a blouse, sundress, playsuit, or halter with left-over fabric.

# ACTIVE SPORTS CLOTHING

Americans have always had a keen interest in active sports. As each sport became more popular, the garments needed to participate became more specialized. Hollywood films had a major impact on the sportswear industry through stars like Dorothy Lamour, Johnny Weissmuller, and Sonja Henie.

## Bicycling

An article in the June 1933 issue of the *Delineator* reported, "Bicycles are back again after all these years — a direct result of all those cruises to Bermuda where you had to ride a bike or stay put on a hotel veranda." This may have been the reason for the renewed interest in bicycling or perhaps it was a reflection of depression frugality. Whatever the case, bicycling was "in" and clothing manufacturers capitalized on this trend by creating cycling garments and accessories.

***Culottes and Shorts***. For safety sake, culottes or shorts paired with a tailored blouse were recommended for the cycling enthusiast. If necessary, the shorts could be easily covered with a matching wraparound skirt when the cyclist reached her destination.

***Bicycle Oxfords***. The "bike" shoe appeared in fashion magazines circa 1934. The tongue of this shoe was made in one piece with the toe. The sides extended forward where they overlapped the sides of the tongue and the toe, similar to a 1930s sneaker. This construction was accentuated when the toe/tongue and the sides were made from contrasting colors. The lacing on bicycle oxfords extended low over a part of the vamp (the area over the toe cleavage). On the most athletic high-top models, the laces were threaded through four or five pairs of eyelets, then looped around three or four pairs of hooks at the top. The bicycle shoe was made with heels ranging from low to Cuban.

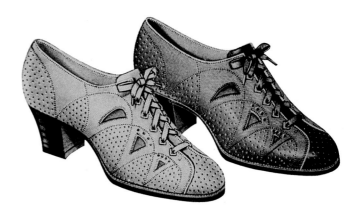

Montgomery Ward (1935) offered these elk-skin bicycle oxfords in white, or beige with brown tongue and toe, "cool cut-outs," and a built-up heel.

***Shoulder-strap Bags***. The July 1936 issue of *Delineator* magazine featured sports clothing and accessories for bicycling. The article recommended the long-handled "sling bag" (shoulder-strap bag). When this practical bag was suspended diagonally over the torso from the opposite shoulder, it left the hands free to maneuver the bicycle.

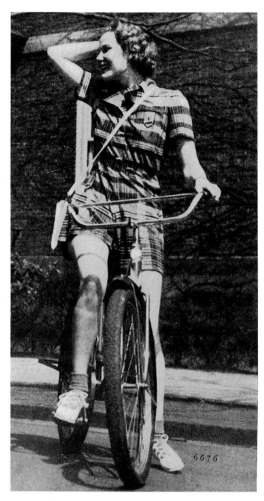

This bicycling ensemble, pictured in *Delineator* (7/36), includes a white sling bag, cotton plaid playsuit, and *gillie* oxfords.

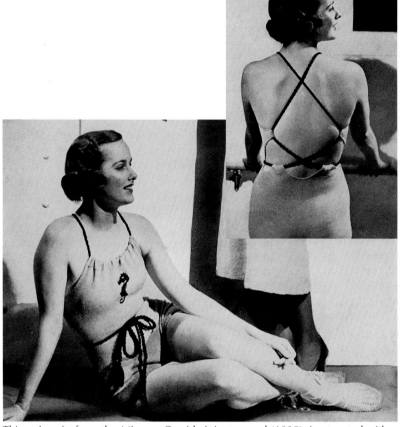

This swimsuit, from the Minerva Capri knitting manual (1935), is accented with a seahorse design. The bodice is held in place by contrasting cord which crisscrosses the back several times, then ties in front. Note: mesh sandals with leg lacing.

## Bathing and Basking

Until the 1920s, ladies were extremely careful to protect their lily-white skin from the sun, as tanned skin was associated with laborers who toiled in the fields. Chanel was one of the first to realize that tanned skin could actually become a status symbol, as only the wealthy could afford the time and the money to acquire a tan off season. As suntanned skin became universally accepted, bathing suits became increasingly briefer, exposing more and more skin to the tanning rays of the sun.

The June 1933 issue of *Delineator* cautioned, "Don't get a wool jersey bathing suit—the wool suit isn't enjoying its usual popularity. It has rivals. The rubber bathing suit and the cotton ones are making it look sick." This fashion commentator was referring to swimsuits made of a revolutionary new elastic fabric called "Lastex." This fabric was made of yarn with a rubber core covered with a cotton, wool, or rayon fiber. Lastex could be woven or knit into fabric with two-way stretch, which was ideal for swimwear. This new fabric clung to the contours of the body, smoothing out bulges in much the same way as a Lastex corset. Suits of Lastex absorbed less water and therefore dried quicker than woolen suits. (For a photo of a satin Lastex swimsuit, see Children's wear, Chapter 15.)

***Maillot.*** The California all-wool, rib-knit tank suit or *maillot* (one-piece suit) was made in solid colors or wide horizontal stripes. Some two-toned models had one color on top and a contrasting color below. This style was often accented at the waist with a white knitted belt or girdle. Some suits resembled a tank top, while others had narrow straps which crisscrossed the back. Low-cut "sun back" or "sunburn back" suits were popular throughout the decade. Knit suits often contained vertical gathers between the breasts for shaping. One piece knit suits were available in wool, cotton, and Lastex.

***Bandanna Suit.*** In the mid-1930s, knit suits with halter-style tops were introduced. The simplest of these halters, called the "bandanna," consisted of a triangle of fabric, often in stripes or a color to contrast with the trunks. The point at the top of the triangle was folded down and stitched to create a tunnel through which a cord was passed. This cord was then tied around the back of the neck. The remaining two points of the triangle were tied in the middle of the back. The halter and the trunks were joined across the front of the suit or merely at the center front which revealed a bit of the midriff on either side. Some suits were decorated with geometric-style appliqués. The most common colors for knit suits were jade green, red, blue, peacock, and navy.

***Dressmaker Suit.*** The dressmaker-style bathing suit, which resembled a short dress with a slightly flared skirt, became popular in the late '30s and '40s. It often had two long, vertical, princess-style seams which ran from neckline to hem in front and back. Dressmaker suits were made of knit or woven fabrics such as chintz, piqué, and other cotton fabrics.

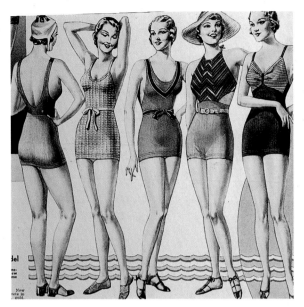

Butler Brothers swimsuit ad (1934) featuring: *(1)* Sun-back wool-knit *maillot*. *(2)* Wool-knit *maillot*. *(3)* Two-toned sun-back wool-knit *maillot*, contrasting trim and girdle. *(4)* Wool bandanna-top swimsuit (ties behind the neck and center back), knit belt. *(5)* High-waisted wool *maillot*, gathered at bust.

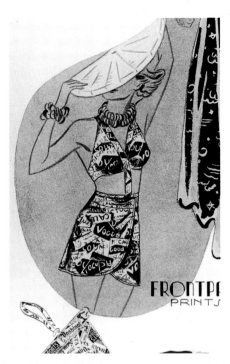

Illustration from *Vogue* (1936) featuring a two-piece bathing suit consisting of a halter top and *lava-lava* made of a collage print containing the names of fashion magazines. Note: wooden beach jewelry, wide-brim hat, and beach bag.

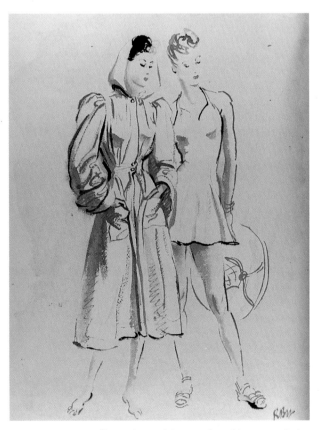

*Vogue* sportswear illustration (7/1/39). *Left:* White terry cloth beach coat with hood. *Right:* White cotton-piqué dress-maker bathing suit.

***Two-piece Suits.*** Circa 1934, some venturesome souls were seen on beaches in the new two-piece bare-midriff swimsuits consisting of a brassière top and shorts. Also introduced at this time were Polynesian-style suits consisting of a bra top and a "*lava-lava*" (short wraparound skirt) with attached trunks below. Island-style fashions were usually made of large floral or undersea prints in bright colors. Two-piece suits, of this kind, were popular into the 1940s.

Swimsuits were made of wool challis, wool knit, cotton knit, rayon jersey, *matelassé*, elastic lace, sharkskin, sateen, and Lastex. Mini prints in florals, geometric shapes, and nautical motifs were popular along with colorful stripes.

Fashion designers who created swimwear during the 1930s were Jean Patou, Edward Molyneux, Lucien Lelong, and Elsa Schiaparelli. Manufacturers of swimwear included Jantzen, Catalina, Izod, and B.V.D.

***Wraparound Skirts.*** Swimsuits were frequently offered with a matching wraparound over skirt. These skirts were ideal for strolling on the boardwalk or browsing in seaside shops. They were anywhere from knee to calf length, and appeared in all the fashion magazines and mail-order catalogues. Early wrap skirts contained a row of buttons down the center front. However, as more and more of the buttons were left undone, designers soon did away with them entirely, retaining only one to fasten the waistband.

The sarong was a long, slender wraparound skirt, worn by both men and women in Malaysia and Indonesia. It was made of four to five yards of brightly-colored floral-print fabric (often batik) and varied in length from the knee to the ankle. It was introduced in 1936 by Dorothy Lamour in the movie *The Jungle Princess*. She continued to wear the exotic wrap in numerous

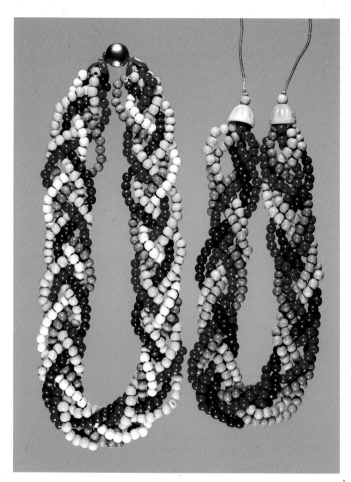

Czechoslovakian wooden-bead necklaces of this kind were often worn as "beach jewelry." They contain three of the most popular bathing suit colors: red, blue, and green. $25-$40 ea.

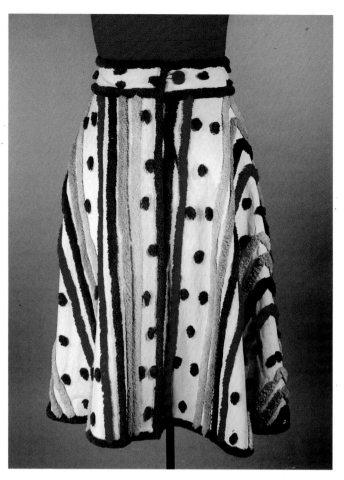

Versatile cotton wraparound skirt decorated with colorful chenille. Designed to coordinate with the popular swimsuit colors. $40-$60.

jungle movies of the late '30s and '40s. This inspired the sarong-style swimsuits and beach coverups worn during the late '30s and '40s.

**Beach Jackets, Coats, Robes, and Capes.** Suits made of woven fabric in colorful prints were often accompanied by a matching thigh-length beach jacket lined with absorbent terry cloth. Terry-cloth beach robes, which resembled tailored bathrobes, were also popular as they absorbed moisture from the wet skin and suit. They were made with notched collars, long sleeves, sash, and occasionally a hood. Slender ankle-length beach coats, with buttons down the center front, were also designed for the beach. Capes worn loose over the shoulders were another option.

**Beach Pajamas.** Colorful beach or resort pajamas were introduced by Chanel in the late 1920s. They conformed to the prevailing dropped-waist style by featuring a long top which ended at the hips. In 1930, the dropped waist became *passé*, as emphasis shifted back to the natural waist once again. Pajamas of the 1930s conformed to this new trend by adding a belt at the natural waist or by tucking the top into the pants. Pajama tops were usually sleeveless and often backless with such voluminous pants that they resembled long skirts. One-piece pajamas, resembling the contemporary jumpsuit, were another option.

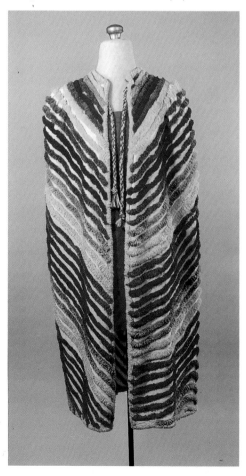

Cotton beach cape decorated with rows of multicolored chenille and braided tie. *Courtesy of Mary Anne Faust (Yesterday's Delights).* $40-$60.

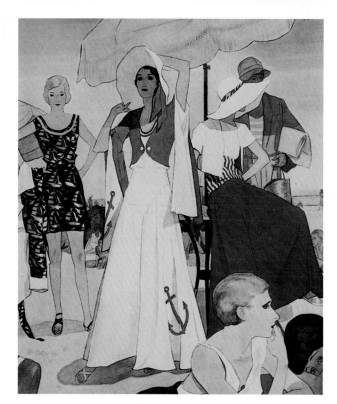

*Harper's Bazaar* sportswear illustration (1/31) featuring: *(1)* Two-piece swim suit in sailboat print, beach jacket lined with white terry-cloth, by Worth. *(2)* High-fashion white silk-crêpe beach pajamas with enormous legs, blue crepe jacket. *(3)* White sleeveless top, red wide-leg pants, striped sash, and white bolero. Note: wide-brim straw hats.

Beach pajamas and lounging pajamas were often used interchangeably during this period. (For more information and examples of lounging pajamas see Lingerie, Chapter 2). Pajamas were made of linen, rayon, sailcloth, cotton jersey, broadcloth, and cotton crinkle crepe. They were made of solid or printed fabrics in florals, polka-dots, checks, and plaids. Pajamas were eventually replaced by the briefer playsuit or beach suit.

**Beach Hats.** Tailored hats with ultra-wide brims were frequently used for the beach. They were made of straw with rigid "cart wheel" or soft floppy brims and were often held on with ribbon tied under the chin.

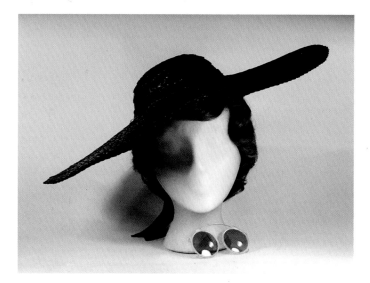

Black straw beach hat with shallow crown and wide brim, black grosgrain band and streamers. Label: John Wanamaker, Philadelphia. *Courtesy of Mary Anne Faust (Yesterday's Delights).* $40-$50. Oxford clip-on sunglasses with round celluloid rims. $15-$20.

**Bathing Caps**. Aviator-style rubber bathing caps with adjustable/ detachable straps were popular for those women who liked to take the big plunge. The U.S. Howland cap featured an exclusive patented suction band on the inside of the cap to "keep the hair dry and the water out of the ears." Some caps had a design embossed in the rubber, while others had fancy rubber appliqués. Caps were available in the popular bathing suit colors: red, blue, green, canary, and white.

**Bathing Shoes.** Rubber bathing shoes were still worn by some women to protect the feet from sharp shells and hot sand. They were produced in the same colors as bathing caps and often came in matching sets with similar embossed designs on each.

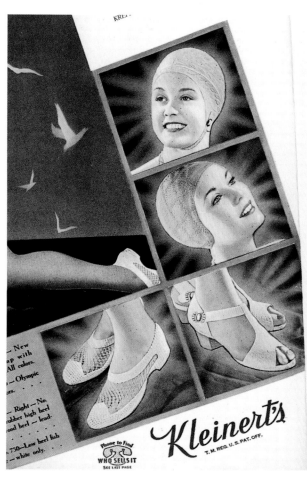

*Harper's Bazaar* advertisement (7/37) for Kleinert's beach accessories. *(1 & 2)* Rubber bathing caps. *(3)* Low-heel rubber fish-net shoes. *(4)* Rubber sandal with wooden heels.

## Golf

The hemline for golf dresses followed daytime styles, dropping to the calf in the early '30s, then rising again to the knee towards the end of the decade. They were made in the tailored shirt-waist style with long or short sleeves and long slender skirts. Golf dresses often featured a belt and two to four patch pockets. Long, slender skirts made of wool plaid or tweed fabric were often worn in cooler weather with a tailored blouse and cardigan sweater or perhaps a short-sleeve pullover. Fringed kiltie oxfords or *gillies* and a beret or Tyrolean-style hat completed the outfit.

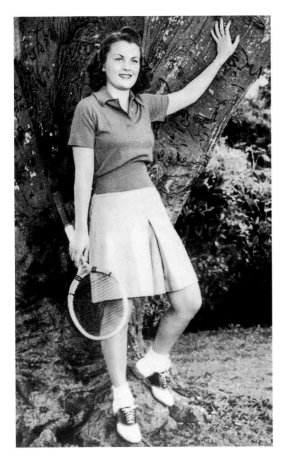

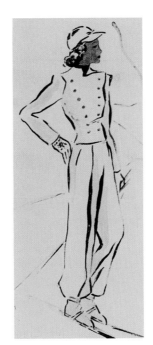

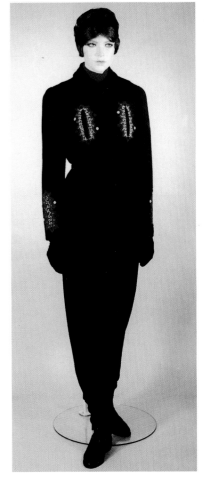

*Harper's Bazaar* published this advertisement (3/1/38) for a tennis outfit consisting of polo shirt, culottes, white socks, and saddle shoes.

Navy-blue wool-flannel ski suit - pointed collar, gathered waist peasant-style embroidery on bodice and sleeves, late '30s. *Courtesy of Pam Coghlan (Odds and Ads).* $150-$200. *Insert:* Ski suit with cadet-style jacket and visor cap.

## Tennis

Tennis skirts remained short, when other hems dropped in the early '30s. Influenced in the late '20s and early '30s by Spanish tennis star Lili de Alvares, many women began to wear culottes cut just below the knee. In 1933, Alice Marble played at Wimbledon in shorts just above the knee. Short-sleeved polo shirts were universally worn from the early thirties.

## Skiing

*Ski Suits.* Two-piece ski suits featuring a jacket and full knickers called "plus fours" were a carry-over from the preceding decade. Knickers were soon replaced by long, full-cut pants which were gathered into rib-knit cuffs at the ankles. They often had zipper closings at the bottom of the leg for ease when dressing.

Ski jackets were made in two lengths. The first ended at the hip and featured a belt at the natural waist. The second ended approximately two inches below the fitted waist. Single-breasted jackets featured zipper closures, while the double-breasted versions had either a notched collar or a high military-band collar. The latter style was called a "cadet" or "bell hop" jacket. No doubt many of these warm suits also doubled as skating outfits.

Ski suits were often two-toned or featured a solid color with a coordinating plaid. Sometimes the jacket was plaid, while the pants were a coordinating solid. Or the jacket might be a red and navy plaid, while the collar, cuffs, pockets, belt, and pants were solid navy or vice versa. The fabrics commonly used for ski suits were wool (solids, plaids, and tweeds), gabardine, wool fleece, corduroy, and a new high-gloss fabric called ski satin. Ski suits were usually lined with cotton flannel.

*Ski Caps.* Popular hockey-style knit hats were made from a knitted tube gathered together on one end where a large pompon was attached. A visor was added to this style to create an Alpine ski cap. Another style was made of woven fabric with a visor and ear flaps which could be worn up or down over the ears. Skiers wore heavy wool mittens with full *gauntlets* which were pulled up over the end of the sleeves to keep out the cold.

## Skating

The popular Norwegian figure skater, Sonja Henie, was world champion for ten years and won the Olympics at three consecutive games. She starred in twelve Hollywood ice musicals from 1936 to 1948, which did much to popularize the sport of figure skating. Her movies were a pleasant distraction from the hardships of the depression, and her grace and beauty made her the "Fred Astaire of the ice." Henie wore many glamorous skating costumes featuring short mid-thigh length skirts for ease of movement.

The November 1938 issue of *Woman's Home Companion* featured a skating costume consisting of a red rib-knit turtleneck sweater and a black knee-length jumper embroidered over the bodice with red and white yarn. Sears, Roebuck's skating costume for the winter of 1939 included a fitted jacket of quilted velveteen and a circular skating skirt ending just below the knee. Colorful wool mittens and a warm hockey-style knitted cap completed the outfit.

## Horseback Riding

The informal riding habit consisted of a hacking jacket and either *jodhpurs* or breeches (brE-chez.) The snug-fitting jacket resembled a man-tailored blazer of wool tweed or subdued check. Both pants styles were puffed out over the hips, then fitted from the knee to the ankle. *Jodhpurs* had a cuff at the ankle and were worn over riding boots. Breeches, however, had buttons from the knee down with no cuffs and were worn inside of riding boots. Breeches and *jodhpurs* were held down with stirrup straps, which passed under the arch of the foot or boot. *Jodhpurs* and breeches were made of sturdy cotton cavalry twill, cotton whipcord, or gabardine and the inside of the knees were reinforced with suede-leather knee guards. Common colors were tan, brown, navy, stone, dark green, and black. Either a hard bowler or a mannish Tyrolean-style hat and black or brown riding boots completed the ensemble.

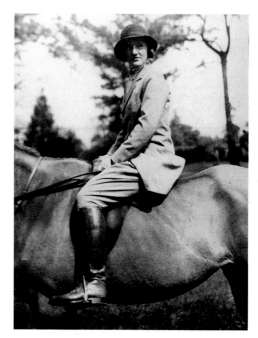

*Town and Country* photograph of an informal riding habit consisting of knock-about hat, hacking jacket, breeches, and riding boots, c. 1934.

## CLOTH COATS

Outerwear of the 1930s was produced in a variety of silhouettes. The surplice, polo, and reefer-style coats all projected a similar long, slender silhouette. In contrast, the roomy swagger coat introduced a wide, flared line. In the late 1930s, the hourglass-style princess-line coat and the broad square box coat were introduced. Coat hems dropped below the calf in 1930-31, then rose again to the knee in 1937, where they remained through the Second World War.

"Railroad" stitching was the most popular form of detailing used on collars, lapels, cuffs, pocket flaps, yokes, and belts throughout the decade. It consisted of numerous parallel rows of closely-spaced topstitching. Topstitching was taken to new heights, in the late 1930s, with the revival of a decorative form of quilting called "trapunto." By stuffing cotton batting into small areas outlined with topstitching, a raised design could be created on collars, lapels, and cuffs. This technique was also used on housecoats, dresses, suits, evening gowns, and handbags. (For further information and examples of trapunto see Chapters 2, 4, and 9.)

Shoulders became broader and more masculine as the decade progressed. Collars and lapels also grew wider, often extending beyond the armseye. Enormous fur collars were at the height of popularity throughout the decade.

An ephemeral style, which began c. 1936-37, featured a row of closely-spaced covered buttons across the collar, along the shoulder seam, down the outside of the sleeves (from the shoulder to the wrist), or along the front edges of the coat (from neck to hem). Rows of buttons were similarly employed on dresses and suits of the period and were strictly ornamental.

## 1930-1931

**Surplice-Style Coats.** Coats during the first two years of the decade were a carry-over from the 1920s. They featured the surplice closing, a style in which the right front overlapped the left front and buttoned at the waist on the left side of the coat. The edge of the left side was fastened with a tie to the inside of the right side seam, drawing it smooth against the body. Most 1930s coats featured a self-fabric belt emphasizing the natural waist. All of the interest was centered on the collar and the unusual sleeve treatment, rather than on the slender skirt which ended below the calf.

These early coats often featured stylish funnel-shaped "gauntlet" or "mousquetaire" cuffs, which flared out towards the elbow similar to a 17th-century musketeer's *gauntlet* (glove). The opposite was true of the cuffless "bell" sleeve which widened as it reached the wrist. It usually contained a snug-fitting under sleeve, which protruded two to four inches from the edge of the outer bell. Buttoned tabs at the wrist were popular as a decorative detail.

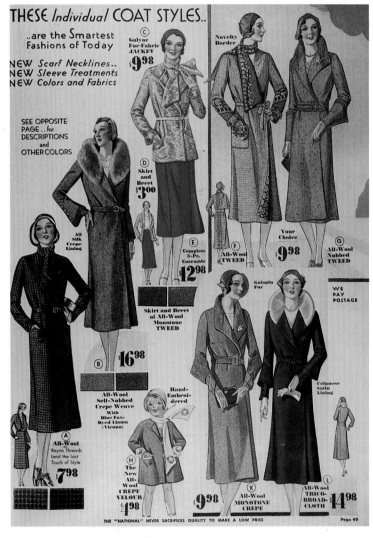

Bellas Hess illustrations (1931) for surplice-style spring coats. *(A)* Ascot collar. *(B)* Tweed with *vicuna* collar, bell sleeves. *(C)* "Fur fabric," throw scarf, *rever* collar. *(F)* Tweed, throw scarf. *(G,K)* Tweed, railroad stitching on *rever* collar, belt, and *gauntlet* cuffs. *(L)* Coney (rabbit) collar, bell sleeves.

The *rever* collar was the most common style used for coats throughout the 1930s. It featured one wide, notchless point on either side of the front neck opening (as opposed to the usual two points of a notched collar). This collar could be worn open or buttoned up around the throat for a "smart" asymmetrical look. The point of the *rever* collar was usually equidistant between the neck and the waist; however, some coats had "wide-angle" collars in which the point was located towards the waist.

Another popular style was the jabot collar which was made of drapeable bias-cut fabric. As the name implies, the collar fabric was allowed to fall in graceful, undulating ripples like jabots on either side of the front opening.

Many coats featured a narrow 30-inch "throw scarf" with diagonally-cut ends. It contained a large buttonhole, slightly off center, through which one of the ends was threaded. The scarf was then turned to the side so that one end fell down the front of the coat and the other down the back. Some surplice coats contained an elbow-length cape attached under the collar.

Winter coats featured enormous fur collars which extended to the outer edges of the shoulders when open. When fastened at the neck they formed a high rolled "bumper" collar which literally enveloped the shoulders, neck, and head (to the ears) in soft, luxurious fur. If matching fur was added to the sleeves, it was usually in the form of a band around the elbow or uniquely spiraled up the arm. (The types of fur used for collars and trim are discussed under fur coats, later in this chapter.)

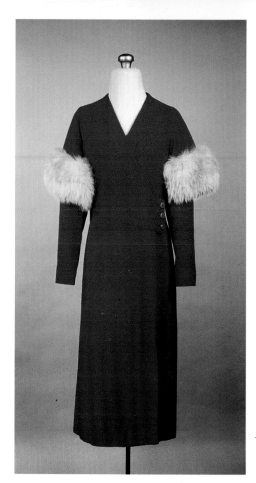

Red/orange wool-crepe surplice-style coat with asymmetrical waist treatment accented by three hollow celluloid buttons, fox fur trim at elbows, c.1933. $150-$200.

# 1932-1937

Notched, *rever*, and jabot collars continued to grow in width, often extending beyond the armseye. In fact, "button back" collars were so large that the tips were buttoned to the coat to hold them in place. Additional width was often achieved by binding the edges of the collar with a contrasting fabric. Many collars styles were designed to be worn up at the back of the neck. Ascots made of self fabric were often provide for added warmth.

There were three common sleeve styles used at this time. The bishop sleeve was full to the elbow, then snug fitting from the elbow to the wrist. The ephemeral "pouch" sleeve concentrated the fullness around the elbow. "Pleat-top" sleeves created width at the shoulders for a more masculine, squared-off look.

Coats were fastened with large "platter" buttons measuring a whopping 2 to 2 1/2 inches in diameter. They were made of celluloid, Bakelite, metal, and wood in interesting colors, shapes, and textures. Buttons with matching mirror-image belt clasps were also common. (Examples of coat buttons appear in Accessories, Chapter 12.)

***Polo Coats.*** The classic polo coat was worn to polo matches by male spectators during the 1920s and was adopted by women during the early '30s. A 1933 Sears, Roebuck and Co. advertisement for the polo coat read, "Marlene Dietrich, Joan Crawford, and Greta Garbo — these stars know the charm of a perfectly tailored coat like this [polo coat]."

This double-breasted sport coat was made of tan camel's hair, *vicuña*, or camel-colored wool and trimmed with four to

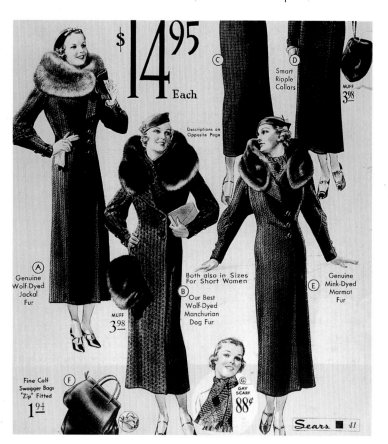

Sears, Roebuck and Co. illustrations (1935) for surplice-style "tree-bark" wool-crepe winter coats, bumper collars, pouch sleeves. Note: matching fur muff. Sears, Roebuck and Co. 1935-36.

six bone buttons. It featured a wide notched collar which could be worn open or closed. The collar gradually widened as the decade progressed.

The sporty raglan sleeves had deep armholes and buttoned cuffs or tabs at the wrists. The pleated "action back" allowed for ease of movement, while the self belt defined the waist. Deep patch or flap-style pockets contributed to its casual look. The seams and edges of the fabric were accented with a single row of top stitching. A wraparound version of the polo coat had no buttons, only a self sash to hold the two sides together.

*Reefer.* The classic reefer was inspired by the U.S. Navy pea jacket. This semi-fitted double-breasted coat was extremely popular for women throughout the 1930s. It featured a notched "two-way" collar which could be worn open or closed. The pleated "action back" was accented with a half belt at the waist.

Circa 1937, hems rose to the knee and skirts took on a gentle flare. Pleat-top sleeves were also popular and created broader, more masculine shoulders. The collars and pocket flaps were often decorated with numerous rows of railroad stitching.

*Swagger Coat.* During the second half of the decade the new loose-fitting "swagger" coat was introduced. The most identifiable characteristic of the swagger was the flared "fishtail" back, which fell (usually from a shoulder yoke) in fluted ripples to the hem. The flared back could be created by the use of three different techniques: the bias cut, a central inverted pleat, or five or six slender gores.

The unfitted front had either a single-breasted or edge-to-edge closing. The most common collars were the small-rolled,

Peter Pan, notched, and the long tuxedo collar which extended the length of the coat. Loose-fitting raglan sleeves were the most common, followed by pouch and straight sleeves.

Swagger coats were produced in two lengths: full (below the calf) and 3/4 (below the knee). The 3/4-length model was frequently offered with a matching calf-length skirt creating a practical "top coat suit." When hem lengths rose to the knee circa 1937, the swagger coat followed suit. Due to the voluminous nature of the swagger coat, one or two models were usually included in the maternity section of mail-order catalogs.

## 1937-1939

*Princess-Style Coat.* The single-breasted "princess-style" coat was introduced in the late 1930s and remained popular through the Second World War. Its nipped-in waist and knee-length flared skirt created a hourglass silhouette. It was cut in long slenderizing gores or panels stretching from the shoulder or the bust line to the hem. No waist seam was necessary. Pleat-top sleeves and heavy padding gave breadth to the shoulders. The wide notched and the small round-rolled collars were the most common. This coat was usually accented with Bakelite buttons and a self or simulated-leather belt.

*Box Coat.* Towards the end of the decade, broad boxy coats were introduced with straight lines and no hint of a waist. The squared-off masculine shoulders were created by the use of pleat-top sleeves and heavy shoulder padding. Common collars were the wide notched and the small round-rolled collar. The box coat also remained popular through the war years.

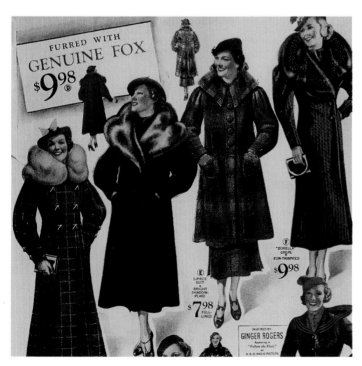

Sears, Roebuck and Co. illustrations (1936-37) for wool coats. *(1)* Reefer, window-pane pattern, pouch sleeves, lamb-fur bumper collar. *(2)* Swagger coat with fishtail back, fox-fur collar. *(3)* Shadow-plaid suit, 3/4 swagger jacket with fishtail back, matching skirt. *(4)* Surplice coat, lamb-fur *jabot* collar, pleat-top sleeves. Note: *pochette*-style bags.

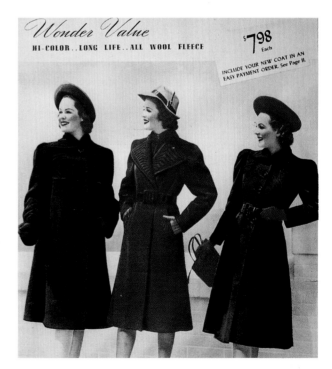

Sears, Roebuck and Co. offered these wool fleece coats in 1939-40. *(1)* Skipper-blue square-shoulder swagger coat. *(2)* Rust coat with trapunto quilting on the *rever* collar and pockets. *(3)* Teal princess-style coat, matching leather belt.

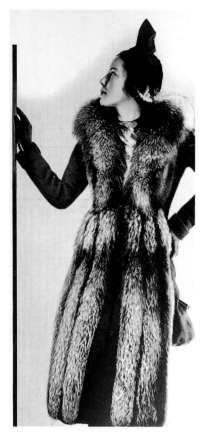

## Coat Fabrics

The most popular fiber for coats of the 1930s was wool used in such fabrics as gabardine, worsted, twill, flannel, homespun, melton, all wool suede fleece, and "pebble" and "tree bark" textured crepes. Bouclé increased in popularity towards the end of the decade. Wool was blended with other fibers such as cotton, silk, and rayon. Cashmere, camel's hair, mohair pile, and silk seal plush were also used for winter coats.

Checks, herringbones, and plaids were popular (including tartans, "shadow" plaids, and "broken" plaids). *Ombré* striped fabric (from the French word meaning shaded) made an appearance during the late 1930s. *Ombré*-stripe fabric was generally monochromatic with each stripe gradually blending to a lighter or darker shade of the same hue.

Practical nubby tweeds were especially popular as indicated by the following poem from the 1939 fall and winter Sears catalog:

> Tweeds that whisper...Tweeds that shout
> Smart for travel...Or knock-about.
> Right for sports, country, city
> Church or tearoom, school committee.
> Warm and sturdy, Rain or shine...
> Tweeds are perfect, ANYTIME! (1939:21)

"Snowflake tweeds" produced in solid colors with flecks of white silk or cotton were at the height of fashion. Other color combinations such as brown flecks on rust, gray on black, or wine on navy were also popular.

The dressy "spring coat" was an important part of the feminine wardrobe. In addition to the fabrics listed above, cottons such as gabardine, twill, waffle-weave piqué, and lace were used. Spring coats were usually unlined.

*Harper's Bazaar* published this ad (1/38) for a princess-style coat by Fromm, trimmed with panels of silver-fox.

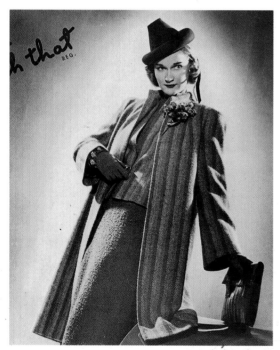

*Harper's Bazaar* published this ad (3/1/38) for a tri-tone *ombré*-striped wool box coat with square shoulders, matching jacket, and coordinating skirt. Note: truncated cone-shaped hat with bumper brim.

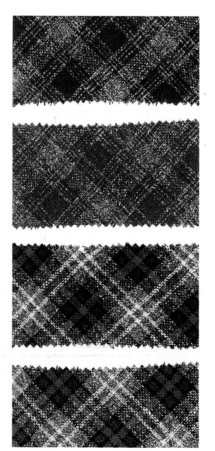

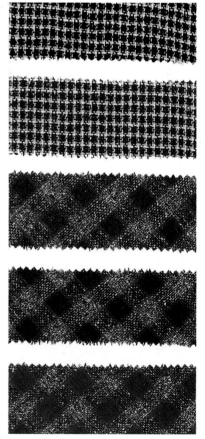

Shadow plaids and checks made of coarse wool-tweed fabric with white silk nubs. Tweeds of this kind were popular for coats and suits during the 1930s.

## Colors

Common colors for coats were tan, black, oxford gray, guardsman blue, navy, beaver brown, dark green, copen blue (medium blue), and copperglo (reddish brown). During the late 1930s, more sophisticated colors like wine (burgundy), American beauty (shocking pink), nuberry (dark purple), russet (rust), teal (deep blue/green), laurel green (dark green), and skipper blue (royal) were introduced.

It was fashionable to wear a hat, handbag, shoes, and gloves all of the same color to complement one's coat. Popular color combinations during the second half of the decade included gold accessories with a laurel green coat, teal with nuberry, nuberry with skipper blue, gold with rust, American beauty with light blue, wine with navy, and rust with teal. The autumn colors rust, gold, and green were often used together as were teal, rust, gold, and brown.

# CAPES

Period movies, released during the 1930s, inspired a revival of Victorian fashions. Capes and matching muffs were an example of this renewed interest in 19th century styles. They were produced in a variety of lengths including elbow, tunic, and the prevailing hem length. Longer capes were often given a full fishtail back similar to the swagger coat. Capes were made of tweed and a variety of furs and fur effect fabrics.

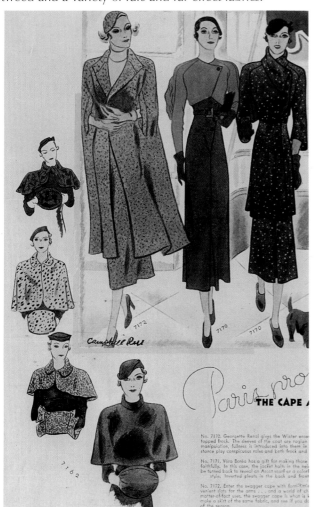

# FUR COATS

Silver fox was the most coveted fur of the 1930s and consequently very expensive. It was actually a mutation created from two red fox parents. The fine under wool was black, covered by heavier black guard hairs tipped with white. Luxurious white fox was often used for evening wraps and coats.

Other costly furs used in a variety of coat and jacket styles were mink, chinchilla, baum marten, lynx, ermine, and mouton. Broadtail, caracul, and krimmer—forms of Persian lamb—were also popular. Krimmer had *ombré* stripes which blended from black, to medium gray, to light gray. Fashionable, yet moderately priced furs included lapin, beaver, nutria, coney (rabbit), muskrat, raccoon, and Manchurian wolf dog.

It was also possible to shear and dye ordinary pelts to resemble more expensive furs such as beaver-dyed French *coney* or Hudson-seal-dyed muskrat. Less expensive fox varieties could be dyed, then "pointed" to resemble genuine silver fox. Pointing was the process by which the heavier silver guard hairs from imperfect pelts were glue into the dyed fox.

Even more economical were "fur-effect" fabrics made to resemble such furs as beaver, broadtail, and leopard. Astrakhan cloth (imitation Persian lamb) and rayon pile were also used.

The furs described here were also used for collars and trim on cloth coats. Fur muffs were frequently offered to match the fur of a collar, scarf, coat, or cape. (An example of a fur muff appears in Handbags, Chapter 9.

# FUR SCARVES

Fur "scarves" or "fur pieces" were glamorous, but impractical status symbols, worn over a coat, suit, or dress. Stone and baum marten, mink, sable, and fox were used in their entireties including the head, paws, and tail. Two or three animals were stitched together, one following the other, forming a line. The first and last animals were fastened together by the wearer in one of the following ways. First, the lead animal contained a clasp-like mouth (similar to a pinch-style clothespin) which could be clamped to the tail of the last animal. Second, the furs could be fastened together by the use of snaps attached to the animals' paws. Third, the body of the lead animal could be passed under a cloth strap fastened to the underside of the last animal. The latter example formed a tighter wrap. (See photos demonstrating each of these methods.)

Fur pieces were familiar, even dear to my childhood friends and me, as we wore our mothers' discarded furs for dress up during the late 1940s and early 1950s. While teaching "History of Costume" at a local community college during the 1980-90s, I brought (among other accessories) three fur pieces for show and tell. Many of my students had never seen a fur piece before. I, therefore, found it most amusing to observe their reactions. Most found it unbelievable that fashion-conscious women would choose to wear these animals around their necks. They

*McCall's* illustration (12/32) for cape patterns, available in a variety of lengths. (Top to bottom) tweed, broadtail, leopard, astrakhan (imitation curly lamb), and beaver. Note: matching muffs.

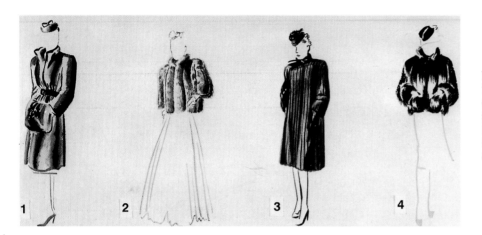

*You* (magazine) illustrations (1938-39) featuring fur coats produced in a wide variety of styles. *(1)* Fitted sheared beaver coat with squared shoulders. *(2)* Short jacket of Guanaco, an inexpensive fur from the South American llama. *(3)* Mink coat in boxy style with vertically arranges pelts. *(4)* Long haired black fox jacket.

Additional fur coat illustrations from *You* (1938-39). *(5)* Scarf of sable, baum, stone marten or Kolinsky with matching fur muff. *(6)* Straight line seal coat. *(7)* Short square jacket of mink or sable-dyed fitch. *(8)* Inexpensive mouton (lamb dyed dark brown) was ideal for college or country wear.

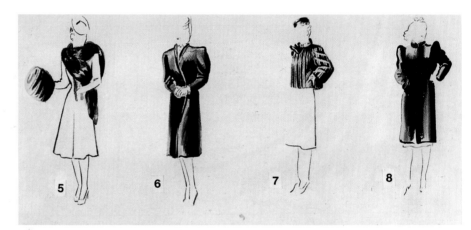

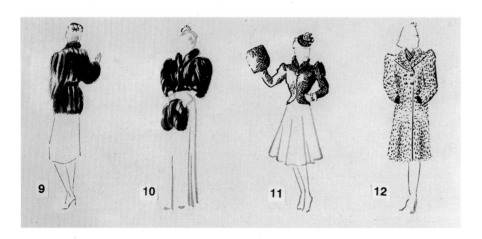

Further illustrations from *You* (1938-39). *(9)* Sable-dyed skunk in a hip-length jacket, suitable for town or country. *(10)* Baum marten in a fitted jacket with matching muff. *(11)* Curly Persian lamb jacket with peplum, hat and muff to match. *(12)* Leopard coat, suitable for informal day and sportswear.

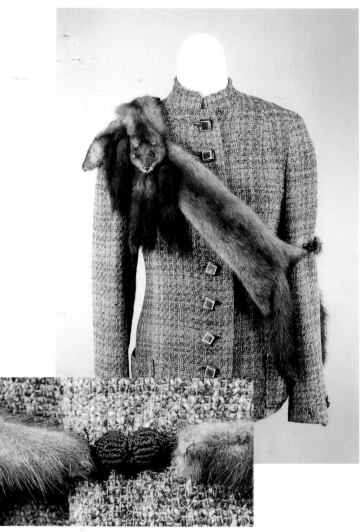

Wool tweed jacket accented with hollow celluloid buttons. *Courtesy of Ethel Bishop.* The three mink fur pieces contain heads with glass eyes, legs, and tails. *Insert:* The animals have been stitched together in back and can be fastened together in front by the use of a snap attached to the paws. Label: Gunther, New York. *Courtesy of Margaret Denio.* $35-$55.

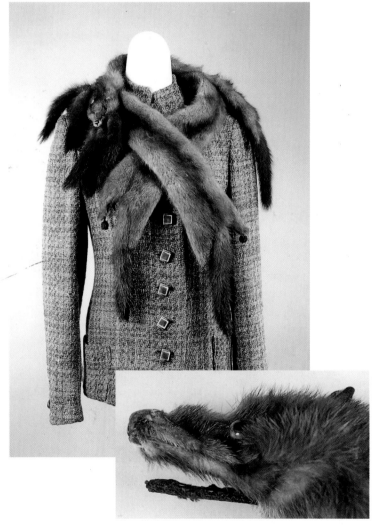

There were also brown grosgrain straps attached to the underside of the two end minks. If the wearer desired a tighter wrap she could slip the mink on one end into the strap on the under side of the mink on the other end. *Insert:* As an alternative way to fasten the animals together, the first mink's spring-loaded mouth could be opened and clamped onto the tail of the last mink in line. *Courtesy of Margaret Denio.*

viewed my furry-faced friends as though they were macabre pieces of "road kill." (On the other hand, fashionable women of the 1930s would certainly have found the tatoos and nose rings worn by my students of the '90s, equally bizarre.)

# EVENING WRAPS

## Coats and Jackets

The most popular outer garments worn for evening affairs were the long columnar black-velvet coats and hip-length jackets, invariably lined in white satin, taffeta, or silk. Two popular collar styles included the small Peter Pan and the "bumper" collar which was shirred to create a large roll around the neck. Collars were often made of white ermine or were trimmed with white ermine tails. Loose-fitting hoods trimmed along the edge with white ermine were also popular. *Rever* collars provided a sophisticated asymmetrical line when closed. Sleeves were either fitted, raglan, or puffed to allow ample room for puffed-sleeve evening gowns beneath.

Tunic-length jackets were made of a variety of fabrics including silk velvet, lamé, and taffeta. Fluffy marabou bed jackets also doubled as evening wraps, particularly for teenage girls. (An example of a marabou jacket appears in Lingerie, Chapter 2.) Evening coats, jackets, and capes were also created from the furs listed above.

For her *"Commedia dell'Arte"* collection in 1938, Schiaparelli designed evening coats made of colorful felt patches. These coats were patterned after the costume worn by Arlecchino in the Italian Renaissance comedy.

## Capes

Elegant velvet taffeta, and satin evening capes often featured fur-trimmed shawl or shirred stand-up collars. Hooded capes of varying lengths became popular towards the end of the decade.

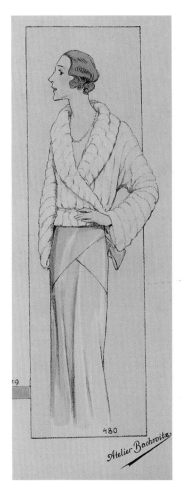

Original French fashion illustration (1931-32) from the Atelier Bachroitz. This short surplice-style evening jacket of white ermine features a shawl collar and bell sleeves.

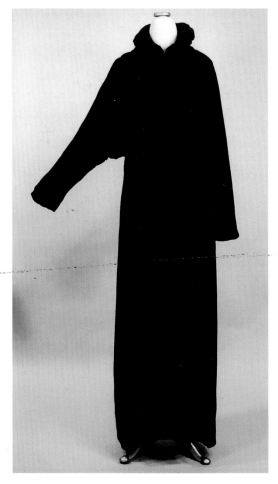

Typical full-length black silk-velvet evening coat featuring batwing sleeves and shirred stand-up collar, lined with white silk satin. Marked: Bloomingdale's New York. $140-$150.

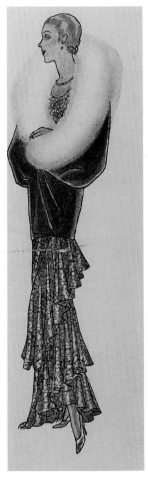

Illustration from *Delineator* (12/32) for a sophisticated evening wrap of jade green rayon velvet with a luxurious white fox collar.

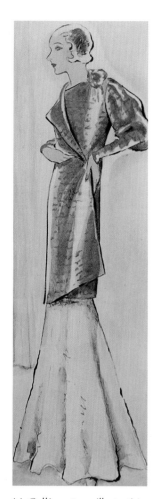

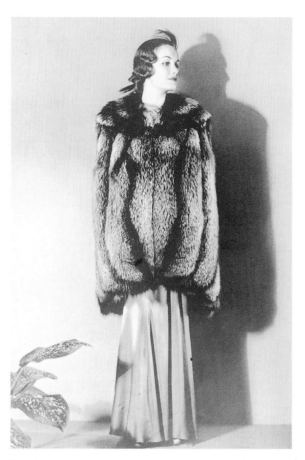

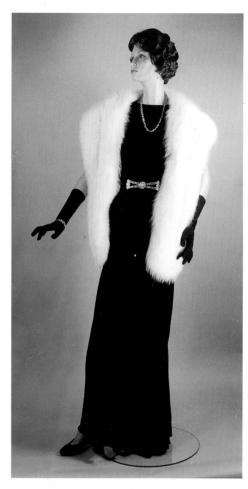

*McCall's* pattern illustration (12/32) for a tunic-length evening coat by Lucile Paray, bishop sleeves, asymmetrical closing, and a matching fabric flower at the shoulder.

This luxurious silver-fox cape by Fromm was advertised in *Harper's Bazaar* (11/37). Note: aigrette (feather ornament) worn in the hair.

White fox stole lined with white satin. Label: Bergdorf Goodman on the Plaza New York. $100-$150.

Schiaparelli became well known for her flamboyant evening capes featuring exquisite hand embroidery by the prestigious firm, the Maison Lesage. In 1938, she created a black-silk cape emblazoned with the Greek sun god, Apollo, riding in a chariot pulled by four galloping horses. This design was inspired by the Apollo fountain in the *Parc de Versailles* and was executed in gold sequins, bugle beads, and metallic thread.

For her astrology collection that same year, Schiaparelli designed a shocking-pink wool cape which she had embroidered with a glittering golden sun. This design was also rendered in gold sequins, beads, and metallic thread.

# Chapter 8

# Hair and Headgear

## HAIR

**Platinum Blonde Hair.** Jean Harlow, the "blonde bomb-shell" of 1930s motion pictures, introduced "platinum blonde" hair, which was a very pale silvery yellow...almost white. The May 1933 issue of *Photoplay* magazine reported: "Jean's platinum halo has probably aroused more comment and curiosity than any one feature of any star. Naturally blonde, Jean encourages whiteness by weekly shampoos with white soap and a final rinse containing a few drops of French bluing. She brushes for softness and sets her waves with water and vinegar."

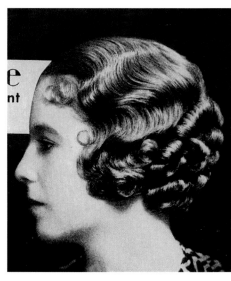

*McCall's* published this ad (4/34) for the Eugène perm featuring waves over the crown with a cluster of curls below.

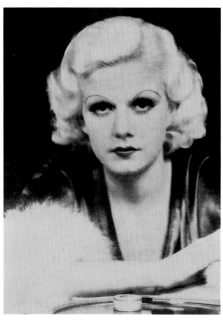

*Photoplay* published this photograph (5/33) of Hollywood sex goddess, Jean Harlow, wearing the platinum-blonde hair which she popularized.

In 1931, Antoine, the world-renowned Paris hair stylist, introduced the unusual fad of bleaching a platinum blonde streak across a dark head of hair.

**Waves.** By the early 1930s, the short "shingle" and severe "Eton-crop" hair styles worn by flappers of the previous decade had disappeared. Hair was now allowed to grow below the ears. There was a prominent part, either on one side or down the center. The hair was styled close to the head with waves over the crown (a carry-over from the 1920s). The ends of the hair, however, were now curled in one long "bologna" roll around the sides and back of the neck, or in a cluster of rolls.

A page or two in each 1930s mail-order catalog was devoted to the myriad of ingenious devices designed to aid women in producing perfectly styled waves and rolls. Old-fashioned curling irons, a carry-over from the teens, were still offered in catalogs along with modern electrified versions.

The "Baldwin Marceler" consisted of a soft, flexible perfumed rubber waver with notches around which to wind the hair. An advertisement touted the waver's ability to "not only wave the hair but curl the ends. [It] can be arranged to make lovely continuous waves all around the head."

U-shaped celluloid wave combs pressed waves into the hair at the top of the head. Each comb had a large attached rubber band which stretched over the forehead to hold the combs in place.

The "Marcelette" hair waver was designed to create two broad 6-inch-wide waves. The light metal frame was fastened like a barrette into wet hair. Six wavers were generally enough to wave the entire head.

**Rolls.** The brown celluloid "Hold-Tite Curlette" roll maker created one neat even roll at the nape of the neck. The ends of the hair were securely clamped between the closed jaws of the Curlette. As the Curlette was rotated, it rolled the hair up into a

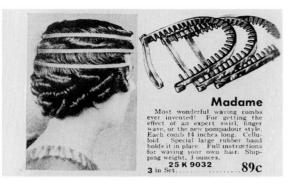

**Madame**

Most wonderful waving combs ever invented! For getting the effect of an expert swirl, finger wave, or the new pompadour style. Each comb 14 inches long. Celluloid. Special large rubber band holds it in place. Full instructions for waving your own hair. Shipping weight, 3 ounces.

25 K 9032
3 in Set..................... **89c**

This Sears, Roebuck and Co. ad (1935-36) illustrates the U-shaped 14-inch long celluloid waving combs with attached rubber bands to hold them in place.

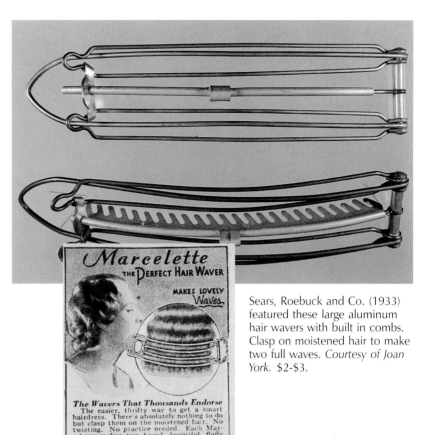

Sears, Roebuck and Co. ad (1933-34) for Baldwin Marceler. Strands of hair were wound around the prongs of the perfumed-rubber waver which not only created waves but end curls as well.

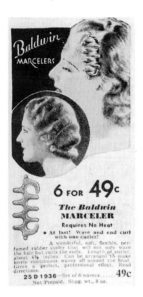

**Baldwin MARCELERS**

**6 FOR 49c**

**The Baldwin MARCELER**

**Requires No Heat**

● At last! Wave and end curl with one curler!

A wonderful, soft, flexible, perfumed rubber curler that will not only wave the hair but curls the ends. Length of curler, about 4½ inches. Can be arranged to make lovely continuous waves all around the head. Gives a perfect, professional effect. Read directions.

25 D 1936—Set of 6 wavers...... **49c**
Net Prepaid. Shpg. wt., 8 oz.

**Marcelette**
THE **PERFECT HAIR WAVER**

MAKES LOVELY
*Waves*

**The Wavers That Thousands Endorse**

The easier, thrifty way to get a smart hairdress. There's absolutely nothing to do but clasp them on the moistened hair. No twisting. No practice needed. Each Marcelette makes two broad, beautiful, fluffy waves, fully 6 inches wide. That's why Marcelette is a thrifty curler. Six are enough to curl most heads. Light metal frame conforms comfortably to shape of head. Shpg. wt., 8 oz. Not Prepaid.

25 D 1937—Set of six Wavers... **49c**

Sears, Roebuck and Co. (1933) featured these large aluminum hair wavers with built in combs. Clasp on moistened hair to make two full waves. *Courtesy of Joan York.* $2-$3.

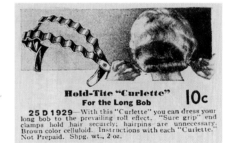

**Hold-Tite "Curlette"**
**For the Long Bob**       **10c**

25 D 1929—With this "Curlette" you can dress your long bob to the prevailing roll effect. "Sure grip" end clamps hold hair securely; hairpins are unnecessary. Brown color celluloid. Instructions with each "Curlette." Not Prepaid. Shpg. wt., 2 oz.

This Sears, Roebuck and Co. advertisement (1931) shows the Hold-Tite "Curlette" roller. The ends of the hair were fastened between the jaws of the clamp, then rolled up.

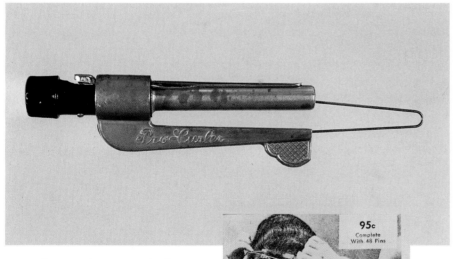

**95c**
Complete
With 48 Pins

**HAVE BEAUTIFUL NATURAL LOOKING CURLS**
**PRO-CURLER Makes Curls Quickly, Invisibly**

Now just one Curler makes all the curls you want! And it's so easy to use. Just spread a bob pin apart, insert it in the end of the handy Pro-Curler, roll hair around curler and pull it out. Presto! the pin slips automatically in place.

Best of all, the pins don't show one speck. You can go anywhere while Bob pins placed by the Pro-Curler invisibly curl your hair. Heavy metal. Strong clamp. Instructions included.

16 A 1160—Ship. wt. 4 oz. Pro-Curler with 48 Pins....... **95c**

This Montgomery Ward ad (1937) illustrates the Pro-curler with bob pin inserted into the holes in the ends. The ends of the hair were fastened under the clamp. The black plastic handle was rotated causing the hair to roll onto the shaft. The Pro-Curler was pulled out leaving the hair roll fastened by the bob pin. Marked: PAT 2,039,789 (1936). *Courtesy of Joan York.* $10-$15.

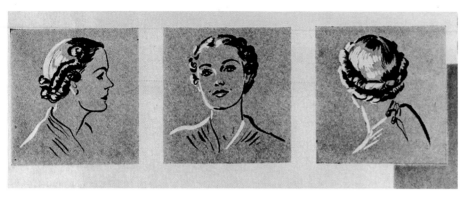

This hair style of the mid-30s was featured in *Ladies' Home Journal* (3/36). It contained a center part, smooth crown, and two rows of "bologna" curls.

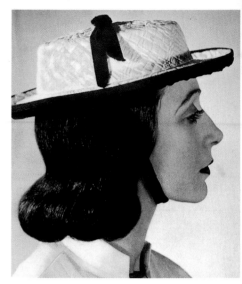

*Harper's Bazaar* advertisement (1937) featuring the page boy hair style topped by a white straw hat with black velour trim by Reboux.

uniform roll. Since the Curlette was then invisible, it could be left in the hair all day.

Only one of the ingenious "Pro-curlers" was needed to curl all of the hair ends. Just spread the "bob" pin apart, insert it into the holes in the end of the curler. Fasten the hair under the metal clamp, rotate the black plastic handle, which rolls the hair around the rod. Withdraw the curler and presto! The roll of hair is automatically fastened with the bob pin.

**Smooth Crown.** Hair became longer as the decade progressed and eventually waves gave way to a smoother look over the crown. The ends could be worn in one or two long continuous rolls, one above the other or in relaxed fluffed-up curls.

**Page Boy.** The "page boy," named for the hair style worn by medieval pages (boys training for knighthood), appeared in fashion magazines circa 1936-37. For this style, shoulder-length hair was worn smooth and straight to the ends which were turned under all around. This style was worn by Greta Garbo during the 1930s and it remained a popular style through the 1940s and 1950s.

**Up Sweep.** By 1938, styles began to emerge which would become trademarks of the war years. The most identifiable characteristic of these styles involved the hair above the ears. This hair was swept up to the top or to the back of the head, thus exposing the ears. A part was created cross the top of the head, from ear to ear. For one style, the hair in front of the part was combed forward into loose, frizzy bangs. The hair behind the part and over the ears was combed to the back where it was arranged in helter-skelter curls.

For another popular style, the hair above the ears was swept up to the top of the head where it was formed into several neat rolls or a cluster of curls. The hair behind the part was swept to the back and arranged into more rolls or curls. These styles are generally attributed to the hair stylist Antoine.

During the late 1930s, many women created rolls by the use of the new "rat-tail" comb. One end of the comb had the usual teeth, while the other end had a long pointed handle. The strands of hair were placed over the index finger. The tail of the comb was used to wind the hair around the finger. The finger was then withdrawn and a bob pin was pushed in place to fasten the roll.

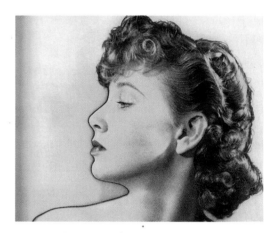

*Harper's Bazaar* illustration (2/37). The hair in front of the side-to-side part is combed forward into fluffy curls or bangs, while the hair over the ears is brushed back into helter-skelter curls.

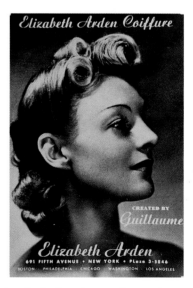

This hair style by Elizabeth Arder was featured in *Harper's Bazaar* (3/15/38). The hair above the ears has been pulled up to the top of the head where it is formed into rolls. Rolls were also created at the nape of the neck.

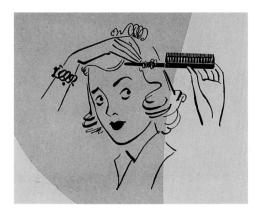

*Woman's Home Companion* (12/39) offered this instructional line drawing on the use of the rat tail comb.

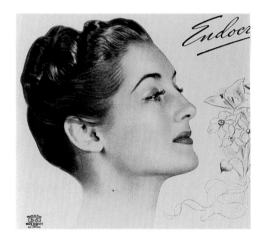

This *Harper's Bazaar* advertisement (3/1/38) shows a typical hair style used for special occasions. The hair is swept to the top of the head where it was formed into rolls. It was introduced in the late '30s and continued through the war years.

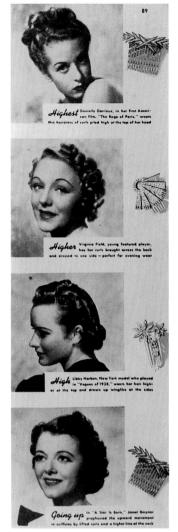

These *McCall's* photographs (6/38) illustrate various hair styles. *(1)* The hair piled high on the head. *(2)* Curls brought across the back and dressed to the right side. *(3)* The hair by the ears is swept up at the sides while the remaining hair is formed into rolls. *(4)* The hair over the forehead is brushed up in a pompadour. Note: decorative rhinestone hair combs.

***Evening Hair Styles.*** During the early '30s, the hair was worn the same for evening as for day. Towards the end of the decade, all of the hair was brushed to the top of the head and curls were formed where they were most effective. Fancy rhinestone studded combs and barrettes were often used to hold the hair in place.

# DAYTIME HATS

During the previous decade, two main hat styles reigned supreme, the *cloche* and the wide-brim hat. As the *cloche* faded from view in the early '30s, an enormous variety of hats in all shapes and sizes, took its place. They ranged from small, close-fitting caps to huge, wide-brimmed "picture" hats. Many were adaptations of men's conservative classics, while others were flamboyant and often a bit outrageous! Some hats were worn for only a brief period while others remained in style for a number of years. This chapter will deal with the most common, most recognizable hat styles. The majority of 1930s hats were quite tailored, even mannish in style and degree of ornamentation. They were often decorated with a simple grosgrain band, a bow, a single quill, or a hat ornament.

Hats of the early '30s were shallow, head hugging, and unobtrusive. The masculine Tyrolean-style hat was introduced circa 1934 and dominated the millinery scene well into the 1940s. It was ideally suited to the masculine broad-shouldered styles worn by women during this period and became one of the trademarks of the decade. Crowns on hats became progressively higher and more tapered as the decade drew to a close.

Hats of the 1930s were primarily made of felt, straw, or fabric. "Velour felt," felt made of fur, was often used for better quality hats. It had a felt side and a soft velvety side. Veils grew in popularity towards the end of the decade and were often embellished with embroidered borders, chenille dots, or sequins. They were either soft and fine, or coarse and stiff. Veils generally ended at either the eyes, the nose, or the chin.

Most hats, from 1932 on, were worn tilted over the right eye. For this reason they required an elastic or back strap to secure the hat to the head. Unlike hats of the preceding decades, 1930s hats were usually unlined.

Many fashionable women of means went directly to a milliner to have a one-of-a-kind hat custom designed on her head while she watched. In this way she could select the perfect style and color to coordinate with a particular ensemble. It was con-

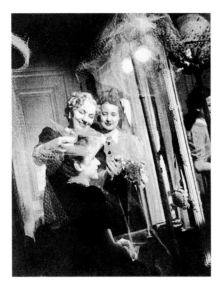

*Harper's Bazaar* (3/15/38) published this photograph of renowned milliner, Madame Suzy, creating a hat for a customer in her Paris salon.

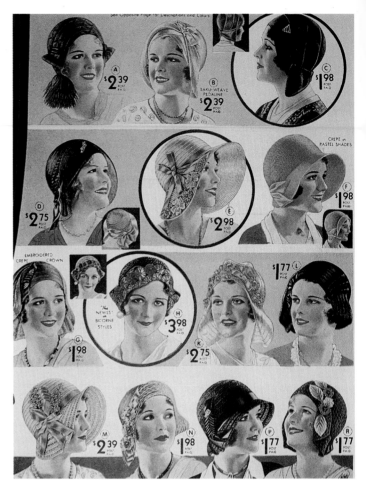

The Bellas Hess catalog (1931) offered these variations of the head-hugging *cloche* decorated with cord, ribbon, feathers, and hat ornaments. *(F,P)* Classic *cloches*. *(B,D,G,K,R)* Off-the-face *cloches* with brims folded up against the crown in front and down in back. *(A,H,L,N)* Brim is folded up against the crown in front and back causing it to bow out at the sides. *(C)* Cloche with no brim. *(E,M)* Wide brim hats.

sidered quite chic to accessorize a dress or coat with a hat, handbag, shoes, and gloves all of the same color.

Americans idolized Hollywood stars of the 1930s and were greatly influenced by the glamorous styles they observed on the silver screen. It is not surprising then that mail-order companies like Sears, Roebuck and Co. hired movie stars to model hats in their catalogs. These hats often contained a label bearing the star's signature.

Concern for consumers' rights intensified during the 1930s. In 1936 the Consumer's Union of the United States was established as an independent non-profit organization which tested and rated products and services. In 1938, manufacturers of products which passed the test earned the right to attach a label to their garments which read "Manufactured Under Fair Labor Standards - Consumer Protection Label." This union is still in existence today; therefore, hats containing this label were made from 1938 to the present day.

## Early Years

*Cloche*. The conventional *cloche*, with its deep crown and narrow down-turned brim, could still be found on the pages of fashion magazines and mail-order catalogs in 1930 and 1931. They also featured a newer version of the *cloche*, called the "off-the-face-hat," which retained the same deep crown. The brim, however, was now folded up against the crown in front and down on the sides and the back of the neck, a style which resembled a Roman legionnaire's helmet. Another style featured a brim which was pushed up against the crown in front and in back which caused the brim to bow out at the sides. Some *cloches* were merely deep crowns with no brims at all.

*Cloches* were made of felt, transparent horsehair, cellophane braid, faille, hemp straw, pedaline straw, baku straw from China, and Toyo (a hat body made of cellophane-coated rice paper). They were trimmed with lace, various types of ribbon, cellophane braid, metallic cord, tinsel, glass beads, and plush or ribbon flowers. They were also accented with decorative hat ornaments made of celluloid, bakelite, or base metal embellished with rhinestones. Common colors were Japanese red, wine, rose, Bermuda green (medium), copen blue (medium), light navy, Lido tan (refers to Lido beach in Venice), beige, Hawaiian brown, black, and white.

*Mad Cap*. In 1930, Schiaparelli designed the head-hugging mad cap which enjoyed immediate and continued success into the late 1930s. Although Schiaparelli's original cap was knitted, the style was copied far and wide in all types of fabric. The mad cap was so easy and economical to make that the home seamstress could create one to match any outfit with just a scrap of left-over fabric. The following instructions for creating a mad cap appeared in the *Home Arts - Needlecraft* magazine, 1936:

"Cut a piece of fabric 10 inches by 22 inches (or whatever your head measurement is) plus a 1 1/2-inch seam allowance. Fold in half crosswise. Sew up one side and one end [creating a pocket]. Finish the open end with a strip of grosgrain ribbon. Turn this under and hemstitch it in place. Place on the head, having the seam run front to back, or side to side. Pleat, drape, or twist whatever way is most becoming. Pin and stitch in position."

This versatile hat could have several different looks depending on how it was arranged on the head. The top seam could be placed front to back, giving the cap the appearance of a pointed cone (from the front). Or for an distinctly different look the seam could be placed side to side, thus resembling pointed ears. Since the cap folded flat, it could easily be carried in a pocket or packed in a suitcase.

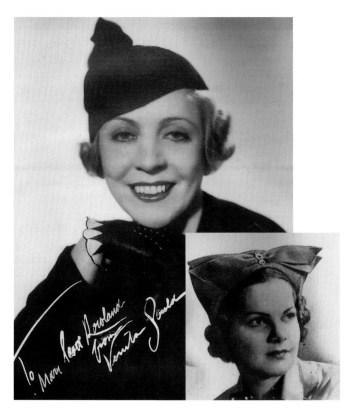

**Beret.** The classic wool felt Basque or "pancake" beret was popular during the early years of the decade, as it conformed to the low head-hugging styles prevalent at that time. Berets were often tilted over the right ear, leaving the left ear uncovered. The beret was one of Greta Garbo's trademarks worn with a belted trench coat and dark glasses. Marlene Dietrich also favored the beret and wore it with a man's sport jacket and trousers. It was a favorite of the infamous Bonnie Parker, gun moll to gangster Clyde Barrow. Berets were offered in mail-order catalogs in felt, wool, velvet, angora, rayon bouclé, and straw in a wide range of colors. They were worn for dress as well as for sport. Handcraft magazines printed instructions for knitting or crocheting berets and various other matching accessories.

Two different views of the madcap introduced by Schiaparelli. Large photo shows top seam - front to back. *Insert:* Montgomery Ward (1937) version shows the same seam - side to side. It is decorated with grosgrain ribbon and a rhinestone ornament.

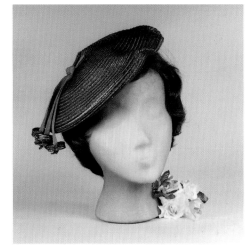

Green straw beret accented with green straw disks suspended from green grosgrain ribbon. $30-$50.

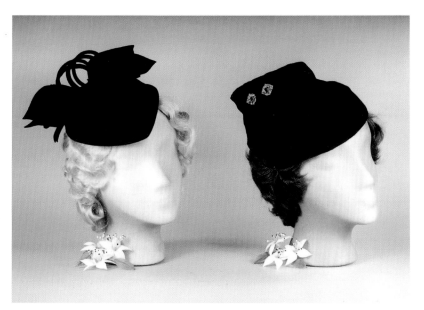

*Left:* Shallow pointed black-felt crown decorated at back with felt-covered coiled wire, felt leaves, and ribbon. *Right:* Black velvet mad cap-style hat with silver-tone hat ornament containing clear and green rhinestones. *Courtesy of Cedar Crest College Alumnae Museum, gift of Ellie Laubner.* $25-$40 ea.

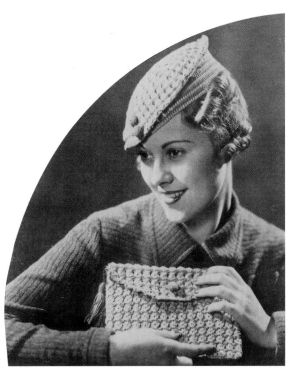

Illustration from the Bucilla crochet manual (1934) for two-tone hand-crocheted shell-stitch beret and matching *pochette. Courtesy of Elaine Cruse.*

**Ribbon Hat**. This small, shallow, head-hugging hat with no brim was popular circa 1932 to 1933. It was composed of strips of ribbon or felt which were fastened together in the front and back only. This allowed a glimpse of hair between the strips. It was worn tipped over the right eye. (An example of a flower girl's ribbon hat appears in Bridal Wear, Chapter 5.)

**Swagger-brim Hat**. This hat had a shallow crown which occasionally featured a raised ridge running from front to back (similar to a man's Panama hat.) The medium-wide "swagger" brim was pulled down over the right eye in front and down in back. This hat was commonly made of crepe, felt, straw, silk, satin, transparent horsehair, transparent pyroxylin hair braid, and piqué. It was decorated with a grosgrain band, *faux* bow, flowers, celluloid or Bakelite hat ornament, or short nose veil. Black, brown, navy, burgundy, sand, and gray were popular colors for fall and winter, while white and pastels were worn in spring and summer.

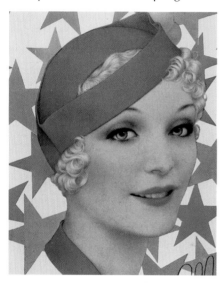

*Delineator* cover illustration (12/32) featuring a hat by Agnès made of red felt strips which allow the hair to peek through the slits. Illustration by Dynevor Rhys.

**Empress Eugénie Hat**. The first to wear this feminine hat during the 1860s was Empress Eugénie, wife of the second French emperor, Louis Napoleon. The shallow crown and narrow up-turned brim were curved to fit the contours of the head (front to back). This feminine style was trimmed with a bow or an ostrich plume which cascaded down the back. Hollywood designer, Gilbert Adrian, revived this style for Greta Garbo, who wore it cocked over one eye in the movie *Romance* (1930). Rose Descat, noted French milliner, is also remembered for her romantic Empress Eugénie hats.

**Pillbox Hat**. The small oval pillbox hat had a flat top, straight sides, and no brim. During the 1930s, it was worn on top of the head and tipped slightly to the right. This hat was popularized by Adrian, who designed one for Greta Garbo in the movie *As You Desire Me* (1932). It was also a favorite of French milliner Mme. Suzy, who often accented her pillbox hats with a *chou* (cabbage flower). This style was made of velvet, felt, or straw and decorated with artificial flowers, bows, feathers, and/or a short nose veil.

## Middle Years

**Tyrolean Hat**. This sporty hat originated in the Alpine Tyrol region of Austria and Bavaria, a favorite vacation spot for wealthy Europeans. It was generally made of soft, dark green felt with a high creased crown and medium-sized brim which was turned down in front and up in back. It was banded with a heavy cord and trimmed with a few short barnyard feathers or bristles.

It was adapted for women, circa 1934, and became the most popular hat style of the decade. It was produced in countless variations. The crown, in particular, took on many diverse shapes through the use of dents, creases, pleats, tucks, ridges, and seams in various configurations. This masculine hat was usually trimmed with a grosgrain band or a lacquered quill. Like so many other hats of the period, it was pulled down over the right eye.

Circa 1936, many Tyrolean hats acquired a wider brim and a high, truncated cone-shaped crown. When this tapered crown had a center crease running front to back, and the brim was

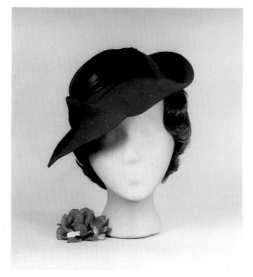

Maroon felt swagger-brim hat with shallow sculptured crown, swagger-brim, black leather over-lay. Label: Made Expressly for R.H. Sterns Co., Boston. $40-$60.

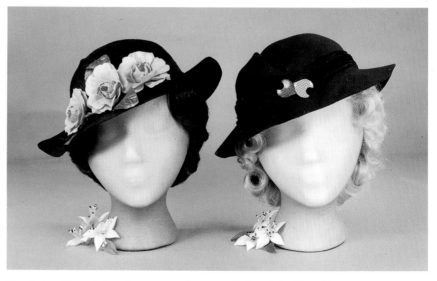

Two hats with sculptured crowns and swagger-brims. *Left:* Navy blue straw, grosgrain band, three pink gardenias. *Right:* Purple felt, chenille band, celluloid pin. $40-$65 ea.

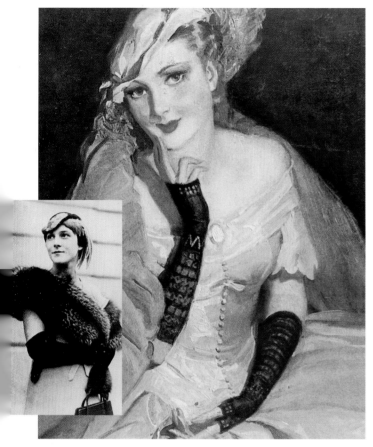

This cover illustration from *Pictorial Review* (2/32) features a Victorian ensemble consisting of an Empress Eugénie hat, "off-the-shoulder" gown with bouffant Winterhalter skirt, decorative brooch, and lace fingerless mitts. Illustration by artist/jewelry designer McClelland Barclay. *Insert: Town and Country* photograph of a feathered Empress Eugénie hat, 1934.

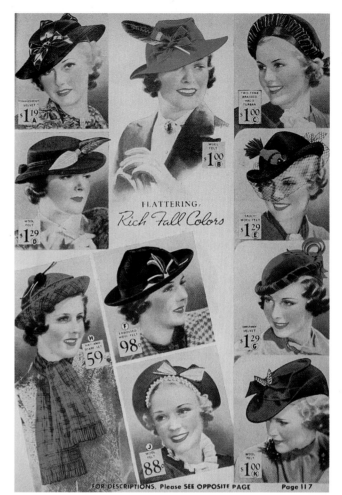

The Chicago Mail Order Co. catalog (1936-37) offered this variety of winter hats including: (A) Swagger-brim hat with a bit of the bandeau back visible under the brim. (B) Tyrolean hat. (D) Kettle brim. (E) Modified fedora. (F,H) Breton sailor. (G) Bumper brim with bandeau back. (J) Modified halo hat. (K) Peak hat.

turned up not only in back but the sides as well, the hat resembled a man's fedora, a style promoted by renowned milliner Lilly Daché. When the crown came to a point and a large quill was added, it became a "Robin Hood" hat. In 1939, some Tyrolean hats featured a long, 6-inch-wide sash in place of the simple band. This sash was made of colorful plaid or striped rayon. Common materials for these styles were wool felt, tweed felt, Panama straw, sisal straw, pedaline braided straw, sharkskin straw, and Toyo. Beige, white, burgundy, brown, rust, violet, navy, green, royal blue, and black were the most common colors.

**Peaked Hat.** Circa 1936, another variation of the Tyrolean hat was introduced. The crown was similar to the Tyrolean; however, the brim was cut away in the back and the sides were rolled up towards the crown, leaving a mannish peak in front. This style was also trimmed with a grosgrain band and a feather.

**Breton Sailor Hat.** First worn by the peasants of Brittany, France, the Breton sailor hat or Breton roller was adopted by women circa 1935. It had a round-flat or dome-shaped crown and a medium-sized brim which was rolled up evenly all around. In 1938-39, a truncated cone-shaped crown was introduced. When worn cocked over the right eye, a back strap, elastic band, or "back bandeau" (stiff extension of the crown under the brim) was often provided. This youthful style was particu-

larly popular with teenage girls who preferred to wear it on the back of the head. When worn in this fashion, the brim framed the face like a halo, thus the nickname "halo" hat. It was produced in felt, straw, velvet, and various other fabrics. The most common colors were white, black, brown, navy, red, burgundy, and spruce green.

**Garden-Party Hat.** The wide-brim garden-party or picture hat was the most common style worn by bridal attendants during the 1930s. These feminine hats featured a shallow, dome-shaped crown and a wide brim which was either turned down evenly all around or drooped in front and back only. (This style is distinguishable from the wide-brims of the 1920s, which drooped at the sides.) They were made of transparent horsehair, cellophane braid, or straw and were often decorated with colorful flowers.

**Cartwheel Hat.** This hat had a shallow crown and a wide, straight brim. It was made of straw and contained some form of stabilizing device at the back to hold it over the forehead.

**Fez.** The Turkish fez was a deep-red felt hat shaped like a truncated cone. It had no brim and a long black silk tassel attached to the center of the crown. It was named after the town of Fez in Morocco. The fez was adapted for women, circa 1933, and was produced in felt and other fabrics in a variety of colors.

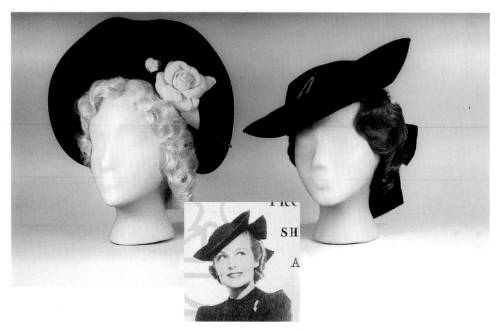

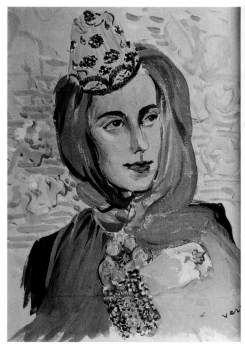

Left: Black felt hat with halo-style up-turned brim accented with a white gardenia. Label: Mfd. Under Fair Labor Standards, c.1938. Right: Black velour-felt Breton sailor hat, grosgrain stabilizing back-strap tied in a decorative bow, silver-toned hat ornament. Label: Edith Kichline, Allentown. Insert: Breton sailor hat from Pictorial Review (2/39). $40-$60.

Harper's Bazaar (3/15/38) published this portrait of Schiaparelli, by Vertès, wearing a pink *fez* encrusted with colored stones and paillette embroidery. From it drift two silken scarves that frame her face. Her bracelet and pendant contain clusters of gold balls.

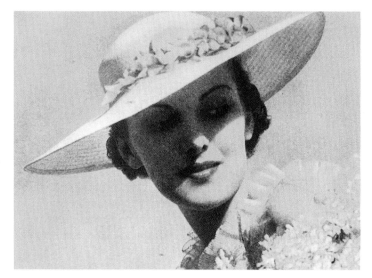

This feminine straw garden-party hat, from the June 1935 issue of the *Delineator* is accented with pastel flowers along the band.

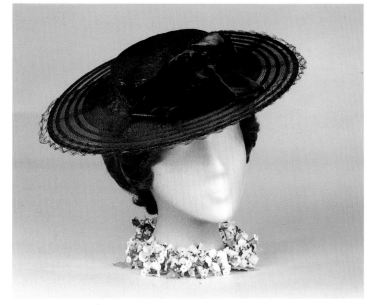

Brown straw cartwheel hat. Shallow flat straw crown, straight brim containing alternating rows of straw and horsehair, brown veil and velvet bow, grosgrain stabilizing back strap. Label: Mfd. Under Fair Labor Standards, Consumers' Protection Label, c. 1938. *Courtesy of Cedar Crest College Alumnae Museum, gift of Ellie Laubner.* $30-$40.

***Tam-o-shanter***. This cap was named after Tam O' Shanter, the main character of a Scottish poem by Robert Burns (1791). Called a "tam" for short, this round, flat cap had a snug-fitting headband and was usually accented in the center with a pompon. It became fashionable for women and children during the 1930s and was worn tilted to the right side of the head. The most common fabrics were wool, wool tartan, felt, cotton piqué, straw, and velvet.

***Tricorne Hat***. This three cornered hat was first worn by men during the 18th century. It had a dome-shaped crown and a brim which was cocked to form three equidistant points, with one point in the center front. Eighteenth-century women wore miniature versions of the hat as part of their riding habit. The *tricorne* hat was revived during the 1930s and was often recommended for the mature woman with a large head size.

***Saucer Hat.*** This hat's shallow crown and narrow, straight brim resembled an inverted saucer. It was often made of straw and decorated with a grosgrain band, flowers, feathers, or a short veil. It was fashionable to wear this style tipped over the right eye and therefore a back strap or an elastic was usually provided.

## Later Years

***Calotte*** (also spelled calot). *Calotte* is the French word for skullcap. It consisted of a small dome-shaped crown with no brim that snugly hugged the back of the head. It was derived from the ancient Greeks and was frequently made in eight pie-shaped sections with a small covered button or loop in the center. A cluster of flowers was often placed on either side over the ears.

***Juliet Cap***. This cap was similar in shape to the *calotte*; however, it was usually made of crocheted or knitted openwork mesh. It was inspired by the Renaissance costume worn by Juliet in Shakespeare's tragedy *Romeo and Juliet*. This style was revived after Adrian designed a Juliet cap for Norma Shearer in the film version (1936). (For another example of a Juliet cap, see Bridal Wear, Chapter 5.)

***Doll Hat***. These amusing miniature hats began with a round or oval, slightly- domed felt form which was commonly decorated with flowers, feathers, or concentric rows of ruffles. Doll hats were perched precariously over the right eye and held in place by an elastic or back strap. (See photo of bridal attendants wearing doll hats in Bridal Wear, Chapter 5.)

***Glengarry Cap***. This Scottish cap was first worn in 1805 by members of the Glengarry clan in Inverness, Scotland. It consisted of a crown with a central pleat running from front to back. This enabled the cap to fold flat like a military "overseas" cap. It was often decorated on the left side with a clan brooch, cockade, or short feathers and black ribbon streamers down the back. The glengarry cap was adopted by women and children circa 1936 and was usually made of felt or wool in solid colors or tartans. (See example of child's Glengarry cap in Children's Wear, Chapter 15.)

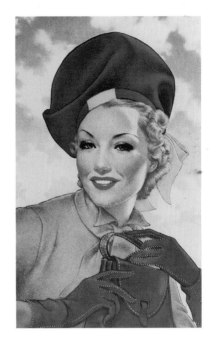

*Woman's Home Companion* illustration (10/37) of a Scottish tam-o'-shanter in rust-colored felt and gold grosgrain ribbon by Agnès. Rust suede gloves and calf bag with beige stitching by Aris. (Rust and gold were popular '30s colors.)

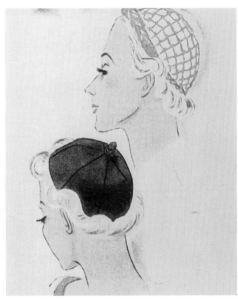

*Woman's Home Companion* illustrations (6/37). *Top:* Renaissance-style mesh Juliet cap inspired by Shakespeare's heroine. *Bottom:* Black felt skullcap.

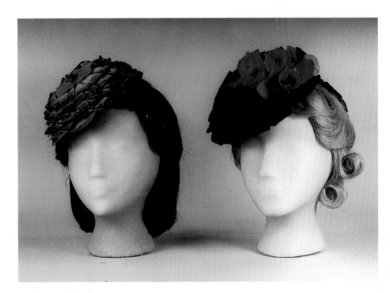

Two doll hats. *Left:* Green velvet gathered ruffles arranged in concentric layers accented by a shocking-pink flower, stabilizing back elastic. *Right:* Black satin ribbon loops arranged in concentric layers, topped with shocking-pink roses, wire stabilizing hoop in back, c. late '30s-early '40s. $50-$70.

**Turban.** Commonly worn by Muslim men, the turban was a long cotton, linen, or silk scarf wound around the head, completely covering the hair. The turban was adapted for women during the early '30s and included any hat body which was draped with fabric. Women's turbans created towards the end of the decade more closely resembled the genuine article. They were made entirely of soft draped fabric, which was usually fastened in a knot or loop over the forehead. The amount of hair covered by the turban was up to the individual wearer. Schiaparelli had a passion for turbans and preferred to tuck all of her hair inside.

**Snood.** Called a *résille* in French, the snood was an openwork mesh hairnet worn during the 1850s-60s to confine a woman's hair at the back of the neck. Hollywood designer, Gilbert Adrian, revived the Victorian snood for actress Hedy Lamarr in *I Take This Woman* (1939). A snood was also worn by Olivia de Havilland as Melanie in *Gone With the Wind* (1939). Snoods made of chenille or silk cord appeared in the Paris collections of 1939 and remained in style through World War II. They were

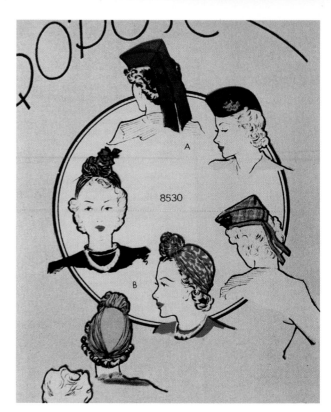

*La Presse* advertisement (12/30/39). *A)* Scotch Glengarry caps accented with feathers and ribbon streamers. *B)* Turban-style headdresses culminating in decorative knots.

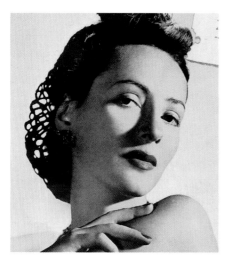

This photo published in *You* (1938-39) features a coarse-net snood.

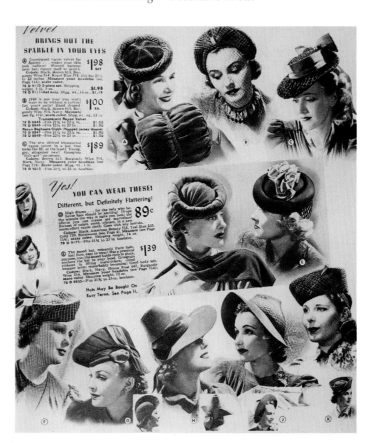

Sears, Roebuck and Co. catalog page (1939-40) devoted to hats.
*(A)* Velvet bumper-brim hat with back strap and matching muff.
*(B)* Draped velvet turban. *(C)* Shirred velvet hat with grosgrain band and streamers. *(D)* Rayon bumper-brim hat with attached wimple.
*(E)* Felt bumper brim-hat with attached snood and flowers.
*(F)* Glengarry-style felt hat with veil. *(G)* Profile hat. *(H)* Felt hat with high truncated crown. *(J)* Felt bonnet converts to halo hat.
*(K)* Velvet *toque.*

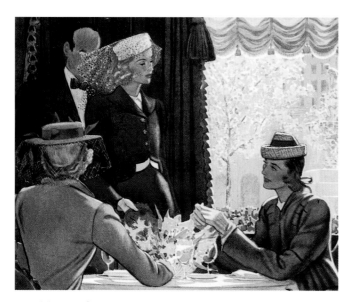

Ad featured in *Harper's Bazaar* (3/1/38). *Top:* Pale blue pillbox hat with a spotted veil. *Left:* Dusty-rose inverted-saucer hat with wine-color band and back strap, rose veil. *Right:* Tan straw bumper-brim hat with truncated cone-shaped crown, green band and back strap.

108

particularly popular with women working in war plants as they prevented long hair from catching in the machinery. Snoods were also attached to the backs of hats.

**Bumper Brim**. Introduced circa 1937, the bumper brim was curved under to form a thick, uniform roll all around the hat. This brim was often used in conjunction with a round-flat or truncated cone-shaped crown. It was usually made of felt or velvet and was held over the forehead by a back strap.

**Wimple.** Originally worn by Medieval women, the wimple consisted of a piece of white silk or linen fabric fastened to the hair in back and draped under the chin in front, covering the neck and throat. In the late '30s, Schiaparelli and John-Frederics created updated versions of the wimple, consisting of a soft strip of jersey fabric 12 inches or slightly longer. The ends of the wimple were fastened to opposite sides of a hat, and the center was draped over the throat. An alternative arrangement called for the attachment of one end of the wimple to the hat, while the other end was draped over the opposite shoulder.

**Hat Ornaments**. Created mainly for decoration, hat ornaments should not be confused with hat pins, which were primarily used to secure a hat to a woman's hair.

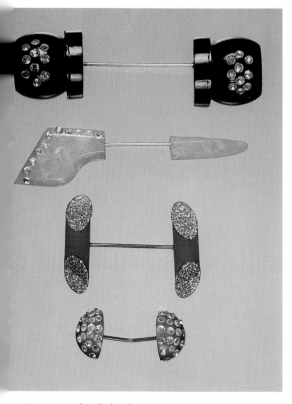

Four typical Bakelite hat ornaments accented with rhinestones and sequins. *Courtesy of Ina Stoudt (Antique Treasures)* $10-$30 ea.

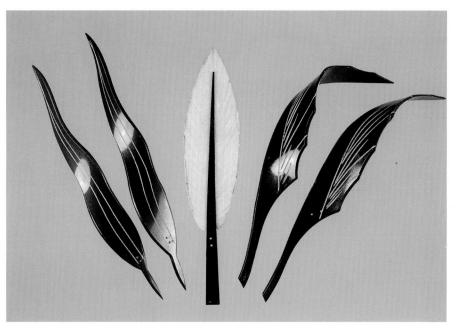

Bakelite leaf and celluloid feather decorations for hats with holes for stitching. *Courtesy of Mary Anne Faust (Yesterday's Delights).* $8-$15 ea.

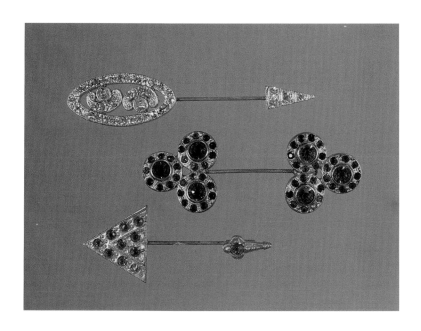

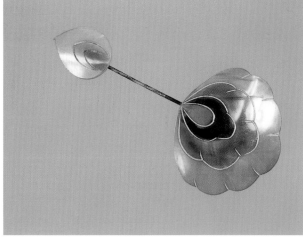

Above: Scalloped celluloid and enamel hat ornament. $20-$25.

Left: Three base-metal and rhinestone hat ornaments. *Courtesy of Mary Anne Faust (Yesterday's Delights).* $8-$15 ea.

Renowned jeweler, Pierre Cartier, began making *cliquet* pins (also known as stickpins, lapel pins, or jabot pins) shortly before the First World War. They became the obvious choice to decorate hats of the 1920s-30s. These double-headed pins contained two usually Art Deco-style heads on either end of a short pointed metal shaft with threads. The heads could look alike or one head could be larger than the other. One head was unscrewed and the shaft was inserted into, then out of the hat. When the head was returned to the shaft, only the decorative heads were visible, creating the impression of two separate pins. Fine jewelers fashioned hat ornaments from platinum, onyx, and precious gems. Modestly-priced hat ornaments were made of inexpensive materials such as base metal, celluloid, or bakelite and decorated with rhinestones, marcasites, enamel, or glass *cabochons*. Other hat ornament styles resembled feathers, volutes (spirals or question marks), and knots.

**Babushka.** Circa 1938, the Russian peasant-style babushka or kerchief became a popular head covering for sports. It remained popular through the war years and into the 1950s. These square scarves were folded diagonally, then tied under the chin. Women's sewing magazines of the late 1930s encouraged women to make babushkas to match their sports ensembles with left-over fabric.

# RENOWNED MILLINERS

**Lilly Daché.** Born in France, Daché was apprenticed to the prestigious Parisian milliner Carolyn Reboux and then to Suzanne Talbot. She moved to New York and by 1937 owned her own building which housed her workrooms and boutique. She is best known for her draped turbans.

**Rose Valois.** Also trained under Caroline Reboux, Valois opened her own salon on the Rue Royale in Paris in 1927. She will be remembered for her *cloches*, Eugénie hats, fedoras, turbans, Tyrolean hats, and opulent dinner hats.

**Agnès.** This leading French milliner of the 1920-30s listed among her friends such Cubist painters as Léger, Mondrian, and Delaunay. She often utilized their fabric designs in her *avant-garde* creations. She was known for her turbans and her experimentation with new and unusual materials such as cellophane.

**Rose Descat.** Another prominent French hat designer of the period was Rose Descat. She will be remembered for her Empress Eugénie hats, silk turbans, pillbox hats, fedoras, and Tyrolean hats.

**Legroux Soeurs.** The Legroux sisters opened their Parisian millinery house in 1917. They were widely known for their off-the-face sport hats and their wide-brim picture hats.

**John-Frederics.** German-born milliner John Harburger (later known as Mr. John) attended the Sorbonne and the *École des Beaux-Arts* in Paris. In 1929, he and Frederic Hirst opened a salon on Madison Avenue in New York City under the name John-Frederics. They created hats for stars like Gloria Swanson and Marlene Dietrich and will be remembered for their whimsical doll hats, skullcaps, and hats with wimples.

**Sally Victor.** American designer, Sally Victor, learned her trade while working in her aunt's millinery shop in New York City. She married Sergiv Victor, the head of a wholesale milli-

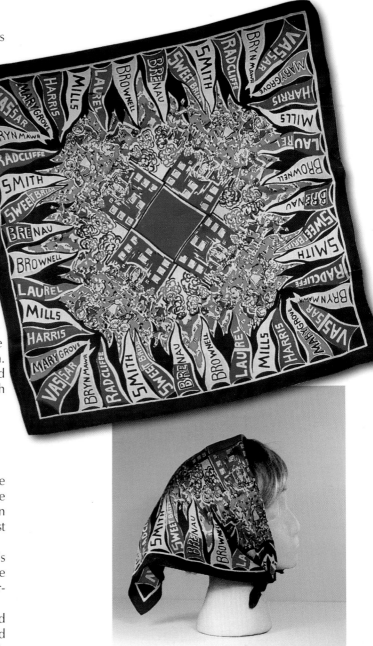

This scarf featuring pennants from various all-girl colleges is typical of the novelty prints offered during the 1930s. $50-$80.

nery company called Serge. Victor soon became the company's head designer. In 1934, she opened a millinery shop and designed hats under her own name. She specialized in pillboxes and Breton sailor hats.

**Elsa Schiaparelli.** Surrealism was characterized by the juxtaposition of objects which would not ordinarily be placed together and also by objects which were made to resemble something entirely different. Schiaparelli was an enthusiastic devotee of Surrealism and a personal friend to many of the Surrealist painters of her day. She frequently called upon them to design for her. Salvador Dali, for example, designed her famous "shoe" hat, which resembled a black inverted shoe. Her other bizarre hats included a lamb chop hat with a white frill (1938), a weather vane hat with a gyrating weather cock, a bird cage hat with a singing bird, a regal crown, a cone-shaped clown hat (1938), a

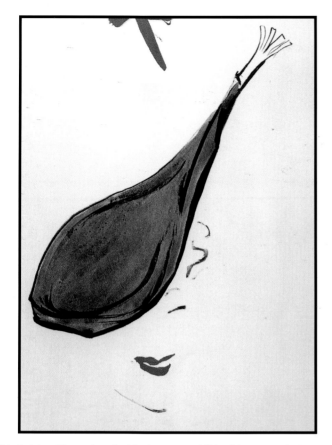

This fashion illustration, by Vertès, was published in *Harper's Bazaar* (1/38). It features Schiaparelli's "mutton-chop" beret with white patent-leather frill.

chicken in a basket hat, a windmill hat, an ice cream cone hat, and an inkwell hat, complete with a quill pen (1938). Her whimsical hats created a diversion from the hard times brought on by the depression and helped to establish her as a designer with whit and a sense of fun.

## CARE OF HATS

When purchasing a vintage hat, it is important to consider its condition. It is advisable to pass up hats which are crushed or misshapen, as it is often difficult to restore them to their original shape. Flower petals can often be revived and reshaped by steaming and their wired leaves can be rearranged in whatever way is becoming.

Ideally, each hat should be stored in its own hat box lined with acid free paper. (Ordinary paper, cardboard, and wood contain acid which can burn textiles with which they come in contact for any length of time.) Be sure that the shape of the hat is not altered by the way it is stored. The crown of a hat should be stuffed with enough acid free tissue paper to hold its shape.

## EVENING HEADGEAR

**Headbands.** Glittering diamond and beaded *bandeaux* were worn over the forehead during the early 1920s as part of an elegant evening ensemble. By 1925, the *bandeau* began to lose favor. In its place were headbands worn over the top of the head, ear to ear. This style continued into the 1930s; yet, it never achieved the popularity of the forehead *bandeau*.

Headbands were made of precious metal accented with glittering gems or plated base metal decorated with rhinestones. An inexpensive headband advertised in the Sears, Roebuck and Co. catalog consisted of a single row of overlapping leaves, reminiscent of an ancient laurel wreath. These bands were made of gold or silver "metal-covered cloth" with rhinestone ornamentation. Another wreath, suitable for bridal attendants and first communicants, was topped with dainty rosebuds in white, blue, orchid, or pink. Chanel often wore a simple ribbon tied in a bow over the top of her head.

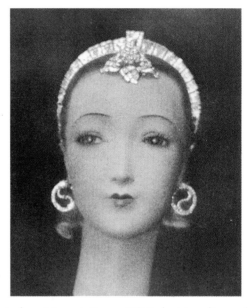

This photo from *Harper's Bazaar* (1/31) depicts a diamond headband by Cartier, featuring flexible floral and foliate ornament.

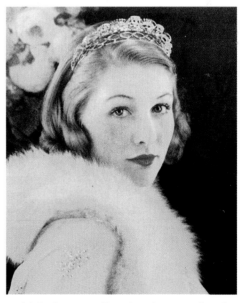

This photo published in *McCall's* (5/34) features a headband worn for formal evening affairs.

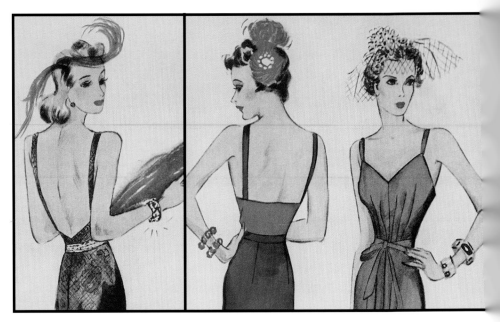

These fashion drawings from *McCall's* (1/38) illustrate a variety of evening headgear. *Left:* Sweeping plumes. *Middle:* Two red feather pompons. *Right:* Stiff-net veil topped by cluster of yellow flowers.

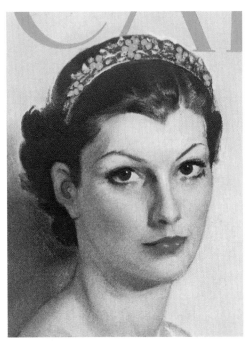

This cover illustration from *McCall's* (4/34) depicts a headband made of gold metal in foliate design set with turquoise-colored stones.

**Combs.** Tortoise-colored celluloid side combs were available from the beginning of the decade and were often decorated with rhinestones, artificial flowers, or berry clusters. Fancy "bob" pins embellished with rhinestone were also offered.

**Skull and Juliet Caps.** Fancy skullcaps were worn as part of a cocktail or dinner ensemble during the second half of the decade. They were often decorated with sequins, feathers, artificial flowers, and small veils. Evening versions of the mesh Juliet cap were often decorated with pearls and *faux* jewels. (An example of a crocheted Juliet cap appears in Bridal Wear, Chapter 5.)

**Flowers and Feathers.** A small bouquet of flowers was often placed on top of the head, accented by a short, stiff eye-level veil. Plumes were also fastened to the hair in sweeping, asymmetrical arrangements.

**Snoods.** Evening snoods could be seen in fashion magazines as early as 1936. They were often accented with colorful flowers or shiny beads and were fastened to the hair with decorative rhinestone-studded hair pins or combs.

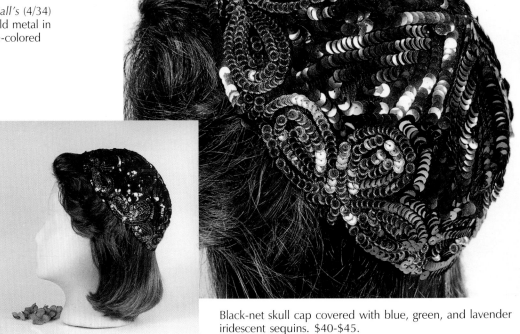

Black-net skull cap covered with blue, green, and lavender iridescent sequins. $40-$45.

# Chapter 9

# Handbags, Vanities, & Compacts

## HANDBAGS

Daytime handbags were evolving from the small dainty purses of the 1920s to the enormous 15-19 inch bags of the 1940s. Bags were made of genuine or imitation leather, suede, cloth, crocheted gimp, or wooden beads. Smaller mesh or glass-beaded bags were reserved for dressy afternoon and evening affairs.

Most daytime bags contained one, two, or three internal compartments, one of which was often closed by a "zip" (later called a zipper). Many purses came with a small change purse fastened by a cord to the inside of the bag. "Double-frame" bags contained a small inner change purse swinging from the hinges on the inside of the larger bag.

Standard colors for handbags during the first half of the decade were black, brown, navy, white, red, and tan. During the later years, more sophisticated colors were added such as marine blue, purple, burgundy, olive, rust, and American beauty (shocking pink).

Fashion magazines encouraged readers to color coordinate their ensembles by wearing a hat, handbag, and shoes of the same color to complement a coat, dress, or suit. There was a custom handbag department in most fine department stores where a customer could special order a bag to match a particular dress or ensemble. Monograms were a fashionable craze during the 1930s and specially designed block letters could be applied to a bag at the time of purchase.

Handbag, vanity, and compact styles were often manufactured for more than one year. It should, therefore, be noted that a particular handbag style may also have been produced before and/or after the circa date which is indicated in this chapter.

### Handbag Styles

**Pochette Handbag.** The most common handbag of the late 1920s and 1930s was the *pochette*, which means "small pocket" in French. This flat, rectangular bag featured sleek, uncluttered lines which rendered it ideal for modern Art Deco-style ornamentation. There were many types of *pochettes*: the flap-top envelope style, the zipper-top style, and those with a metal frame and twisted-knob clasp at the top. Strap-handle *pochettes* contained either a very short top-strap handle with just enough room for the fingers, a vertical strap handle on the back of the bag, or no strap at all. (Vertical back straps were unique to the late 1920s and '30s and are a valuable tool for dating handbags of this period.)

Pochettes were called by several different names in English, relating to the manner in which they were carried. They were tucked under one arm (thus the name "underarm bag"), clutched in the hand (thus the name "clutch bag"), held by the back strap (thus the name "back-strap bag"), or held by the top strap. *Pochettes* were made of leather, mesh, fabric, or crocheted gimp and were decorated with beads and various forms of needlework. They often featured the wearer's initials in bold, Art Deco-style block letters.

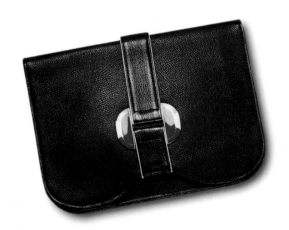

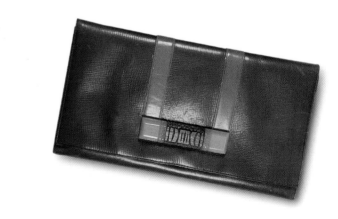

Leather envelope-style *pochettes*. *Top:* Navy blue leather, vertical strap with white piping in front and back, blue and white *champlevé* enameled ornament. *Bottom:* Brown leather with tan leather trim and butterscotch Bakelite and wood ornament, leather back strap. *Courtesy of Gerry Meza.* $75-$85 ea.

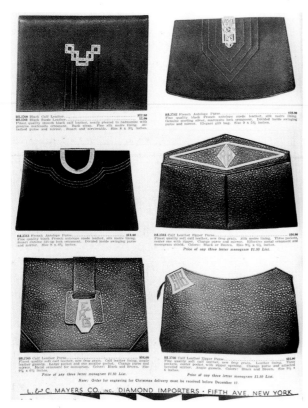

L & C Mayers Co. advertisement (1933) devoted to Art Deco-style *pochettes* in French antelope suede and frog-grained calf leather. *Top two:* marcasite ornaments. *Bottom three:* monogrammed metal escutcheon.

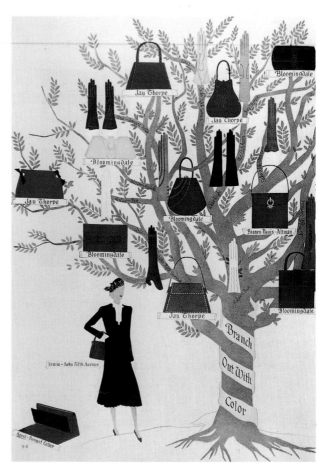

Colorful illustration from *Harper's Bazaar* (1/38) featuring an accessories tree displaying top-handle bags and *pochettes*.

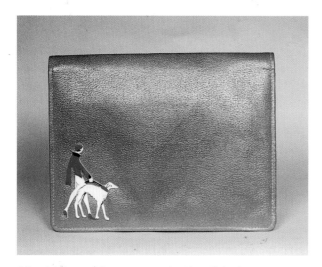

Olive leather *pochette* accented with celluloid ornament in the popular woman-walking-a-borzois motif, late '20s-early-'30s. *Courtesy of Roxanne Stuart.* $100-$110.

***Hard-Sided Handbag.*** Smooth, hard-sided bags with top-strap handles were designed for daytime use. They were made with a metal frame and clasp and the tapered, triangular sides contained gussets for expansion.

In 1935, Hermés, the prestigious French firm specializing in hand-crafted leather goods, introduced a hard-sided hand-bag based on a saddle bag. This bag was later named the "Kelly" bag after American actress Grace Kelly, who frequently used this style.

***Dual-Strap Handbag.*** This style of handbag appeared circa 1936. It was a medium-sized bag with two strap handles and two open compartments on either side of the center zippered section. This classic style is still in use today.

***Pouch-Style Handbag.*** Pouch-style bags were available throughout the decade and featured a body which was gathered to a frame or to a wide yoke at the top of the bag. They were made of soft leather or cloth and were produced in both *pochette* and top-strap models.

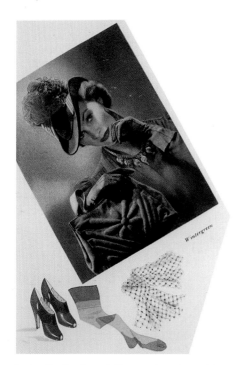

Sears, Roebuck and Co. catalog photo (1939-40) featuring a color-coordinated outfit in popular late '30s color combination. Olive sculptured-suede (trapunto) purse. Note: cluster necklace.

**Shoulder-Strap Handbag.** The July 1936 issue of *Delineator* magazine featured sports clothing and accessories recommended for bicycling, including a practical, long-handled "sling bag." When this bag was suspended from one shoulder diagonally over the torso, it left the hands free to maneuver the bicycle. This style would prove very useful during World War II, when many women were forced to ride a bicycle, due to gas rationing. It was universally accepted and was worn by service women and civilians alike. (An example of a shoulder-strap bag appears in Sportswear, Chapter 6.)

In 1938, Schiaparelli commissioned Jean Clément to make long-handled bags in leather for sport, tortoise-look for day, and lamé for evening. She called them *bandoulière*, which means "shoulder-strap" bag in French.

## Handbag Materials

### Leather

There was a wide variety of leather used for handbags during the 1930s. Steerhide, calfskin, seal, antelope suede, pigskin, snakeskin, alligator, and Moroccan leather (goatskin) were all common. Less expensive simulated leather called leatherette was grained to look like genuine animal skins. White saddle stitching was a popular detail for sports bags.

**Embossed Leather Bags.** Leather handbags with hand-tooled designs became popular during the Arts and Crafts movement, around the turn of the 20th century. This movement promoted handmade decorative arts in lieu of mass-produced, machine-made items. These "Art Craft" bags, as they were called, featured free-flowing *Art Nouveau* designs incorporating objects from nature. Swirling vines and flowers with long flowing tendrils were the most common motifs.

Lower priced bags were machine embossed, rather than hand tooled, and were labeled "tooled-effect" in mail-order

catalogs. They were mass produced in a variety of styles, including medium-length top-strap bags, or rectangular *pochettes* in the short top-strap and back-strap models. They were made of heavy, durable Spanish or English steerhide with frames of dull-gray gun metal or simulated tortoise shell. Many bags featured a turn-latch clasp which opened with a twist of the latch tab. The seams and edges were hand laced with goatskin and the insides were lined with suede or heavy moiré fabric. Hand coloring or gold leaf were often applied to the design for enrichment.

These popular bags remained in style for nearly four decades and were finally phased out circa 1935 or 1936. It is also interesting to note that they remained popular well after the end of the *Art Nouveau* period and through the height of the Art Deco movement (1925-1935). It should be noted that some of the later bags featured a combination of *Art Nouveau*-style tooling and Art Deco-style ornamentation on the frame, clasp, or turn-lock tab. The patent date was often stamped on the inside of the frame.

**Leather Link Bags.** Handbags made of leather links were introduced in the early 1930s. They were referred to as "braided" or "handwoven" bags in period catalogs; however, they were actually made of interlocking leather links. Each link had two oval-shaped holes on each end. Each link was folded in half (crosswise), lining up the holes. The end of the next link was

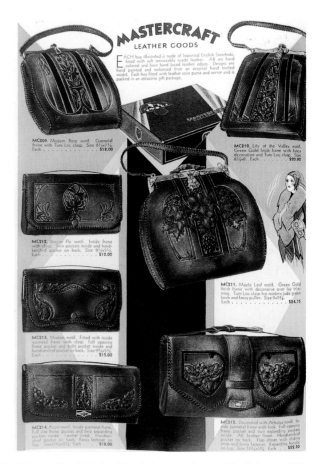

E.L. Rice & Co. (1931) offered these embossed English-steerhide art-craft bags with embossed hand-painted Art-Nouveau-style motifs (rose, lily of the valley, dragon fly, maple leaf, and acorn), hand-laced edges, gunmetal and gold-plated frames with medium and short top-strap handles.

threaded through both holes and folded...and so on. They were usually made of calfskin in the envelope and zipper-top *pochette* styles, plus an unusual round rosette model. Common colors were black, navy, white, brown, red, and tan. Belts were also made with this leather-link technique and were frequently sold in sets with a matching purse. (Examples of leather-link belts appear in Accessories and Related Items, Chapter 12.)

**Plain and Sculptured Suede Handbags**. Many attractive handbags were made of antelope suede which was especially soft to the touch. During the late 1930s, the trapunto technique was used to create raised or sculptured designs on suede handbags. Inexpensive imitations of this sculptured effect were created by embossing designs in simulated leather. (Further information and examples of trapunto appear in Chapters 2, 4, and 7).

## Fabric

**Tapestry Bags**. Handbags made of tapestry were produced in the zipper-top *pochette* and top-strap styles which contained metal or simulated tortoise-shell frames. Tapestry bags were also available with the unusual "double-hinged" metal frame, which contained two pairs of hinges. When opened, this frame expanded to form a wide, square opening.

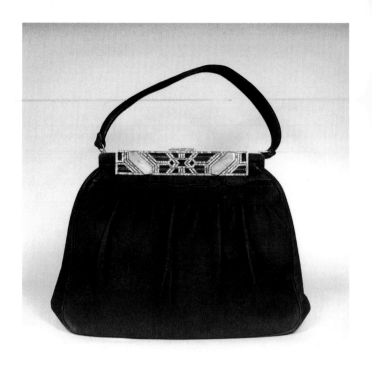

Black suede top-strap bag, frame decorated with lavender glass and marcasite. *Courtesy of Roxanne Stuart.* $65-$95.

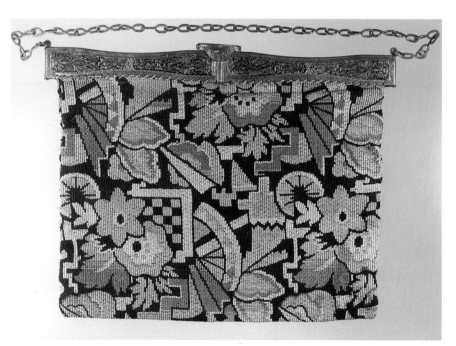

Multicolored tapestry bag with Art Deco-style floral pattern, dye-stamped double-hinged frame, c. late '20s-'30s. *Courtesy of Betsey Pacini.* $125-$150.

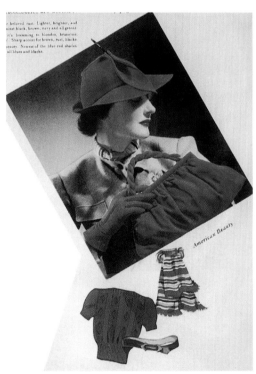

Sears, Roebuck and Co. catalog photo (1939-40) offering a felt hat, pouch-style wool purse, and gloves in the color "American-beauty," (Sear's answer to Schiaparelli's shocking pink).

116

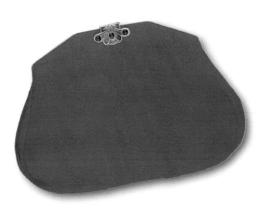

Red crepe *pochette* with gold-plated frame and clasp set with three red-glass cabochons. *Courtesy of Gerry Meza.* $40-$60.

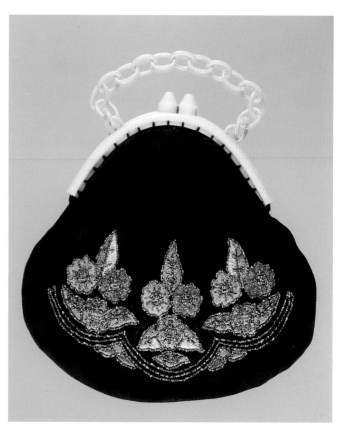

Black faille bag with celluloid frame and handle, decorated with pastel embroidered flowers outlined in cut-steel beads. *Courtesy of Michele V. Weaber.* $80-$100.

**Cloth Bags**. In 1937, Sears, Roebuck and Co. offered a summer envelope-style *pochette* with a linen cover which could be removed for cleaning. It was available in white, maize, pink, wine, or navy blue and was decorated with embroidery. For an extra fifty cents the bag could be embroidered with the owners initials. Handbags were also made of crêpe, wool, and various other types of fabric.

**Needlework Bags**. Handcraft magazines carried instructions and advertisements for do-it-yourself kits to create colorful handbags using embroidery, crewel, needlepoint, and appliqué. Machine embroidered bags were also available.

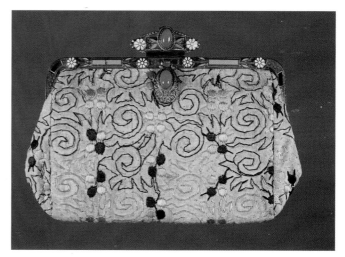

Machine embroidered *pochette* with fancy enameled frame containing two green glass cabochons, vertical back strap. *Courtesy of Sue Steiner.* $120-$150.

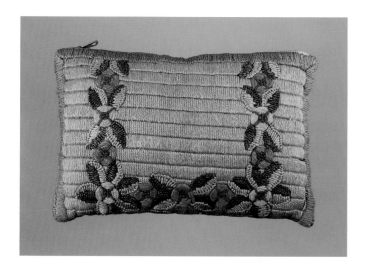

Needlepoint *pochette* in typical Art-Deco stylized floral motif, zipper closing. *Courtesy of Gerry Meza.* $50-$60.

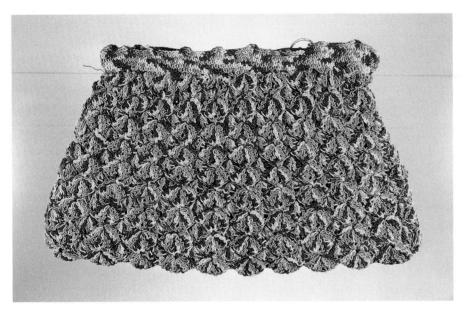

*Pochette* of varigated crocheted-cord in the four popular 1930s colors: rust, gold, green, and blue. $25-$35. *Courtesy of Rose Jamieson.*

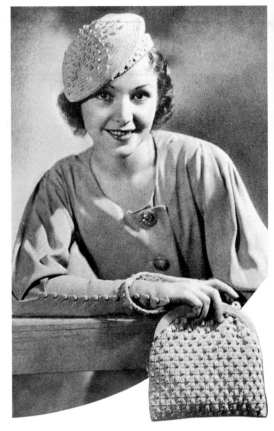

The Bucilla crochet manual (1934) offered this hand-crocheted beret and matching handbag in the popcorn stitch. Note: closely-spaced buttons on sleeve. *Courtesy of Elaine Cruse.*

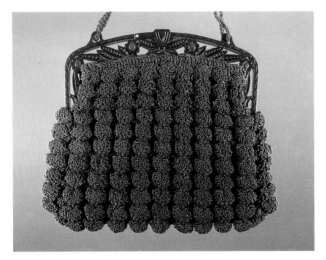

Blue crocheted-cord bag in popcorn stitch, molded plastic open-work frame with articulated clasp. $30-$40.

***Crocheted Bags*.** Handbags crocheted of yarn or cord were popular items during the depression and war years. The bodies of these bags were often crocheted in the popular "shell" or "popcorn" stitches characterized by even rows of raised bumps. They were attached to an openwork plastic frame which often included a handle in its design. The handy housewife could create her own bag and a matching hat by using the patterns provided in handcraft magazines or kits sold in craft shops.

During the second half of the decade, wide-flat-rectangular or fan-shaped crocheted bags were popular and were produced primarily in black. These broad bags remained stylish into the 1940s and reached a whopping 15 to 19 inches in width. Crocheted bags were usually lined with heavy rayon taffeta and in the late 1930s-40s featured clear Prystal bangle-bracelet handles and zipper pulls. The word Prystal is a combination of the words plastic and crystal. It was a product of the Catalin Corporation, makers of Catalin, a phenolic resin

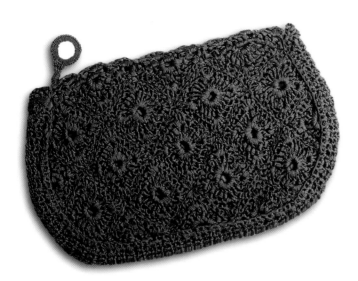

Large crocheted *pochette* made of brown flat braid in an interesting pattern. $40-$50.

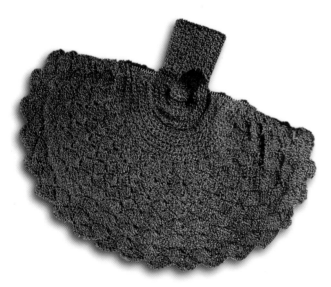

*Art Needlework* (1936-37) illustration of a large fan-shaped crocheted-cord bag with strap handle and zipper closure.

similar to Bakelite.

## Beads

*Glass-Beaded Bags*. Small afternoon or evening bags decorated with glass beads were commonly imported from Belgium and Czechoslovakia. Clear seed beads, simulated seed pearls, and clear bugle beads were used to create patterns, usually geometric in design. (Many of these clear beads were lined with silver to enhance their sparkle. Over the years the silver has tarnished, thereby giving these beads a dark gray appearance.) The cloth handle was also decorated with beads, and the zipper usually contained a short ball-chain pull. They were lined with ivory faille and contained a pocket for a small mirror. A cloth label marked "Made in Czechoslovakia" or "Made in Belgium" was usually stitched to the pocket.

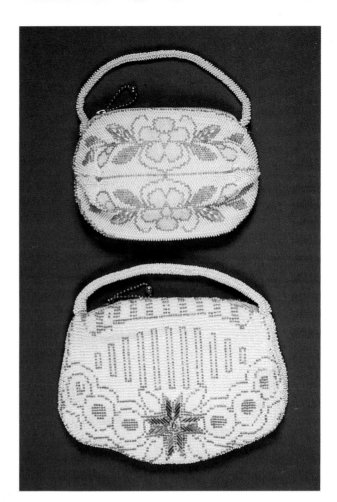

Evening bags decorated in floral and geometric designs with white, *faux* pearl, and (once-clear) seed and bugle beads. Label: Made in Czechoslovakia. $20-$25.

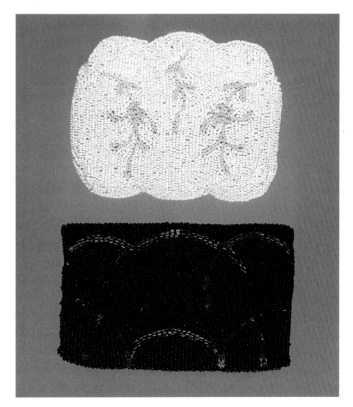

Glass-bead evening *pochettes* with vertical back straps and snap closings, c.1932. Labels: Hand Made in Belgium. *Courtesy of Margaretha J. Laubner.* $15-$20.

119

Romantic French "*beauvais*" bags were machine embroidered with delicate pastel flowers using the tambour (chain) stitch. The background was then filled in with white, pearl, or black seed beads. *Beauvais* bags were usually labeled "Made in France."

***Wooden-Beaded Bags***. Hand-made bags covered with larger multicolored wooden beads were also imported from Czechoslovakia, beginning in the early 1930s. They were advertised as "Summer's favorite bags that go with any costume." These bags were produced in a variety of styles, including the *pochette* and top-strap models. Some were made with celluloid or metal frames. The spherical, elongated, and cube-shaped beads were produced in "gay colors" such as red, yellow, brown, dark blue/gray, black, and white. The varied shapes and colors formed many different patterns including Mexican peasant stripes, zigzags, chevrons, concentric circles, and six-pointed stars. Wooden-beaded bags were also available in multicolored pastels as well as solid colors including black, natural, brown, red, or white. Smaller *pochettes* were designed for afternoon or evening. The rayon lining usually contained a pocket for a small mirror.

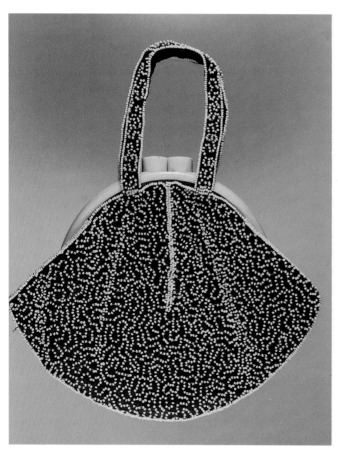

Brown cloth bag covered with white seed beads in the vermicelli (pasta like spaghetti) pattern, celluloid frame. *Courtesy of Rose Jamieson.* $40-$60.

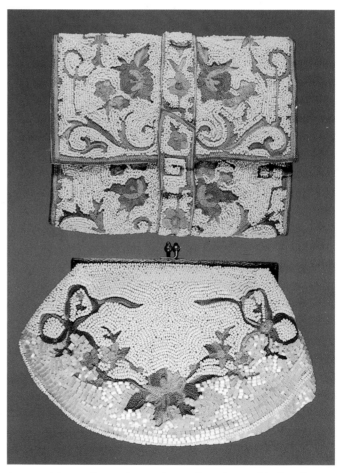

Imported *beauvais* evening *pochettes* featuring multicolored tambour-embroidered flowers with a background of white seed beads, back-strap handles. *Top:* Envelope-style with snap closing. *Bottom:* Gold-plated frame and additional frosted bugle beads. Both marked: Made in France. $45-$60.

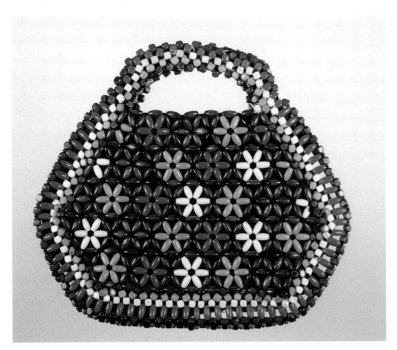

Six-sided bag covered with colorful wooden beads in stripe and star motif. *Courtesy of Rose Jamieson.* $40-$50.

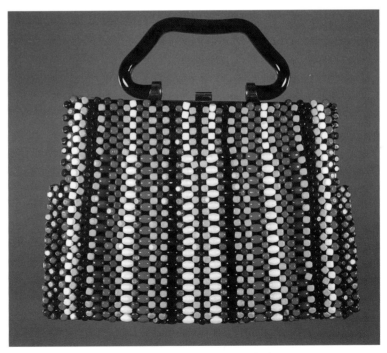

Handbag with gold tone frame, black Bakelite handle, vertical rows of colored wooden beads. Marked: Jemco, USA PAT, 1,915,313 (1933). $40-$50.

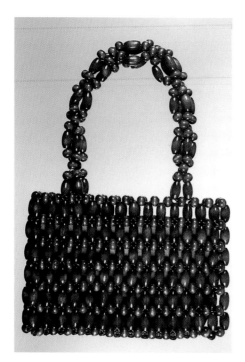

Brown handbag made from round and oval wooden beads, zipper closing. *Courtesy of Rose Jamieson.* $30-$40.

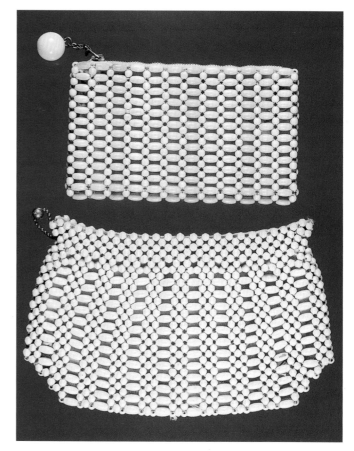

White and pastel wooden-bead *pochettes* for summer wear, zipper closings and vertical back strap. $25-$35.

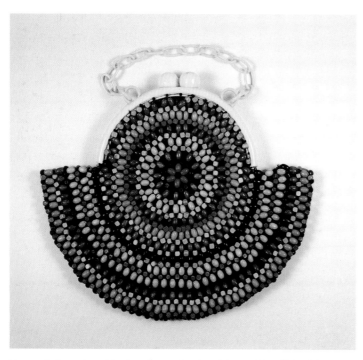

Unusual-shaped multicolored wooden-bead bag with celluloid frame and chain handle. *Courtesy of Gerry Meza.* $50-$60.

## Fur

Numerous period movies released during the 1930s triggered an interest in Victorian fashion, accessories, and jewelry. A good example of this trend was the revival of the Victorian muff. The muff was originally used as protection for the hands against the cold. Muffs of the late '30s contained a handy zippered compartment for small necessities. Muffs were frequently designed to match a coat, cape, hat, or fur collar. They were made of velvet, wool, astrakhan, and a variety of furs and were usually stuffed with kapok.

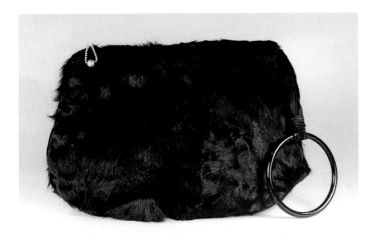

Black *swakara*-lamb muff with zippered compartment, black Bakelite bracelet handle attached with satin strap. *Courtesy of Michele V. Weaber.* $50-$75.

## Mesh

Both ring and armor-mesh bags were immensely popular during the 1920s and continued to appear in fashion magazines and wholesale jewelry catalogs of the early 1930s. They were advertised in Sears, Roebuck and Co. catalogs as: "a proper accessory for smart afternoon and evening wear." The five main types of mesh used in the production of handbags during the 1930s were "ring," "armor," "beadlite," "tile," and *"baguette"* mesh. Frames for mesh bags were usually die-stamped and then plated with gold, silver, or chrome. Many ornate Mandalian frames were enameled in colors to match their mesh bodies or were set with colored stones.

***Ring-Mesh Bags***. Thousands of tiny interlocking rings, resembling the chain mail worn by medieval knights, were used in the production of ring mesh bags. They were originally assembled by hand. However, in 1909, A.C. Pratt invented a mesh-making machine which led to the mass production of these bags in a fraction of the time and at more affordable prices.

A man by the name of Dresden subsequently invented a machine which could manufacture minute rings used in the production of "fine" or "baby fine" mesh bags. As many as 100,000 of these fine rings were needed to produce one fine-mesh bag. Since these rings were so delicate, many bag manufacturers offered soldered fine ring-mesh bags at an additional charge. As incredible as it may seem, each tiny ring was individually soldered to provide a stronger, more durable bag.

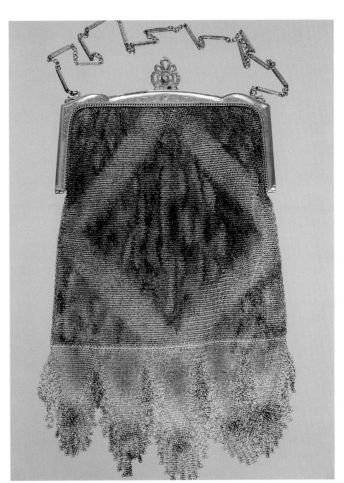

Enameled Dresden ring-mesh bag, gold-plated frame and *baton*-link chain, elaborate chain fringe, silk lining and mirror, c.1930-31. Marked: Whiting & Davis. *Courtesy of Arlene Rabin Antiques.* $150-$225.

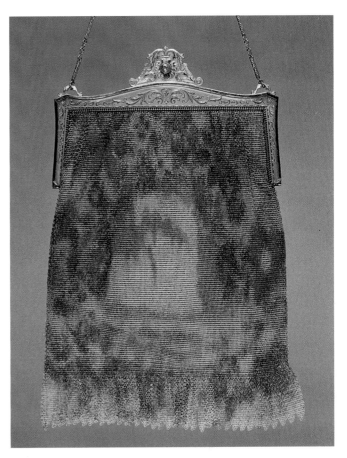

Beautiful Dresden ring-mesh bag with ornate gold-plated frame and *baton*-link chain, silk lining, mirror. Marked: Whiting & Davis, early '30s. *Courtesy of Arlene Rabin Antiques.* $250-$275.

"Dresden" mesh bags (named after the inventor of the fine-mesh-making machine) were created by stenciling colored enamels onto the fine ring mesh. This procedure resulted in designs with a soft, blurred appearance, similar to *chiné* fabric.

**Armor-Mesh Bags.** Tiny metal links resembling multiplication signs (when used on the straight) or plus signs (when used on the bias) were used in the creation of armor mesh bags. The four points of each link were bent, then hooked into adjacent rings on the reverse side of the bag. Armor mesh was available in sizes ranging from baby-fine to medium.

Armor-mesh bags were stenciled with colored enamels in stylized floral designs and geometric patterns typical of the Art Deco period.

The "Gloria" armor-mesh bag by Mandalian featured the new patented "self opening" frame. A flick of the tab clasp and the spring-loaded, segmented frame popped open like a frog's mouth. These frames were used in conjunction with baby-fine armor mesh. During the late 1920s and early '30s, the Mandalian company offered bags enameled with a new "Lustro-Pearl" finish.

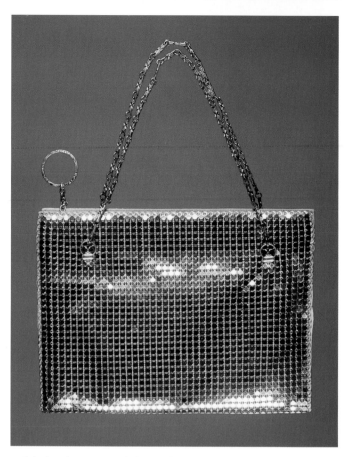

Gold-plated armor mesh bag with delicate chain handles and pull chain with finger ring. Marked: Whiting & Davis. $25-$30.

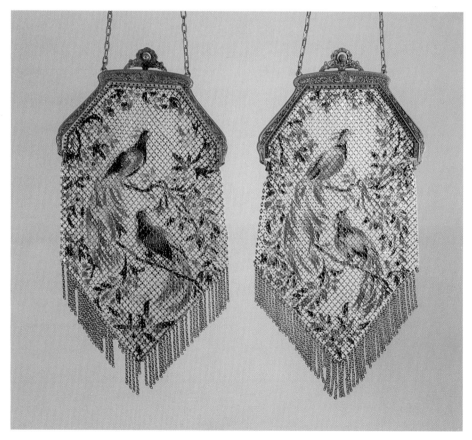

Two fine armor-mesh bags, produced with identical bird motifs but in different color schemes, 1930-31. Marked: Mandalian Mfg. Co. *Courtesy of Arlene Rabin Antiques.* $200-$275 ea.

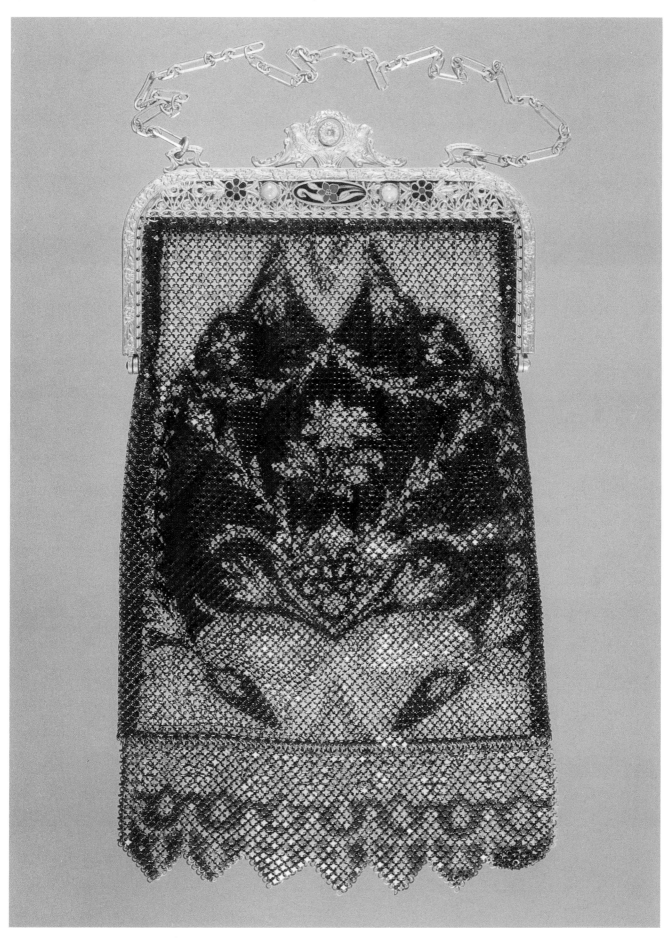

Ornate gold-plated filigree frame decorated with enamel and turquoise glass cabochons, medium-fine enameled armor mesh, late '20s-early '30s. Marked: Mandalian Mfg. Co. U.S.A. *Courtesy of Arlene Rabin Antiques.* $250-$300.

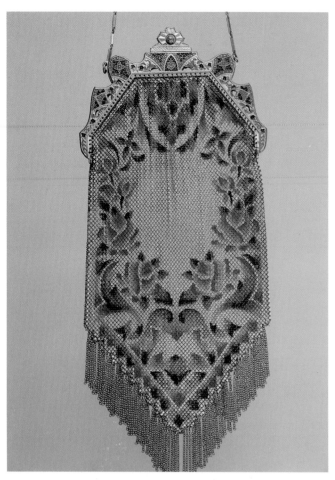

Armor-mesh bag with enameled frame, stylized rose motif stenciled in Lustro-Pearl enamel finish on baby-fine mesh links, chain fringe, 1931. Marked: Mandalian Mfg. Co. *Courtesy of Arlene Rabin Antiques.* $250-$350.

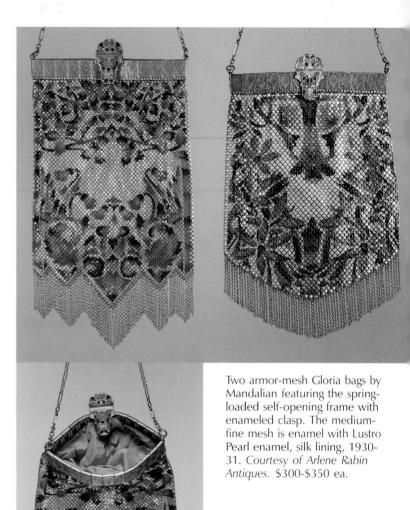

Two armor-mesh Gloria bags by Mandalian featuring the spring-loaded self-opening frame with enameled clasp. The medium-fine mesh is enamel with Lustro Pearl enamel, silk lining, 1930-31. *Courtesy of Arlene Rabin Antiques.* $300-$350 ea.

**Beadlite-Mesh Bags**. A variation of armor mesh, known as beadlite mesh, was introduced in the late 1920s. Each small link contained a raised dome-shaped center which, from a distance, resembled a small bead. These bags were enameled in patterns or solid colors. One very common summer-style bag featured an off-white beadlite-mesh pouch attached to an off-white celluloid frame with a celluloid chain handle.

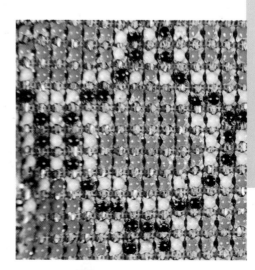

Small beadlite-mesh bag in enameled fish-scale pattern with silver-plated frame. Marked: Whiting & Davis. / Close-up of beadlite links, late '20s-early '30s. *Courtesy of Arlene Rabin Antiques.* $100-$125.

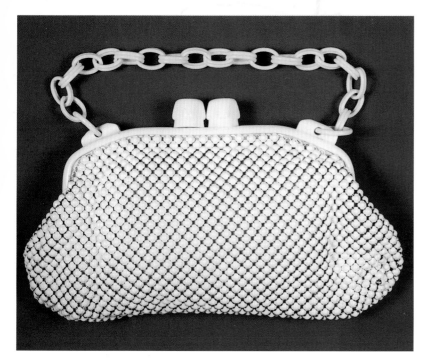

The popular beadlite-mesh summer bag with creamy white enameled links, celluloid frame and chain handle. *Courtesy of Betsey Pacini.* $40-$50.

**Tile-Mesh Bags**. Another variation of armor mesh, known as tile mesh, was composed of square links which were larger and flatter then those of the past. They were made with a metal frame and chain handle or with a new arch-shaped rigid-metal handle which was plated with nickel silver. Zipper-top and envelope-style *pochettes* were also available and often contained a back strap. Tile-mesh bags were generally stenciled with Art-Deco-style geometric or stylized floral motifs; however, they were also produced in solid colors.

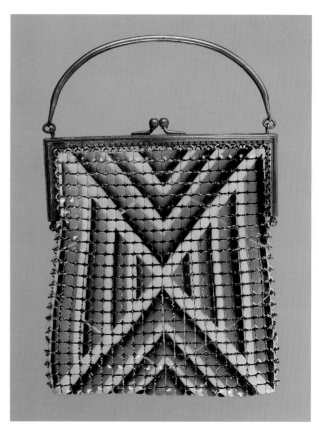

Tile-mesh bag containing large square tile links enameled in a mono-chromatic Art Deco design, arched rigid-metal handle and frame plated with nickel silver, 1933-35. *Courtesy of Arlene Rabin Antiques.* $75-$100.

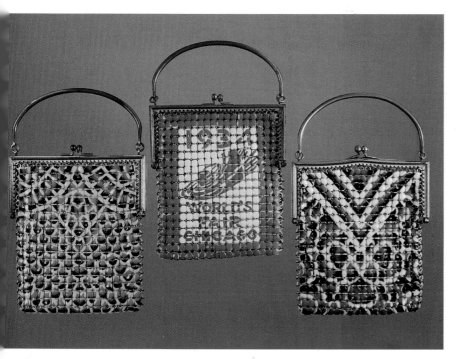

Above: Three tile-mesh bags with large square tile links, enameled in geometric patterns and 1933-34 Chicago World's Fair motif, rigid-metal handles and frames plated with nickel silver, 1933-35. *Courtesy of Arlene Rabin Antiques.* Left and right - $75-$100. Center - $200-$250.

Right: Tile-mesh bag enameled in rose design, rigid-metal handle and frame plated with nickel silver, 1933-35. *Courtesy of Arlene Rabin Antiques.* $75-$100.

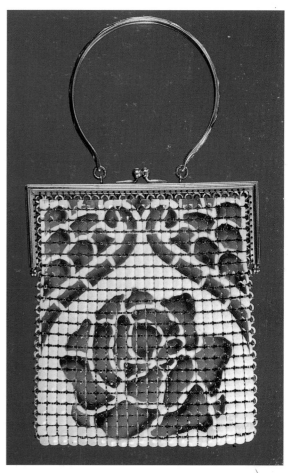

**Baguette-Mesh Bags.** Square links, used in the production of *baguette*-mesh bags, contained two raised *baguette*-shaped bars resembling equal signs. This style of mesh was used on the straight or the bias and was silver-plated or enameled. *Baguette* mesh was used for zipper-top *pochettes* and top-handle framed bags.

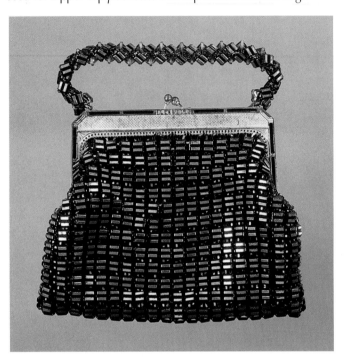

Body and handle of this *baguette*-mesh bag made of unusual square links each containing two *baguette*-shaped silver-plated bars, c. 1935. Marked: Whiting & Davis. *Courtesy of Arlene Rabin Antiques.* $75-$100.

# MAJOR MESH BAG MANUFACTURERS

The **Whiting & Davis Company** which originated in Plainville, Massachusetts, has been a leading manufacturer of mesh bags from 1892 to the present. This company is known for its ring, Dresden, and armor-mesh bags which often featured a zigzag hem end.

Whiting & Davis bags were stamped with the company logo on the inside of the frame or they contained a tiny metal logo tag attached to the inside of the bag. Paper logo tags were also used, although they were often discarded, leaving some Whiting & Davis bags unmarked.

The **Mandalian Manufacturing Company** was founded by Turkish emigrant Sahatiel Mandalian circa 1898. This company is best known for its armor-mesh bags which were enameled in wonderful rich color combinations. The most common motifs were stylized flowers, birds, and patterns resembling Oriental rugs (a reflection of Mandalian's Turkish ancestry). Many of these high-quality bags contained ornate filigree or openwork frames which were often enameled or encrusted with glass or semi-precious stones.

The hem ends of 1930s Mandalian bags were usually zig-zag, step, or V-shaped. The hems were then decorated with fine chain fringe or enameled teardrop-shaped weights. These bags were stamped Mandalian Mfg.Co. on the inside of the frame. The Mandalian Company was acquired by Whiting & Davis in 1944.

## Novelty Bags

**Watch Bags.** Circa 1936, there was a brief fad for watch bags produced by the Graceline and Westclox manufacturing companies. A small round or square watch was recessed into the front of various handbag styles. Some models by Westclox contained watches which could be removed from the bags and displayed on any smooth surface using the stand mechanism incorporated in the design.

**Schiaparelli.** Jean Clément, the creative French accessories designer, was commissioned by Schiaparelli to create original plastic handbags to coordinate with her theme collections. Particularly memorable were the handbags designed for her music collection. One music-box handbag played a tune when it was opened. Another bag resembled an accordion, while a third had a frame resembling piano keys.

# COSMETICS

The relatively new practice of applying makeup was established by flappers during the preceding decade. Cosmetics became an important tool in the beautification process, designed to attract the few eligible bachelors remaining after the First World War. Following the lead of 1930s Hollywood stars like Jean Harlow, women applied powder for a smooth, flawless complexion and rouge for a rosy glow. Red lipstick was used to define the lips and mascara to darken and thicken the eyelashes. Women plucked the lower hairs from their eyebrows, producing a high, narrow arch. This fine line was then emphasized with eyebrow pencil. Some women removed their eyebrows entirely, then relocated them with pencil.

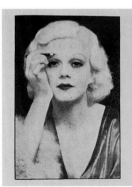 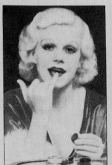 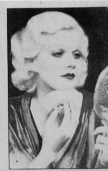

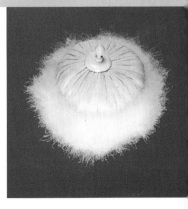

Photos published in *Photoplay* (5/33) reveal beauty secrets, demonstrated by sex symbol, Jean Harlow. *(1)* Her natural eyebrows are plucked away and thin arched brows penciled in. *(2)* "True red" lip rouge applied with the finger. *(3)* "Skin-tone" powder applied with down puff. *Insert:* puff of down, silk, and celluloid.

Stylish vanity bags, vanity cases, carryalls, and compacts were in great demand to carry these indispensable beauty aids. There were numerous designs suitable for every taste and every pocketbook. Exquisite examples were created from precious metals, glittering gems, and enamel by world renowned jewelry houses like Cartier, Van Cleef and Arpel, Fabergé, and Boucheron.

Manufacturers like Evans, Volupté, Elgin American, M. J. Fisher, Marathon, McRae Keeler, Bourjois, and Henriette mass-produced "smart" imitations of these cosmetic accessories for the more modest budget. In addition, cosmetic firms such as Coty, Max Factor, Houbigant, Elizabeth Arden, Helena Rubinstein, Yardley, and Richard Hudnut packaged their cosmetics in attractive, refillable compacts and vanity cases, also at affordable prices. These cosmetic accessories were sold in drug stores, department stores, jewelry stores, and mail-order catalogs.

# VANITY BAGS

Dainty mesh vanity bags of the '20s and '30s were used for afternoon or evening affairs. Vanity bags featured a compact as an integral part of the lid or frame. They usually had two openings, one into the compact portion which contained powder, a mirror and often times rouge. The second opening led into the body of the bag which, because of its small size, could only hold a few of the following items: a small comb, a hankie, perfume, coins, or "bob" pins.

# VANITY CASES

The vanity case was a receptacle designed to hold powder, rouge, puffs, and a mirror. They were either made of sterling or plated with gold, silver, or chrome. Vanity cases were available in a variety of shapes including (but not limited to) the circle, square, rectangle, pentagon, hexagon, barrel, shield, and modifications of these forms.

Many vanity cases contained some form of carry chain and by the 1930s there were numerous variations to choose from. Enameled "baton-link" chains were frequently used as well as fancy twisted chains. The ends of the chain were connected at two different locations on the case or both ends were fastened to a loop at the clasp, forming a wrist chain. The popular "tango chain" was fastened to the case on one end and to a finger ring on the other. When a matching lipstick was introduced, it was often connected to the case by a tango chain. Another style featured a lipstick which was fastened to the compact by a chain in an inverted-V formation. The decoration of vanity cases fell into two dissimilar categories: romantic and Art Deco.

***Romantic-Style Vanity Cases***. Vanity cases in the romantic-style were decorated with pastel *guilloché* enameling. Machine engravings called "engine-turnings" were incised into metal objects such as compacts, vanity bags, vanity cases, cigarette cases, and lighters. Typical patterns were sunrays, basket weaves, concentric circles, kaleidoscopes, and rows of dots, circles, squares, diamonds, waves, and stripes. Engine-turnings were

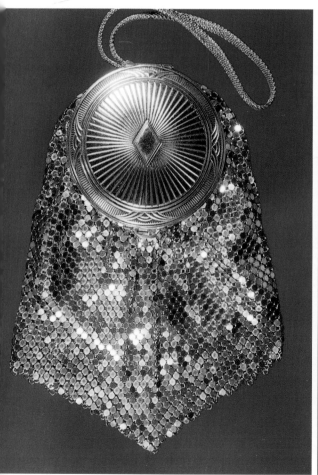
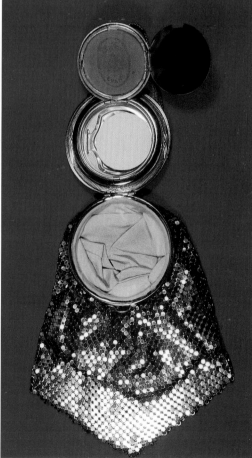

Armor mesh vanity bag. *Exterior* - lid contains raised Art Deco sunburst with diamond center. *Interior* - lid contains powder and rouge compartments plus a polished steel mirror. Marked: May Fair by Evans (in rouge.) $100-$150.

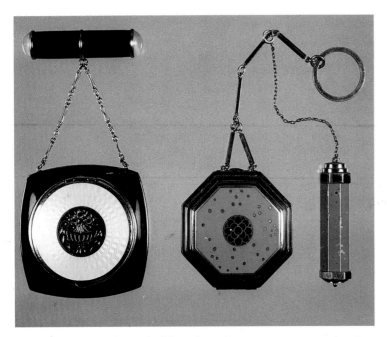

Vanity cases with attached lipsticks. *Left:* Exterior - romantic, hand-engraved flowers in urn surrounded by black *champlevé* enameling, encircled by white *guilloché* enameling. Interior - powder, rouge. Marked: May Fair by Evans, PAT 1624784 (1927), 1869983 (1932). *Courtesy of Eleanore Miller. Right:* Exterior - gold plate, green and black cloisonné enameling, *baton*-link tango chain, attached lipstick. Interior - powder, rouge. Marked: le Début Richard Hudnut. c. 1928-29. *Courtesy of Gerry Meza.* $125-$150 each.

applied over the entire object or used as decorative borders. These engravings were then covered with translucent enamel which permitted the engraved grooves to show through. Delicate pink roses, blue forget-me-nots, or baskets of these flowers decorated with blue ribbon bows were the dainty feminine designs most often hand painted over the *guilloché*. Finally, an application of clear enamel was added for a protective coating.

Another decorating technique called *champlevé* enameling was employed in the decoration of metal objects. Areas on the surface of the object were etched or routed out, then filled in with enamel.

The Marathon Company offered numerous romantic vanity cases with dainty silhouettes of 18th-century men and women, a motif frequently used during the 1920s.

***Art Deco-Style Vanity Cases.*** In sharp contrast, Art Deco-style vanity cases were decorated in modernistic, eye-catching designs. These designs featured step patterns, sunrays, star bursts, lightning bolts, bubbles, concentric circles, pie wedges, chevrons, and grids which were used alone or in combination to provide a bold, dramatic effect. Stylized exotic birds were another popular motif. These cases were often enameled in dynamic Art Deco color schemes such as black and red, black and white, or black with Nile green. Cases were occasionally decorated with genuine marcasites or with a "marcasite effect" (small bumps embossed in the metal). Many cases featured a rectangular *cartouche* suitable for engraving one's initials.

Art Deco chrome-plated vanity cases. *Left:* Exterior - Red and maroon enamel, "marcasite effect" bumps. Lipstick attached with tango chain. Interior - tap-sift powder and rouge. *Right:* Exterior - Engine turnings, *champlevé* enameling. Interior - powder sifter, rouge. Marked: EAM (Elgin American Manufacturing Co.) $125-$150.

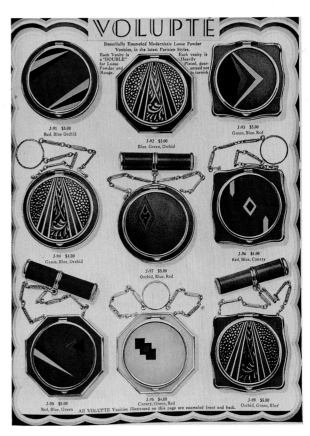

Volupté advertisement for vanity cases enameled in Art Deco-style modernistic designs. Each contains loose powder and rouge cake, 1931.

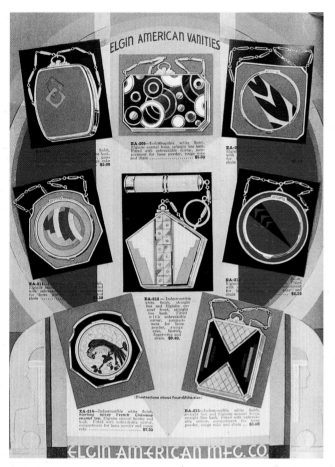

Elgin American Art Deco vanity cases. Each case contains loose powder and rouge cake, 1931.

ELGIN AMERICAN VANITIES

*Pouch-style Vanity Cases*. Pouch-style vanity cases were also patterned after the turn-of-the-20th-century tam-o-shanter coin purse. During the 1930s, the pouch portion was made of gold or silver-plated armor mesh or leather. The lids were often decorated with *guilloché* enameling or petit point. These vanities contained two openings. One exposed the interior of the lid which contained powder, rouge, and a mirror. The other revealed the inside of the tiny mesh pouch which was generally lined with fabric.

*Souvenir Vanity Cases*. Some of the most popular souvenir compacts from the 1930s are those commemorating the two World's Fairs. Mementos of the 1933-34 Chicago World's Fair featured either fair pavilions or the whirling star Arcturus with the motto "A Century of Progress." The Trylon and Perisphere logo appears on compacts and vanity cases from the New York World's Fair in 1939. These items are "cross-over" collectibles, meaning they are sought after by compact collectors and World's Fair enthusiasts alike.

*Commemorative Vanity Cases.* Yardley designed a motif to commemorate the coronation of King George VI (May 12, 1937). The company's gold-plated vanity cases featured raised and recessed plumes (the symbol of the Prince of Wales), embellished with red, white, and blue enameling (English patriotic colors). This motif was used into the 1940s.

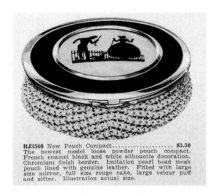

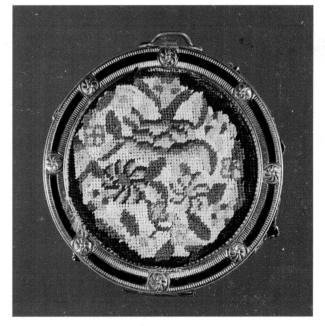

Two tam-o-shanter style compacts. *Side view:* L. & C. Mayers Co. (1933) chrome with black and white enameled silhouette, beadlite-mesh pouch. $75-$100. *Top view:* Petit-point lid, gold-plated mesh pouch. Marked: Richard Hudnut. *Courtesy of Sue Steiner.*

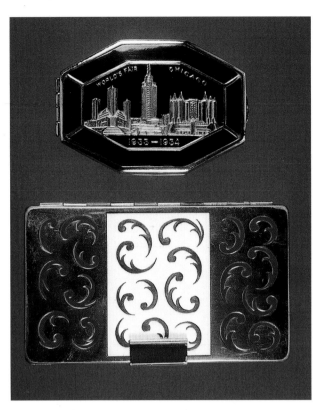

**Novelty Vanity Cases.** The Surrealist movement influenced many phases of the decorative arts and was often characterized by objects which were not as they seemed or as you would expect them to be. Schiaparelli collaborated with Surrealist painters to design objects resembling totally unrelated items. A good example of this was her telephone vanity case, inspired by Salvador Dali. It was made of chrome-plated metal and black enamel and opened when a number was dialed.

The Fillkwik Co. produced an unusual vanity case which resembled a camera. It not only contained compartments for powder, rouge, and lipstick, but perfume as well. Other clever vanity cases resembled a piece of luggage decorated with travel stickers, an envelope with a canceled stamp, or a parcel with *faux* twine, address label, and stamp.

# COMPACTS

The compact was a small receptacle containing loose or pressed powder, a powder puff, and a small mirror. Loose powder compacts usually contained revolving sifters which regulated the flow of powder from the well beneath. Pressed powder compacts contained replaceable pressed-powder refills. Like the colorful enameled vanity cases described above, compacts were available in both romantic floral and modernistic Art Deco motifs. Compacts and lipsticks were frequently produced in matching sets.

**Petit Point Compacts.** Another popular form of decoration appearing on 1930s compacts was petit point. These beautifully executed floral designs contained as many as 1850 stitches to the square inch.

Souvenir and commemorative vanity cases containing powder, rouge, and mirror. *Top:* Embossed chrome-plated fair pavilions and the words "Chicago World's Fair, 1933-1934," black *champlevé* enameling. *Bottom:* Gold-plated case commemorating coronation of George VI. Raised and recessed plumes in red, white, and blue enamel. c. 5/12/37. Marked: Yardley. $125-$150.

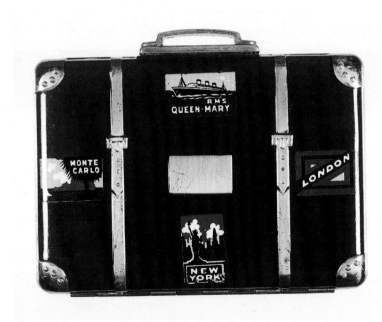

Vanity case resembling suitcase, green enamel with colorful travel stickers, gold-plated straps, corners, and central *cartouche* for monogram. Contains powder, rouge, and mirror. Marked: PAT 1,883,793 (1932). $125-$150.

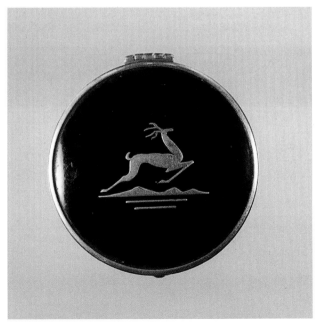

Small chrome-plated compact, embossed Art Deco leaping stag surrounded by black enamel. Contains mirror and powder compartment with concave door for puff. Marked: House of Tre-Jur Inc. $60-$75.

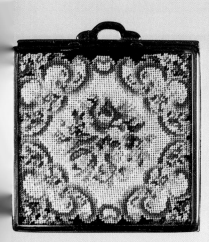
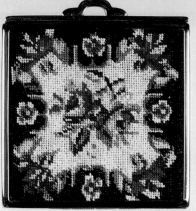

Two gold-plated compacts with intricate petit-point designs. Contain loose powder well, puff, and mirror. Sticker reads: 1850 stitches to the square inch. Both marked: PAT 1,802,796 (1931) Made in USA. $40-$60.

**Whoopee Compacts.** The McRae & Keeler Company introduced the hexagonal-shaped "Whoopee" compact. This style featured an articulated metal handle through which the three middle fingers could be placed. The handle also served as a stand to hold the compact's mirror at the proper viewing angle on a table. This style was produced in the late '20s and early '30s.

# MINAUDIÈRE

A fashionable American woman arrived at Van Cleef and Arpels in Paris, circa 1930. In her hand she carried an ordinary cigarette tin in which she had placed her lipstick, compact, cigarettes, lighter, and keys. Charles Arpels noted her makeshift carrying case and recognized its possibilities. He set to work designing an elegant jeweled box with multiple compartments in which a woman could carry numerous essential items. This box, patented the *Minaudière*, became the inspiration for the many carryalls that followed well into the 1950s.

# CARRYALLS

Many less-expensive imitations of the Minaudière, called carryalls, were mass-produced by such makers as Evans, Volupté, Elgin, Park Lane, and Mondaine. They were usually rectangular in shape and their compact interiors were fitted with compartments for some of the following items: powder, rouge, lipstick, mirror, comb, card or money clip (bills), coins, keys, stamps, cigarettes, lighter, and telescoping cigarette holder. Mother-of-pearl was a popular form of decoration used in checkerboard or other marquetry designs. Imitation mother-of-pearl, referred to in period catalogs as the "pearl effect," was manufactured from plastic for less expensive gold tone carryalls.

In 1938, Elgin American advertised a compact rectangular carryall decorated with pearl-effect plastic and rhinestones. Its compact interior contained a lipstick, powder and pill compartments, a money holder, a cigarette case, and a mirror. The wearer had the option of attaching the handy wrist chain handle or slipping the carryall into its black moiré carry case with the convenient moiré handle. (Carry cases were also made of faille, satin, suede, or brocade.) In addition, this carryall could be mounted on the top of a smart black-leather boxy evening bag with two articulated handles.

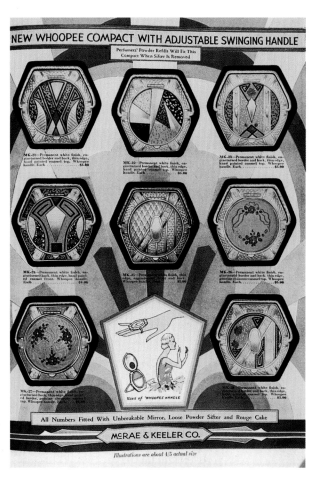

"Whoopee" vanity cases by McRae & Keeler which show the typical overlapping of Art Deco geometric and romantic floral designs. Each contain swing handle, loose powder, and rouge cake, 1931.

133

# Chapter 10

# Footwear

The average Victorian or Edwardian woman had little need for decorative shoes as they remained hidden beneath her long, street-sweeping skirts and layers of frothy white petticoats. Shoes finally emerged as a fashion accessory during World War I, when women engaged in war-related work were forced to wear shorter, more practical skirts. Shoe manufacturers soon realized the potential these newly visible accessories represented and supplied the modern flapper with a wide variety of decorative styles from which to choose.

Shoes of the late '20s and early '30s were extremely busy, as if shoe designers were making up for lost time. In the past, a single row of broguings (perforations) along the edge of the leather was considered sufficient. During the 1930s, however, too many broguings were never enough! Multitudes of tiny perforations were strategically arranged to form stripes, chevrons, sunrays, circles, scallops, arches, and swirling arabesques.

In addition, scores of cut-outs in the shape of circles—called "portholes," ovals, teardrops, crescents, triangles, squares (in lattice design), and rectangles (in ladder formation) were also punched out of the leather. In fact, it was not uncommon to combine cut-outs and perforations in the same shoe. Summer shoes were particularly susceptible to this form of decoration, as hole punching was taken to dizzying new heights, for the sake of ventilation. *Huaraches* and Lido sandals, made of woven strips of leather (often two-toned), provided yet another form of texture and pattern.

Textured materials also contributed to the over-all busyness of 1930s shoes. There was a noticeable trend in the late '20s and early '30s toward the use of reptilian skins such as lizard, alligator, crocodile, and snakeskin. For the modest budget, simulated reptile (leather embossed with a reptile texture) was offered. Leather was also available in other embossed patterns, called "Art Grains." These included basket weaves (called *basquette*), tree bark, swirls, ripples, waves, and pebbles. "Suede prints" featuring shiny dots, fishscales, grids, or waves on a matte suede background were also popular. Dressy shoes were made of such patterned fabrics as satin brocade, moiré, embroidered velvet, and paisley prints.

Shoe manufacturers often combined two or three contrasting materials in the same shoe. The quarter, instep, and toe might be made in a color or texture which contrasted with the rest of the shoe. Geometric Art-Deco overlays (appliqués) were applied as a trim, while contrasting underlays were visible through decorative cutouts. Typical combinations were kid on reptile, alligator on patent, kid on suede, or patent on suede.

The terms used for various parts of a shoe include:
quarter - covering the back of the heel
heel - under the heel of the foot
shank - under the arch
vamp - over the toe cleavage
instep - over the sloped part of the foot
toe - over the big toe

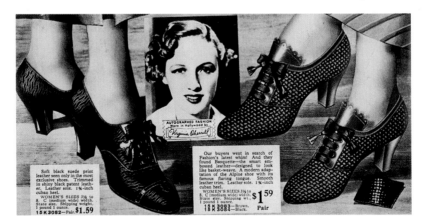

Sears, Roebuck and Co. ad (1935-36) for oxford shoe styles with tasseled laces. *Left:* Black "suede print" oxford with wave pattern rendered in black suede and patent leather. *Right:* Brown "art grain" embossed-leather oxford in the *basquette* (basket-weave) pattern, wide pinked tongue.

The following is a list of the common 1930s heel styles and their heights ranging from the lowest to the highest. (The heel height is measured at the front or "breast" of the heel.)

Low heel (1 inch)
Wide walking heel (1 1/4 inches)
Thick military heel (1 1/2 inches)
Chunky Cuban heel (1 3/4 inches)
Slender "spike" or "skyscraper" heel (2-3 inches)

"Stacked" or "built-up" heels made of thin layers of polished leather were extremely popular during the 1930s. Crepe rubber soles and heels were introduced during World War I and were used for many of the active sportswear styles.

Shoes, in general, were evolving from the dainty feminine styles of the 1920s to the bulky masculine shoes of the 1940s. Long delicate tapered toes gave way to broad round "snub" or "box" toes, which gave the feet a short, stubby appearance. Ankle straps created a horizontal line, making the leg look shorter and thicker. Shoe straps became noticeably wider during the second half of the decade. This effected the instep-strap, the vertical portion of the T-strap, and the horizontal straps of the monk and the kiltie oxfords.

Styles of the first half of the decade were primarily carry-overs from the 1920s. After 1935 new features emerged including open-toes, platform soles, wedge heels, and draped vamps which carried over into the 1940s.

Standard colors for shoes during the 1930s were black, brown, navy, white, red, and tan. More sophisticated colors such as marine blue, purple, burgundy, forest green, rust, and American beauty were added during the second half of the decade. Burgundy and navy was a popular color combination. One fashion magazine suggested: "For those who must buy carefully, it is in perfect taste to wear brown or black with the new wines or greens." Matching handbags occasionally accompanied shoes in mail-order catalogs of the period.

# EVENING SHOES

Evening shoes of the 1930s were dainty, feminine, even sensual. They had either slender spike, baby spike, or low 1 1/4-inch heels.

The instep-strap shoe (bar shoe in the U.K.), a carry-over from the 1910s and 1920s, was fastened with a small buckle at either the side of the shoe or at the center of the strap. (A few token strap styles retained shoe buttons; however, these were considered *passé*.) Instep-trap shoes were made with Cuban or spike heels. They were often made with decorative cut-outs where the strap met the shoe.

The pump (court shoe in U.K.) and the one-eyelet tie shoe (carry-overs from the 1920s) were available in evening shoe styles as well. The graceful T-strap evening sandal, another popular carry-over, had delicate straps and provocative open sides. Some versions had triangular-shaped openings cut from the quarter where the straps were attached. The vamp often consisted of a series of slender side-to-side, crisscross, or radiating straps. During the late '30s, evening shoes featured a "draped" vamp made of pleated fabric, or gold or silver kid which was draped across the vamp. Another new style featured open sides with horizontal side straps connecting the vamp and the quarter. Evening shoes were usually made of satin, crepe, or silver or gold kid.

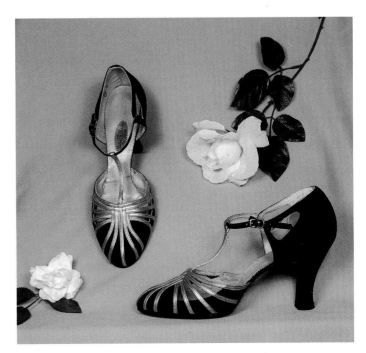

Black faille T-strap evening shoes, slender silver-kid straps, spike heels, c.1934. Label: Perfect Poise. *Courtesy of Mary Whitehouse.* $60-$75.

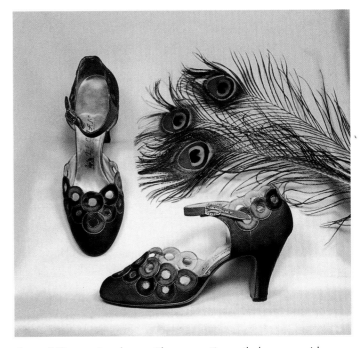

Green faille evening shoes with green satin portholes, open sides, ankle strap with small rhinestone buckle, and spike heels. Labels: Delman, New York, Chicago, London, and Paris. Bergdorf Goodman. $75-$100.

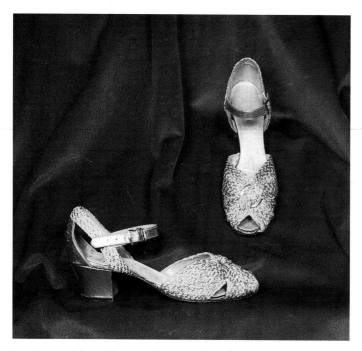

Evening sandals, gold and white draped braid passes through gold-metal rings, gold kid military heel, ankle straps attached to open quarter. Late '30s-early '40s. $50-$75.

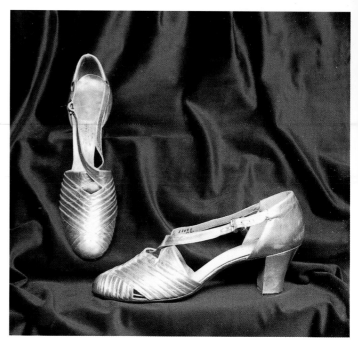

Silver-kid evening shoes with round toes, crisscross-draped vamp, open sides with horizontal straps, Cuban heels, late '30s. Label: Farr Ahead. *Courtesy of Cedar Crest Alumnae Museum, gift of Ellie Laubner.* $80-$110.

## Shoe Button/Buckle Covers

Decorative shoe button/buckle covers were created to convert a plain shoe to a dressy shoe. They were designed for instep-strap and T-strap shoes and were sold in pairs. To attach the cover to the shoe, the shoe strap was threaded through the bracket on the reverse side of the cover and the shoe button or buckle was fastened. The cover was then pushed over the button or buckle. Covers were made of brass, silver-plated base metal, or cut steel and decorated with enamel or rhinestones. Given the Art Deco-style designs on many of these covers and the continuing popularity of strap shoes, it seems fair to assume that shoe-button covers were worn into the early '30s.

Shoe ornaments which clipped over the edge of the vamp were another way of enhancing a plain pair of pumps. These could be made of cut steel or base metal set with rhinestones.

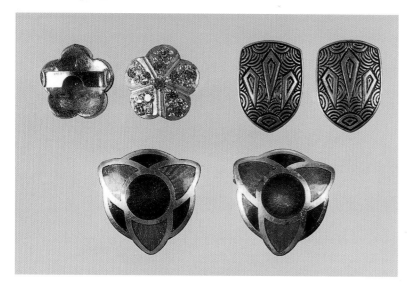

Shoe button/buckle covers. *Left:* Rhinestones set in base metal (reverse side reveals bracket). *Right:* Art Deco, brass with black *champlevé* enameling. *Bottom:* Gold-plate with brown and rust *guilloché* enameling, late '20s-early '30s. $25-$65.

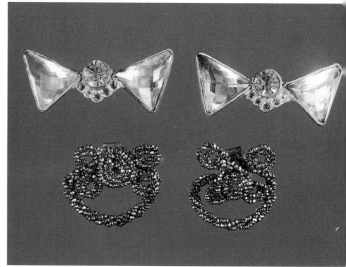

Rhinestone and cut-steel-bead shoe ornaments. *Courtesy of Suzanne M. Checksfield.* Top $45-$65. Bottom $25-$35.

# DAY SHOES

## Oxfords

An oxford is a shoe which laces over the instep. It was first worn by Oxford University students, circa 1640. It became a popular style for women in the late 1920s and '30s. As a rule, 1930s oxfords were fastened with soft, flat tasseled laces. Many oxford styles of the '30s featured a pointed tongue which protruded above the lacing. During the second half of the decade, the tongue took on a rounded "Alpine flare" and was often pinked, scalloped, or fringed along the edge.

Oxfords were made with a variety of heels ranging from the low to the spike heel. Elderly people tend to resist change, clinging to the old familiar styles of the past. As I was growing up in the 1950s, I noticed older women wearing laced oxford shoes with stout Cuban heels. At the time, we thought of them as "old lady" or "mamma" shoes. However, it is interesting to note that these same shoes were considered quite chic during the 1930s, when these women were young and style conscious. The following are variations of the oxford, which were popular during the 1930s.

***Kiltie-tongue Oxford***. The Scottish kiltie oxford, a carry-over from the 1920s, featured a long fold-over tongue with fringed ends, which flared out over the instep. Shoe laces were threaded through the eyelets of the shoe, then through two holes in the tongue, and tied in a bow on top of the tongue. Some kiltie oxfords had a strap which passed over the tongue and fasten with a buckle on the side of the shoe. Other models came with two different colored interchangeable tongues. They were generally made with a low, a military, or a Cuban heel and were often decorated with perforations. This classic shoe is still worn today by both men and women.

***Moccasin-Vamp Oxford***. A simulated moccasin was created when a U-shaped raised seam or tuck was top stitched around the edge of the vamp and the toe. The apron, or inner portion of the U, was often made of a color or texture to contrast with the rest of the shoe. It often featured a low rubber sole and heel. The moccasin-toe was revived in the 1970s for both men and women.

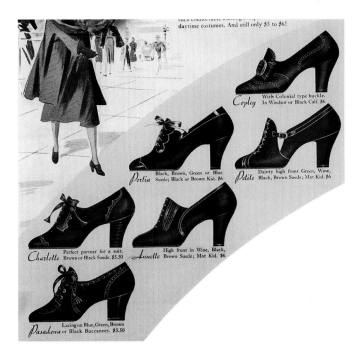

Enna Jetticks ad from *Woman's Home Companion* (10/37). Suede or calf daytime shoes in typical '30s colors. / Rust colonial pump. / Green monk shoe. / Black, brown, wine, and navy oxfords. Note: five spike heels and one Cuban heel.

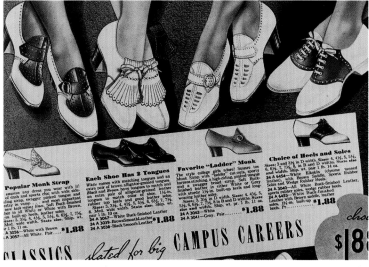

Montgomery Ward catalog illustrations (1937) featuring sport shoes with built up heels. *(1)* Monk shoe with side-buckling strap and moccasin-style vamp. *(2)* Kiltie oxfords with extra pair of interchangeable fringed tongues. *(3)* Square-toed monk oxford with pinked tongue and ladder cutouts. *(4)* Saddle oxfords of white buckskin and brown calf with choice of heel.

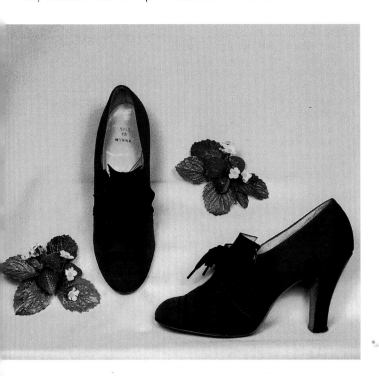

Maroon twill oxford with black patent leather tongue and spike heel, accented with double rows of black braid. Marked: Myrna PAT NO. 1,953,048 (1934). $95-$125.

**Saddle Oxford.** The classic two-toned "saddle" oxford was introduced in the 1920s and remained a popular sport shoe through the 1950s. This shoe was usually offered in white buckskin with a contrasting black or brown calf saddle and quarter. Other options were white buckskin with a reptile or smoke-colored calfskin saddle. The saddle shoe was decorated with perforations along the edges of the dark leather.

**Gillie-Tie Oxford** (also spelled *ghillie*). This Scottish dancing shoe was originally worn with a kilt. The Prince of Wales (later known as the Duke of Windsor) introduced it on his visit to the United States during the 1920s. For this reason it is also known as the "Prince of Wales" shoe. It had no tongue and round laces which were threaded through leather loops rather than through eyelets. These laces were then crisscrossed up the leg and tied over the ankle.

**Tongueless Oxford.** A very popular variation of the *gillie* was the tongueless oxford which featured soft flat tasseled laces threaded through eyelets. Many had additional cutouts on either side of the laces, creating a very holey instep.

**One-Eyelet Tie Oxford.** This afternoon or evening shoe (formerly the Theo of the 1910s and '20s) resembled a tap-dancing shoe. It had an instep strap which was fastened together in the center by a ribbon laced through one pair of eyelets and tied in a bow. These shoes were revived for teenage girls during the 1970s. At this time they were called "Ruby Keelers" after the popular tap dancer of 1930s movies. Keeler made a stage comeback in 1971 in a revival of the 1917 Broadway musical, *No, No Nanette*.

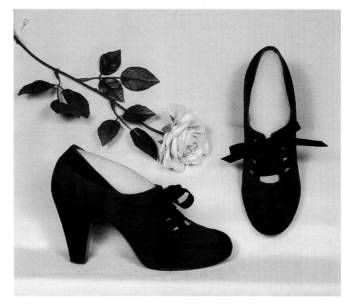

Wine suede tongueless oxfords with navy grosgrain toes, upper quarters, and heels. Marked: Fanchon. $95-$125.

Kedette whipcord-twill sport shoes (4/38). *(1)* Green kiltie oxford. *(2)* Navy *gillie. (3)* Yellow open-toe monk shoe. *(4)* Red moccasin-vamp oxford with pinked tongue and vamp. *(5)* Brown and white oxford. Note: the perforations and the striped soles on many of the models.

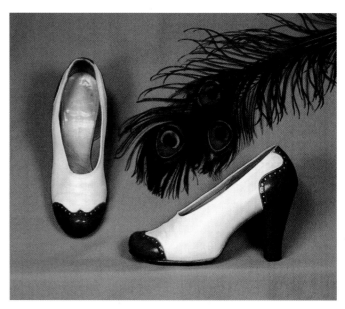

Spectators with wall toes, white buckskin with brown wing tips, quarters, and spike heels, late '30s-early '40s. *Courtesy of Rose Jamieson.* $50-$60.

## Monk Shoes

The monk shoe and its many variations emerged during the second half of the decade. It was a plain shoe with a high, wide tongue over the instep. A strap passed across the tongue and buckled at the outer side of the instep. In a later variation, the strap was threaded through two vertical slits in the tongue, then buckled at the side. When the tongue was narrow, a narrow strap (or in some cases a shoelace) bridged the gap between the tongue and the side of the shoe, creating a small opening below the strap or lace. This shoe was usually made with round, square, or wall toes and low, military, or Cuban heels. It remained popular for men and women through World War II and was revived again in the late 1960s and 1970s.

## Spectators

Introduced in the 1920s, the two-toned spectator shoe was known as a "co-respondent" in the U.K. This white buckskin shoe had a contrasting wing tip, quarter, and heel usually made of navy, brown, or black kid with perforations along the edges. Spectators were made in the pump, oxford, instep-strap, kiltie-tongue, and tongueless-oxford styles. In some versions, the edges of the darker leather were pinked. This classic shoe is still worn today.

## Sandals

Shoes labeled sandals, during the first half of the decade, were merely oxfords or instep-strap models with numerous cut-outs. Circa 1935, open T-strap sandals appeared. These airy summer shoes had open sides and backs. One popular style featured a broad "T" which was made in one with the instep and vamp. Another style featured a narrow "T" with side-to-side or diagonal straps which crisscrossed the vamp. Most sandals were covered with countless cutouts in the form of circles called portholes, squares, rectangles, and diamonds. The heels varied from low to Cuban. White was the most common color followed by tan, red, navy, pink, black, and multicolored. Sandals were worn with sundresses, shorts, and beach clothing including lounging pajamas.

***Huaraches and Lido Sandals.*** Hand-made peasant-style *huaraches*, made of narrow, closely woven strips of calfskin, were imported from Mexico beginning in the 1920s. Another sum-

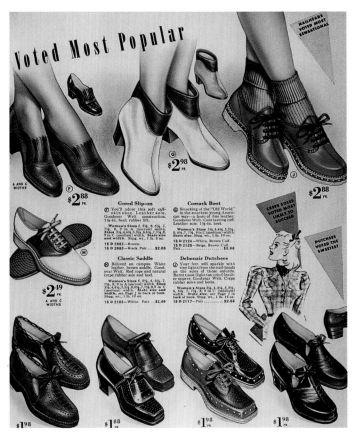

Sears, Roebuck and Co. catalog page (1939-40). *Clockwise from top left. (1)* Gored slip-on. *(2)* Cossack boot. *(3)* "Dutchees," crêpe platform soles with nail studs, wall toe. *(4)* Monk shoe, wall toe. *(5)* Square wall-toe oxford. *(6)* Shawl tongue, wall toe. *(7)* Monk shoe. *(8)* Saddle shoe.

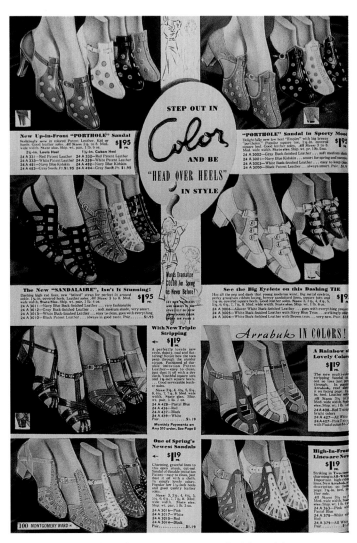

Montgomery Ward catalog page featuring colorful sandals. *(Row 1)* Round cut-outs called portholes. *(Row 2)* Square cutouts and oxfords with slits. *(Row 3)* T-straps. *(Row 4)* T-straps, pinked edges, geometric cut-outs. Montgomery Ward, 1937.

mertime favorite was the Lido sandal, named for the popular Lido Beach in Venice. Both of these sandals were made in a wide variety of styles including (but not limited to) the oxford, tongueless oxford, instep strap, T-strap, and ankle-strap models. As a rule, they were made in white or natural tan; two-toned models were also made in tan and brown, white and black patent, or beige and blue.

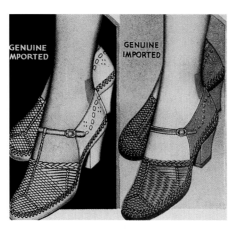

Sears, Roebuck and Co. catalog illustration (1931). T-strap and instep-strap Lido sandals made of woven strips of calfskin with a 1 1/2 inch military heel.

## Espadrilles

Made of esparto grass, *espadrilles,* were first worn by poor Spanish and French farmers of the Mediterranean area. They were adapted for beach wear in the 1930s. The uppers were made of heavy canvas with either rope or crepe rubber soles. Cord-style lacing began at the vamp, crisscrossed the instep, and tied around the ankle.

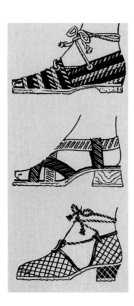

Sport shoe ad which appeared in *Harper's Bazaar* (1/38) - *Top:* Espadrille - in multicolored peasant cloth with open toe, crepe sole, and leg lacing. *Middle:* Sandal - Lastex straps for fit without fastening, crepe sole. *Bottom:* Bathing shoe - Latex treated fish net, with cord leg lacing.

## Pumps

The "opera" pump or "court" shoe, consisted of a plain upper cut from one piece of leather or fabric. Pumps were often decorated with rhinestone clips, bows, cut-steel beads, or "steel effect" buckles.

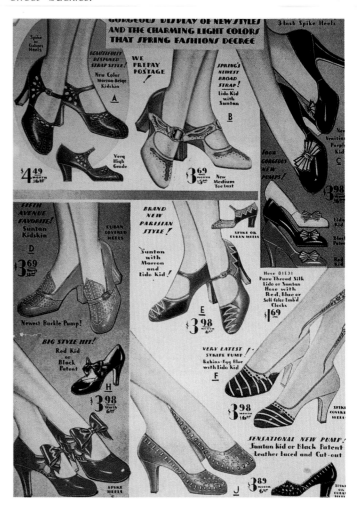

Hamilton Garment Co. shoe advertisement (1930). *(A)* Cutouts, perforations. *(B)* Underlays, center buckle. *(C)* Pumps with butterfly bows. *(D)* Colonial pump. *(E)* Zigzag-modern lightning-bolt overlay. *(F)* Striped overlay. *(H)* One-eyelet-tie shoes. *(J)* Cutouts.

***Colonial Pumps.*** This shoe was a carry-over from the previous two decades and featured a pointed tongue which extended up over the instep of the foot. This style was often decorated with a rectangular metal buckle over the instep. Some high-cut pumps were fitted with triangular elastic gores at the sides of the tongue for a snug comfortable fit.

**Spat Pumps**. Introduced c.1938-39, the spat shoe was an adaptation of Victorian men's spatterdashes. This high-cut shoe was usually made with a black patent-leather toe and heel (representing a shoe). The vamp, instep, and quarter were often made of suede (representing the spat). They were accented with two or three shiny round buttons imitating those of a spat or gaiter.

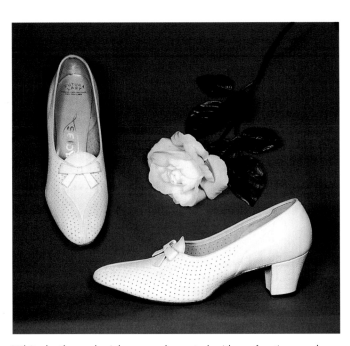

White leather colonial pumps decorated with perforations and a bow over the instep. Label: Selby. *Courtesy Cedar Crest Alumnae Museum, gift of Sue Steiner.* $40-$60.

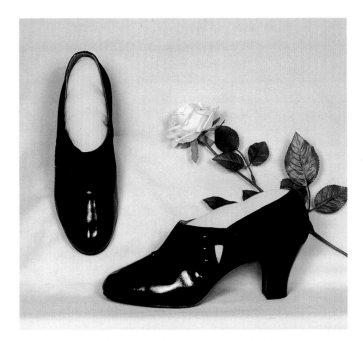

Spat shoes with black patent leather vamps and Cuban heels, black suede insteps, sides, and quarters, accented with three shiny *faux* buttons, 1938-39. $75-$110.

**Sling-Back Pumps**. This pump had an open quarter (back) and was held on by a narrow strap which fit around the heel of the foot. This classic style was produced throughout the 1930s and has been popular ever since.

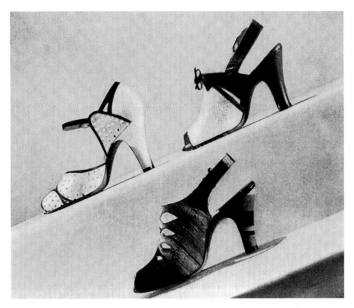

Open-toe sling-back pumps featured in *Harper's Bazaar* (7/37). *(1)* White buckskin outlined in navy, pierced with portholes. *(2)* Striped scarf print. *(3)* Natural-colored mesh vamp, leather heel and strap.

**Side-Strap Pumps**. These shoes had the lower portion of the sides removed, leaving horizontal side straps connecting the vamp and the quarter. This style was introduced circa 1937. (An example of the side-strap shoe appears at the beginning of the chapter under evening shoes.)

## Dress Boots

**Camisole-Tie Boots.** This ankle boot featured a leather drawstring which was threaded through eyelets around the mouth of the boot (similar to the neckline of a chemise or camisole worn by 19th-century women).

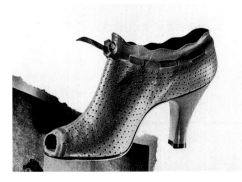

This open-toe boot, featured in *Harper's Bazaar* (3/1/38), contains a camisole-style drawstring neck, a spike heel, and rows of perforations.

**Richelieu Boots.** This ankle-high boot, similar to the monk shoe, had a large fold-over tongue fastened to the sides of the boot with a buckle. This boot was reminiscent of those worn by 17th century musketeers, thus the name Richelieu.

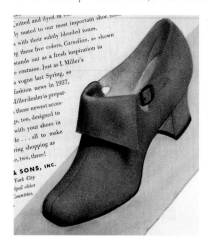

*Harper's Bazaar* advertisement (2/37) featuring a gray suede, square-toe "Richelieu" boot (variation of the monk) with fold-over tongue by I. Miller.

## New Features (1935-1939)

Many of the shoe styles already mentioned were worn into the second half of the decade. They were joined by new features, introduced in the late 1930s, which we commonly associate with the 1940s. These features were used alone, in combination with each other, or combined with earlier shoe styles.

**Wall Toe.** The wall or "box" toe rose vertically from the sole, then turned at a right-angle over the toes, creating a boxy look. It was used for round and square toes alike, giving them a broad stubby appearance.

**Open-Toes.** A toe or two began to peek out of summer sandals circa 1935. Soon a smattering of winter shoes were designed with open toes (called "peep toes" in the U.K.).

**Pleated and Draped Vamps.** In the late '30s, a new shoe style was created by draping pleated fabric or leather crisscross-style over the vamp, often leaving the toes exposed. Ankle straps were fashioned from leather or more of the draped fabric.

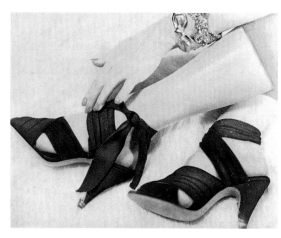

Shoe illustration from *Harper's Bazaar* (1/38), featuring pleated black and blue silk-crepe draped across the vamp and tied around the ankles. (Designed to be worn with a black afternoon dress or dinner suit.)

**Ankle Straps.** Unlike instep straps, which were attached to the sides of the shoe, ankle straps were attached to the quarter or back of the shoe.

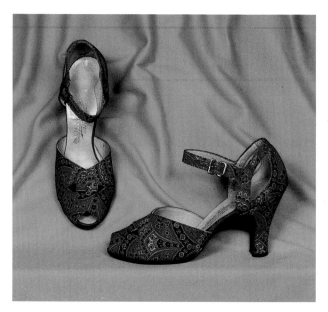

Red paisley shoes with spike-heels, open-toes, and ankle-straps. Marked: Middletown Footwear, Middletown, N.Y. $50-$75.

**Platform Soles.** Prominent Italian shoe designer, Salvatore Ferragamo, introduced platform soles, circa 1935. They varied in height from 1/2 to 2 inches and were used for a variety of sport and dressy shoe styles. These thick soles were made of wood or cork known as "rafts." Cork soles became a popular alternative to rationed leather soles during World War II.

One of Ferragamo's more spectacular sandals, designed in 1938, featured platform soles and heels made from sculptured layers of cork. Each layer was covered in suede of a different bright color topped by gold kid straps. These shoes are now in the costume collection of the Metropolitan Museum of Art.

The March 1938 issue of *Harper's Bazaar* contained six pairs of platform shoes designed for Schiaparelli by the renowned shoe designer André Perugia. They included a *sabot* (clog) and several pairs of eccentric sandals with kinked platform soles and straps.

In 1939, the Sears, Roebuck and Co. catalog featured the "Dutchee," a modern version of a Dutch clog or French peasant's *sabot*. It contained a leather upper which was fastened to a thick crepe rubber sole by the use of decorative metal studs. Platform shoes increased in popularity during the Second World War and were revived again during the late 1960s and 1970s.

**Wedge Heels.** Another shoe feature pioneered by Ferragamo, circa 1935, was the "wedgie." This shoe had a sloped, wedge-shaped heel which was made in one with the sole. The most common material for wedge heels was cork, followed by leather and wood.

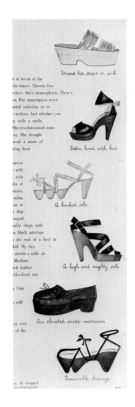

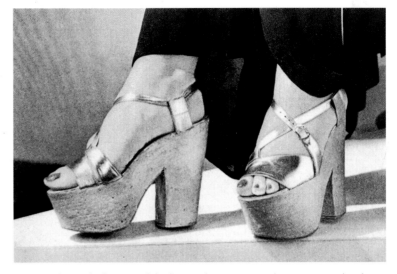

Above: These platform sandals, featured in Vogue (12/37), were made of thick-cork soles and gold kid straps.

Right: These "Little shoes with great soles" appeared in *Harper's Bazaar* (3/15/38). They were designed by André Perugia of Padova for Schiaparelli. *(1)* Thick cork-soled *sabot* (clog). *(2)* Platform shoe with ankle-strap, open-toe, spike heel. *(3)* Kinked sole with narrow straps. *(4)* Platform sole, ankle strap. *(5)* Platform sole, moccasin. *(6)* Kinked sole, narrow ankle straps.

# GALOSHES

Galoshes or ankle boots were worn over the shoes for protection during inclement weather and were removed when the wearer reached her destination. They were fastened with snaps or zippers and were often trimmed along the top with fur.

# CARE OF SHOES

Shoes, like hats, should be stuffed with acid-free tissue paper to retain their shape. This is especially important for strap shoes as thin straps tend to become misshapen without the proper support.

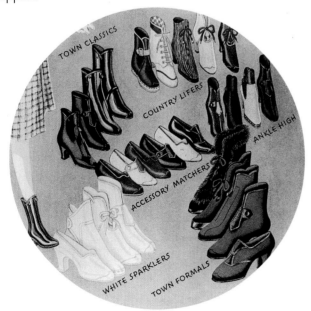

United States Rubber Company offered this wide selection of Gaytees boots and rubbers in 1939.

# WORLD RENOWNED SHOE DESIGNERS

**Salvatore Ferragamo.** By the age of fourteen, Salvatore Ferragamo had six craftsmen working for him in his own shoemaking establishment in Italy. In 1923, he moved his shop from Florence to Hollywood where he began designing shoes for early motion picture stars such as Clara Bow, Mary Pickford, Pola Negri, Gloria Swanson, Marlene Dietrich, and Greta Garbo. Dissatisfied with the caliber of craftsmanship in Hollywood, he returned to Italy in 1927, where he began exporting his elegant creations to prestigious stores in the United States.

**André Perugia.** The noted French shoe designer, Perugia, opened his house on the rue de la Paix in Paris. He designed shoes for his wealthy clientele as well as creative styles to complement Schiaparelli's daring designs.

**Roger Vivier.** His early training in sculpture at the *École des Beaux-Arts* in Paris has been evident in Vivier's work (particularly his innovative heels) for over sixty years. He began his career in workrooms on the *Place Vendôme* in Paris where he created styles for world renowned shoe firms like Pinet, Bally, Rayne, Turner, I. Miller, and Delman. He opened his own salon in 1937 and designed shoes for such entertainers as Marlene Dietrich and Josephine Baker.

# NOTED SHOE MANUFACTURERS

Noted shoe manufacturers of the 1930s included Armstrong, Arnold, Bally, Delman, Enna Jetticks, I. Miller, Naturalizers, Queen Quality Shoes, Rayne, Red Cross Shoes, Selby, and Vitality Shoes.

# Chapter 11
# Jewelry

During the 1930s, there was a major increase in the production of less expensive "non-precious," "costume," or "fashion" jewelry. There were many reasons for this rapid growth.

The wild excessive spending of the 1920s was curtailed following the stock market crash and people at every economic level needed to buy wisely. Many who had spent money lavishly during the '20s, were now forced to cinch in their belts and do without the luxuries to which they had grown accustomed. This had a profound influence on both the fine and the costume jewelry industries.

Fine jewelry houses were suddenly faced with cancellations of orders. Many firms were forced to reduce production and discharge some of their skilled designers and craftsmen. Suddenly out of work, American and European artisans accepted work with American costume jewelry firms at lower wages, in exchange for the assurance of a steady income. This infusion of skilled labor did much to improve the quality of costume jewelry during the 1930s and placed the American costume jewelry industry far ahead of its European counterparts.

Chanel pioneered the use of "high end" costume jewelry during the early '20s. She believed that jewelry was the crowning touch needed to complete her classic look. She commissioned the Maison Gripoix to create *pâte-de-verre* (poured glass) jewelry and the Duke de Verdura to design high-quality fashion jewelry to complement her designs. She made no attempt to disguise these "frankly fake" imitations, in fact their sheer size gave them away.

Schiaparelli promoted whimsical imaginative costume jewelry. She had a keen interest in the arts which was reflected in many of her designs. She drew inspiration from a talented circle of artists who became her friends. The most notable of these artists was Salvador Dali, her collaborator for many zany surrealistic pieces. She commissioned Jean Schlumberger and Jean Clément to execute these designs which often coordinated with her theme collections. Her outrageous designs were exciting conversation pieces, sure to attract attention wherever they were worn.

Chanel, Schiaparelli, Eisenberg, and many other fashion designers helped to make costume jewelry truly chic and respectable enough to accompany their elegant *couture* creations. Their non-precious jewelry was embraced by their rich and famous clientele around the world.

Costume jewelry was and continues to be more closely associated with fashion then fine jewelry. Most costume pieces

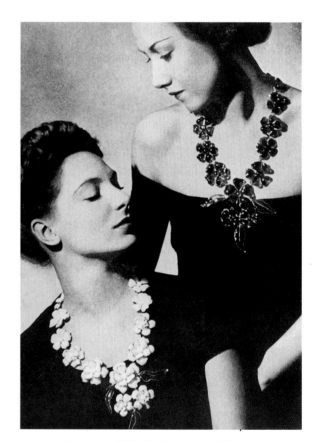

*Harper's Bazaar* published this photo of Chanel's evening leis in March of 1938. *Left:* White porcelain. *Right:* Multicolored glass.

were designed with a particular garment or contemporary look in mind. Since costume jewelry was relatively inexpensive to produce, its designers could afford to follow each fickle whim or fad and consumers had less anxiety about shelving old pieces in favor of new.

Hollywood movies of the 1930s provided an exciting showcase of glamorous fashions accessorized with flamboyant jewelry. Many of the jewelry pieces worn on the screen were made with authentic gem stones. However, Eugene Joseph, the noted costume-jewelry designer, was often commissioned by the major movie studios to design costume jewelry needed for the production of their films. These pieces were imitated by jewelry manufacturers at more affordable prices.

From the Victorian era until the 1930s, jewelry had been mass produced by the die-stamp method. New technological advances in the production of vulcanized rubber led to the use of rubber molds. These molds, used in conjunction with the ancient lost-wax casting process, allowed jewelry manufacturers to mass produce large quantities of jewelry at a fraction of the cost.

Fine jewelry firms began to substitute semi-precious materials in order to reduce costs. Smaller stones were often placed in "illusion settings" to give them a larger appearance. Jewelry designers continued to make interchangeable jewelry which could be converted from one form to another. For example, the much imitated double-clip brooch could be worn as a brooch or pulled apart and worn as two dress clips. A brooch might have a drop which could be removed and worn as a pendant or the center medallion of a bracelet or necklace might be removed and worn as a brooch. As a result of this versatility, the buyer could purchase two pieces of jewelry for the price of one.

Jewelry designs were often marked with the patent number on the reverse side of the piece. Using patent tables it is possible to determine the year in which a particular design was patented. (Invention patents remained in effect for 17 years and design patents for 14 years). Once valuable time and materials were spent on the production of a die or mold, jewelry houses often utilized them for several years. A patent date, therefore, represents the earliest date in which a piece could have been made.

The jewelry in this chapter has been organized into five categories: influences, materials, techniques/styles, motifs, and forms. While placed under only one category, many of the pieces pictured in this chapter could fall under other categories or sub-categories as well.

# INFLUENCES

## Art Deco

The strongest influence on jewelry during the first half of the decade was the Art Deco movement. This style originated in Europe and was promoted by the Bauhaus, the German *avant-garde* school of design. In 1925, the *Parisian Exposition International des Arts Décoratifs et Industriels Modernes*, an international exhibit of modern decorative arts, was held in Paris. This exhibit introduced to the world the new art movement which would later be called "Art Deco." This style dominated the decorative arts from 1925 through 1935. (For further information and photographs on Art Deco see Historical Background, Chapter 1.)

Art Deco-style objects were bold, uncluttered, and devoid of extraneous detail. They were characterized by rigid geometric shapes, parallel lines (both straight and curved), converging lines, broad sweeping lines (resembling comet trails,) concentric circles, half circles, step patterns, zigzags, lightning bolts, sunrays, star bursts, fountains, and stylized flowers, including the "Deco rose." Art Deco designs were usually executed in a symmetrical format, i.e., double-clip brooches and mirror-image clasps.

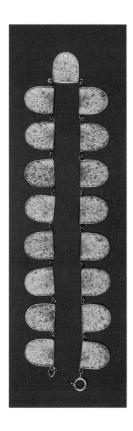

Czechoslovakian Art Deco-style necklace made of brass and mottled pressed-glass segments. *Courtesy of Roxanne Stuart.* $130-$150.

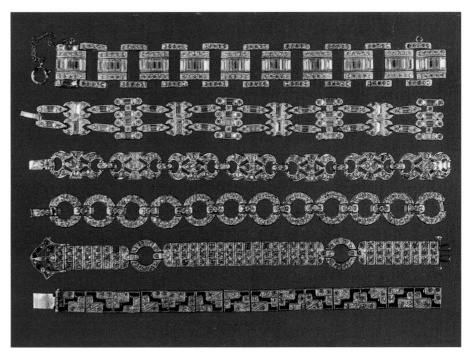

Geometric Art Deco-style segmented bracelets (five all-white) made of base metal with pavé-set clear rhinestones and blue and clear glass *baguettes*. Bottom two - *Courtesy of Betsey Pacini.* $75-$100 ea.

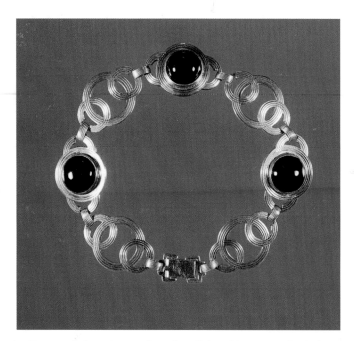

Art Deco-style bracelet, sterling-silver links with concentric-circle engraving and bezel-set black onyx cabochons. *Courtesy of Theresa Schouten.* $75-$100.

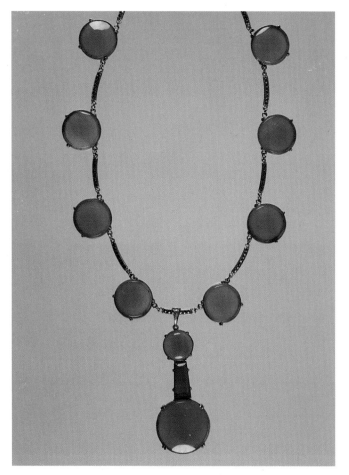

Silver Art Deco-style necklace made of carnelian and marcasite. Marked: Sterling, Germany. *Courtesy of Roxanne Stuart.* $275-$350.

Typical Art-Deco color combinations were achieved in costume jewelry by combining BLACK (onyx, glass, Bakelite, or enamel) with one or more of the colors listed below.

1) WHITE (crystal, clear rhinestones, marcasite, silver, or clear Bakelite.)
2) GREEN (jade, amazonite, chrysoprase, Bakelite, glass, or enamel)
3) CORAL (coral, celluloid, glass, or enamel)
4) RED (celluloid, Bakelite, glass, or enamel)

Other semi-precious stones used at this time were chalcedony (blue/gray), carnelian (orange or red/brown), citrine (yellow), moonstone (light blue opalescent), aquamarine (blue/green), smoky topaz (brown), and stained agate. It was not so much the intrinsic value of the materials which made Art Deco costume jewelry so appealing; it was the clean lines, bold geometric shapes, and dynamic color combinations.

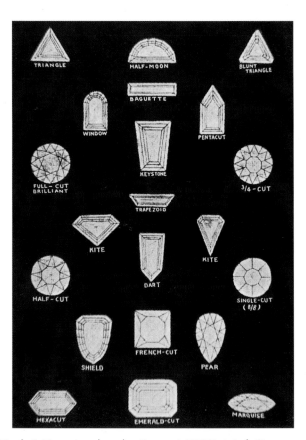

This *Hardy & Hayes* jewelry advertisement (1931) stated, "As an indication of the modern trend in jewelry cutting, we illustrate a few of the unique shapes in which we are having diamonds cut for us."

Stone cuts such as the round, pear (teardrop), emerald (rectangle or square with corners cut off), and marquise-shaped (pointed oval) stones had been used in jewelry since before the turn of the 20th century. Influenced by Cubism and the geometric shapes of Art Deco, precious, semi-precious, and synthetic stones were now cut or molded into additional new shapes. These included the *baguette* (narrow rectangle - meaning long

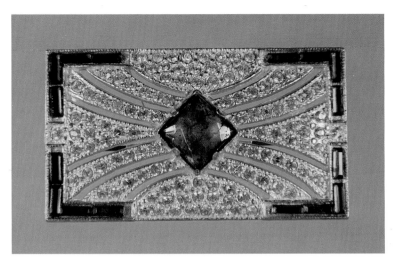

Art Deco-style plaque pin containing square and *baguette*-cut blue and pavé-set clear rhinestones. *Courtesy of Sue Irons (Irons Antiques).* $80-$120.

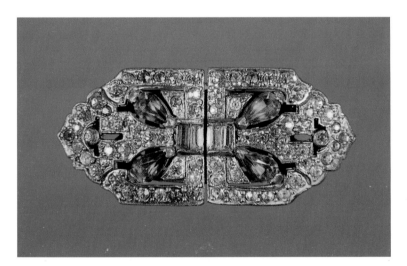

Double dress-clip brooch made of base metal set with green pear-shaped and clear pavé-set rhinestones. Marked: PAT. 2,044,225 (1936). *Courtesy of Sue Irons (Irons Antiques).* $95-$120.

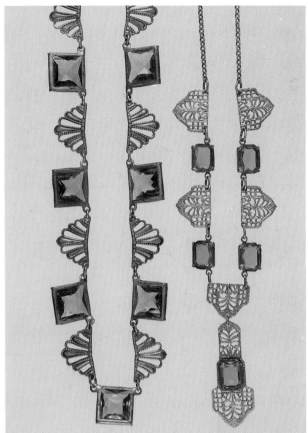

Typical Art Deco-style necklaces and bracelet. Geometric-shaped glass stones alternate with silver, gold, and rhodium-plated filigree segments. $65-$125.

loaf of bread in French), lozenge (diamond), trapeze (trapezoid), demi-lune (half-moon), bullet, triangle, kite, and dart cuts. It was common for Art Deco pieces to contain stones in a variety of shapes, cuts, and sizes.

## Native Jewelry

The Colonial Exhibition in Paris (1931) featured artifacts and jewelry from the French colonies in West Africa and the South Sea Islands. This primitive jewelry included ivory bangle bracelets and necklaces made of such natural materials as semi-precious stones, cork, nuts, seeds, bone, wood, feathers, and shells.

This exhibition sparked a trend for "barbaric," "tribal," or "native" jewelry made from modern materials with a primitive flare. Wide Bakelite bangle bracelets were carved in lush tropical fruit and foliate motifs. Primative-looking beaded necklaces were produced in Czechoslovakia. The imitation carved-ivory beads were made of matte-finish pressed-glass highlighted in the crevices with dark enamel for clarity of design. Brooches resembling African tribal masks and blackamoors were also popular.

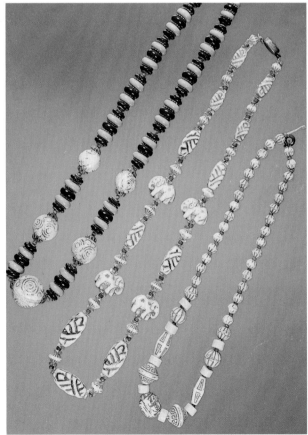

Imitation carved-ivory, barbaric necklaces made of matte-finish pressed-glass beads highlighted with enamel. *Courtesy of Roseann Ettinger (Remember When ...).* $50-$75.

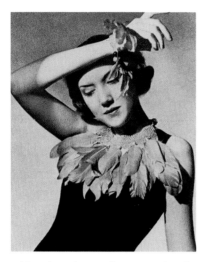

This barbaric necklace by Schiaparelli appeared in the March 1938 issue of *Harper's Bazaar*. It featured pastel feathers dangling from a beaded collar.

Large tribal necklaces featured elongated elements (imitating animal claws, fangs, or spearheads) alternating with small bead spacers. These longer elements were threaded through one end which caused them to radiate from the neck. Schiaparelli was often seen wearing her favorite tribal necklace made of gold claw-like elements and emerald cabochons. Pins in the likeness of Josephine Baker featured feathered headdresses, tribal necklaces, and banana skirts.

## Chinese

Chinese carved jewelry, a carry-over from the 1910s and 1920s, was imported from the Orient until the outbreak of World War II. Pieces of hand-carved and pierced jade, coral, amethyst, lapis, and carnelian were often incorporated in sterling or 14k gold pendants, brooches, rings, bracelets, and earrings. Less expensive imitations made of press-molded glass were imported from Czechoslovakia. Celluloid and bakelite were also molded to resemble Oriental carved stones.

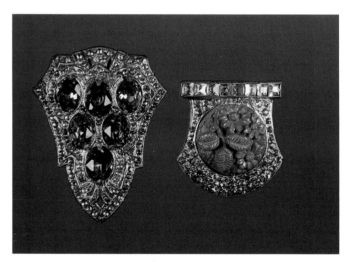

Two silver-plated base metal dress clips containing large blue rhinestones, simulated carved coral, and pavé-set clear rhinestones. *Courtesy of Ethel Bishop.* $40-$60 ea.

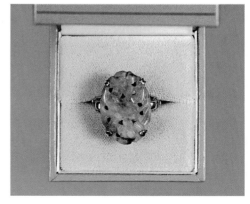

Ring made of 14k gold and carved and pierced jade. *Courtesy of Rose Jamieson.* $125-$150.

A variation of the tribal necklace made of butterscotch Bakelite. The elongated elements are alternated with round beads decorated with purple rhinestones. *Courtesy of Mary Anne Faust (Yesterday's Delights).* $250-$300.

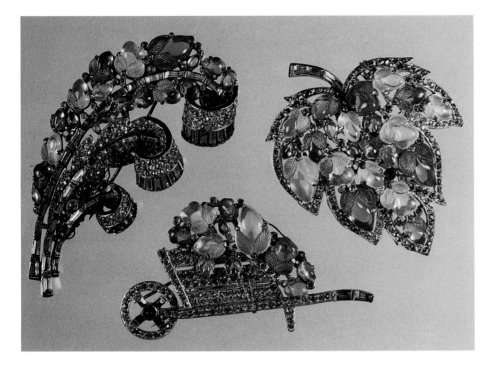

Rhodium-plated fruit-salad fur clips, by Alfred Philippe for Trifari, containing blue and clear Cartier-style press-molded stones with round and *baguette*-shaped pavé-set clear rhinestones, late '30s-early '40s. *Courtesy of Bonny Yankauer (Menagerie)*. $300-$500.

## East Indian

The world renowned French jeweler, Louis Cartier, was commissioned by wealthy Indian moguls to create jewelry using Indian gemstones. These stones were not faceted, but carved to resemble fruits, berries, and leaves. Spherical gems were carved with flutes or longitudinal grooves like cantaloupe, thus the terms "melonized" or "melon-cut" were used. These "melons" were often accented with a small round diamond at the point where the grooves converged. By using carved emeralds, rubies, and sapphires in jewelry for his European and American clientele, Cartier made an exciting contribution not only to fine jewelry but to costume jewelry design as well. Although Cartier was the first modern Western jeweler to use carved gems, Van Cleef and Arpel, Mauboussin, and other fine jewelers followed his lead.

Carved gemstones were imitated in pressed glass for what is now called "Cartier-style" costume jewelry designed by Alfred Philippe for Trifari. Philippe was a French artist who started his career at Van Cleef & Arpels and Cartier. He joined Trifari in 1930 and soon became its chief designer. He incorporated these pressed-glass stones into bracelets, brooches, fur clips, and double-clip brooches resembling floral bouquets, flower baskets, fans, leaves, birds, feathers, cornucopias, and wheel barrows laden with fruits and berries. Due to the fruity nature of the stones, this jewelry is affectionately called "fruit salad" or "tutti-frutti." These Cartier-style costume pieces from the late '30s and early '40s are attractive and highly collectible.

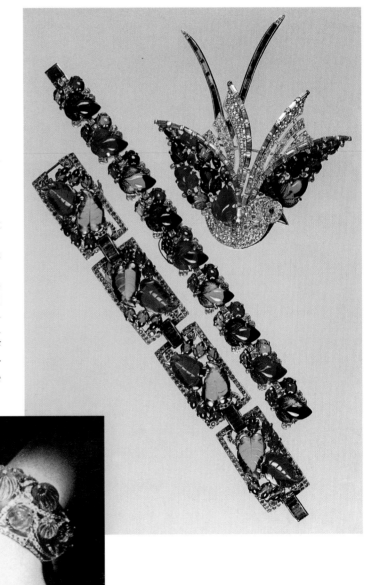

Rhodium-plated fruit-salad jewelry containing red, green, and blue foliate-shaped press molded glass stones, designed by Alfred Philippe for Trifari. Bird and small bracelet marked: Trifari. Late '30s-early '40s. *Courtesy of Bonny Yankauer (Menagerie)*. Bird $2,000-$3,000. / Small $200-$300. / Large $250-$350. *Insert: You* (magazine) 1938-39 photograph of a bracelet set with carved melon-shaped emeralds, by Black Starr & Frost-Gorham.

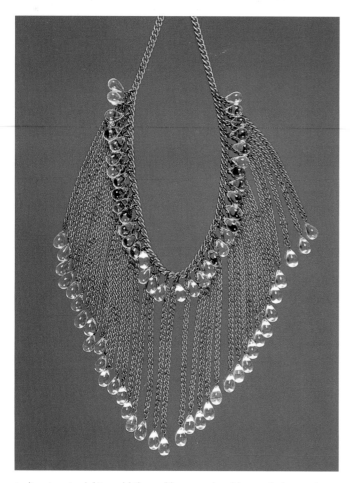

Indian-inspired fringed-bib necklace made of brass chains and crystal teardrops. *Courtesy of Roxanne Stuart.* $100-$150.

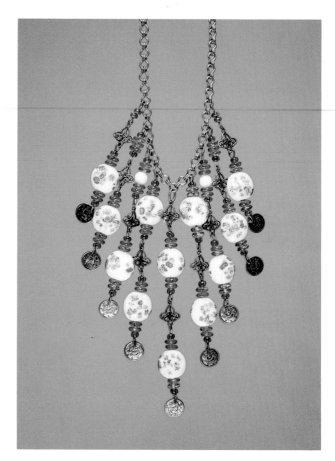

East Indian-style fringed-bib necklace accented with glass beads, rondelles, and filigree. *Courtesy of Roseann Ettinger (Remember When ...).* $200-300.

Also influenced by Indian jewelry were large bib-style necklaces containing beads, pearls, or balls suspended from chain fringe or chain lattice work.

## Retro Modern

The 1935-36 Sears, Roebuck and Co. catalog advertised its engraved "heirloom" bangle bracelets with the comment, "The kind grandmother wore...antique designs are new again."

Period movies like *Anna Karenina* and *Jezebel* sparked a renewed interest in Victorian-fashion. This nostalgia influenced a new artistic style in jewelry, now known as "Retro Modern." As the name implies, Victorian motifs and designs were revived using modern materials, technology, and styling. Although this style emerged during the second half of the decade, it is most often associated with the 1940s.

***Hand Brooches***. Victorian-style female-hand brooches reappeared during the 1930s. These reproductions were not only made of traditional metal, they were now made in such new materials as Bakelite and (in the late '30s and early '40s) Lucite. Some were given a modern spin by the application of red enameled finger nail polish.

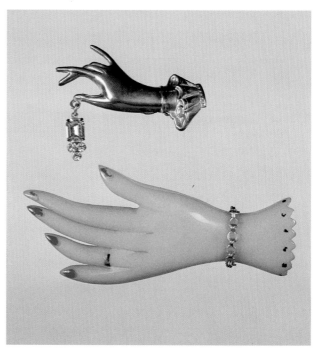

Retro-Modern hand brooches. *Top:* gold-plated brass and glass. $25-$35. *Bottom:* Bakelite with red enameled fingernails. $500+. *Courtesy of Roseann Ettinger (Remember When ...).*

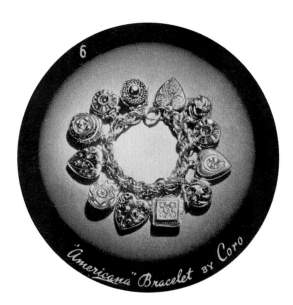

This "Americana" charm bracelet by Coro appeared in the March 1938 issue of *Harper's Bazaar*. It featured reproduction Victorian watch charms, available in gold or silver-plate.

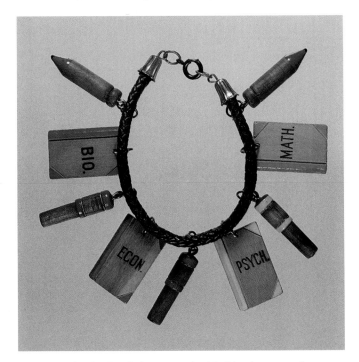

Wooden school-related charms on braided leatherette style bracelet, late '30s, early '40s.

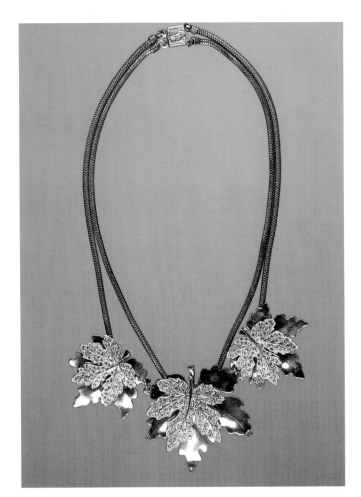

Retro-modern style necklace, shiny gold-plated leaves surmounted by rhodium-plated leaves pavé-set with clear rhinestones on a double mouse-tail chain. Marked: McClelland Barclay. *Courtesy of Rose Jamieson.* $200-$300.

**Charm Bracelets**. Reproductions of Victorian charm bracelets featured metal charms in heart and other assorted shapes. In addition, modern materials such as Bakelite and wood were now used for witty charm bracelets with a theme.

***Chatelaine Pins.*** The 19th-century chatelaine was also given a new twist. The 1930s version consisted of a pair of decorative brooches connected by one or more chains. Both brooches could be worn on one side of a dress or jacket bodice with the chain(s) swagged between them, or the brooches could be placed on either side of a sweater or jacket front using the chain(s) to hold the sides together.

***Mouse-tail Necklaces.*** Also inspired by Victorian jewelry was the choker-style necklace featuring a decorative element suspended on a tubular herringbone-mesh "mouse tail" chain.

These flexible chains were also known as "snake," "gooseneck," or "stovepipe" chains. Mouse-tail jewelry was often produced in suites containing a necklace, bracelet, and earrings to match.

***Cameos and Lockets.*** The classic carved stone or shell cameo was also revived. Modern versions molded from black glass or Bakelite were now available. Sentimental Victorian lockets in the shape of circles, ovals, hearts, and miniature books reappeared. They were hand engraved with floral motifs or machine-engraved with engine-turnings in stripes or patterns. They were often monogrammed with the owner's initials. (See chart with sample monogram styles.)

***Floral Brooches.*** Also reminiscent of 19th-century jewelry were Retro Modern brooches and fur clips. Common naturalistic motifs included light airy floral sprays, birds, fish, and insects. These recreations, however, were larger and more three-dimensional then similar Victorian pieces. Their soft fluid asymmetrical lines were in sharp contrast to the hard-edged geometric symmetry of earlier Art Deco pieces. The majority of these pieces were made of base metal which was electroplated with rhodium to prevent tarnishing. (Rhodium is a metallic element in the platinum family. Its hardness and bright silvery shine made it ideal for plating jewelry). These brooches and clips were then decorated with colored enamels and pavé-set rhinestones or marcasites. Jewelry of this kind was produced by costume jewelry firms such as Trifari, Coro, Boucher, and Mazer and were often signed with the name of the manufacturer on the reverse side of the piece.

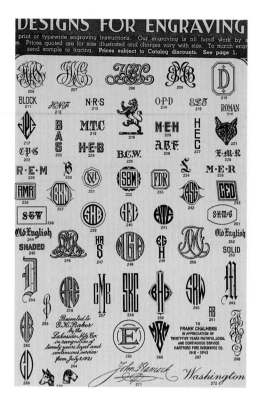

Sample monograms for engraving offered in the L.& C. Mayers wholesale jewelry catalog (1939). Many personal items such as lockets and bangle bracelets contained a cartouche for an engraved monogram. Note: Art Deco examples in which the letters are forced to conform to geometric boundaries.

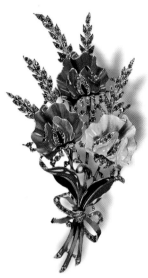

Retro-modern sweet-pea bouquet fur clip with multicolored enameling and rhinestones. Marked: Trifari. *Courtesy of Bonny Yankauer (Menagerie).* $350-$450.

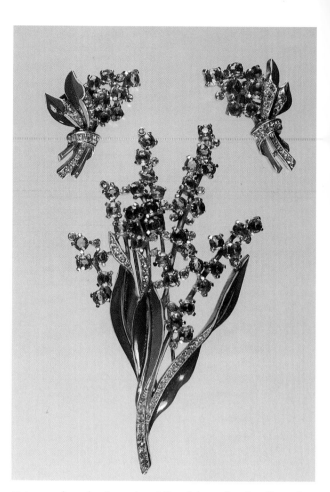

Retro-modern rhodium-plated lily of the valley fur clip and matching earrings featuring amber and clear rhinestones with enameled leaves. Marked: Trifari. *Courtesy of Bonny Yankauer (Menagerie).* $600-$800 set.

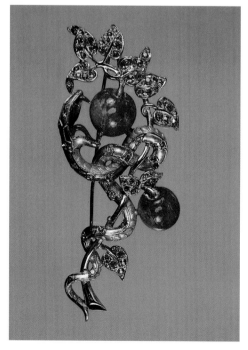

Snake in an apple tree brooch, rhodium-plated base metal, pavé-set rhinestones and enamel. Marked: MB (Marcel Boucher). *Courtesy of Roxanne Stuart.* Rare.

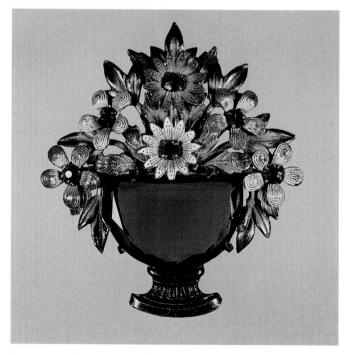

Brooch containing enameled flowers and leaves with purple rhinestone centers, large purple glass vase. *Courtesy of Mary Anne Faust (Yesterday's Delights).* $140-$160.

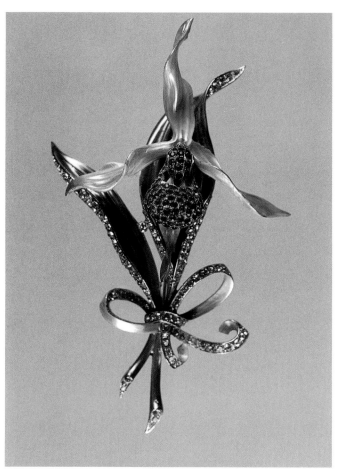

Retro-modern three-dimensional orchid brooch accented with enamel and pavé-set rhinestones. Marked: Mazer. *Courtesy of Bonny Yankauer (Menagerie).* $500-$600.

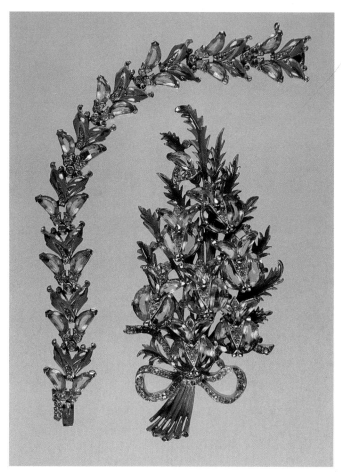

Retro-modern rhodium-plated floral-spray fur clip and watching bracelet featuring *demi-lune* (moon-shaped) aqua glass stones, pavé-set rhinestones, and enamel. Marked: Trifari. *Courtesy Bonny Yankauer (Menagerie).* $600-$800 set.

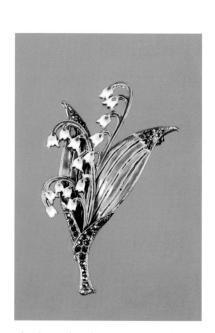

Rhodium-plated Retro-Modern lily-of-the-valley brooch accented with marcasites and enamel. $150-$200.

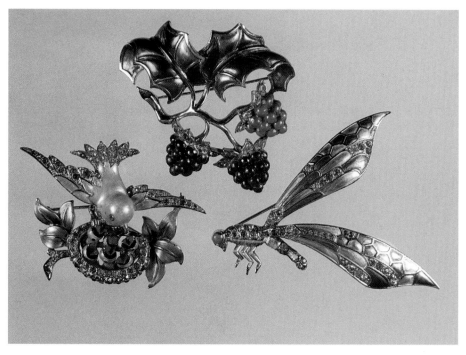

Retro-modern trio of rhodium-plated base-metal pins decorated with enamel and pavé-set rhinestones. All marked: MB (Marcel Boucher). *Courtesy of Bonny Yankauer (Menagerie).* Bird $1,000-$1,200. Berries $400-$500. Bug $1,000-$1,200.

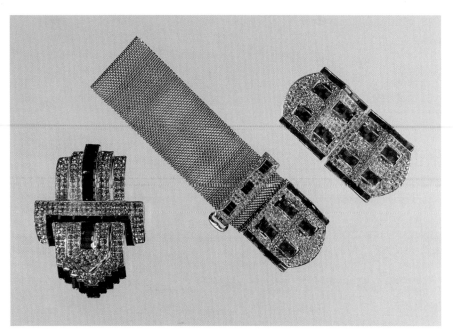

Retro-modern style jewelry made of pavé-set clear rhinestones and red *baguettes*. *Left:* Asymmetrical buckle-shaped duet. Marked: TKF (Trifari, Krussman & Fishel). $200-$300. *Right:* Fine brick-work mesh bracelet and matching duet in imitation of the Victorian garter bracelet. Marked: TKF. $350-$450 set. *Courtesy of Bonny Yankauer (Menagerie).*

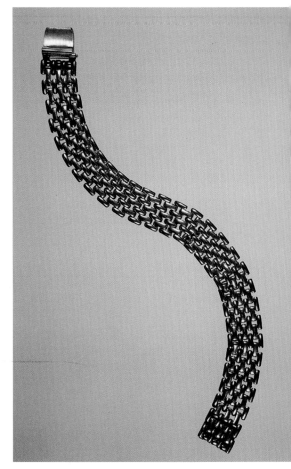

Retro-modern gold-plated brick-work style Ludo bracelet in imitation of the Victorian garter bracelet. $40-$50.

**Ludo Bracelet.** The Victorian "garter bracelet" was reincarnated by Van Cleef & Arpels, c. 1934. This nostalgic style, however, was given a streamlined "machine age" look. Small shiny-gold rectangular links were arranged to form a flexible brick-work-mesh strap, often fastened with a buckle-style clasp. It was named the "Ludo" bracelet after Louis Ludovic Arpels and was widely copied by both fine and costume jewelry designers. It was produced in yellow, green, or rose gold or in more affordable gold-plated metal. This brickwork-style strap was often used for watch bands as well.

**Tank-track Bracelets.** Machine age tank-track style bracelets were similar in design to the brickwork pattern, however, the rectangular links or segments were much longer and larger. These bar-shaped links overlapped one another on the ends only, creating open spaces between the links. In addition to the materials mentioned for the Ludo bracelet, tank-track bracelets were made of colorful Bakelite.

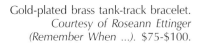

Gold-plated brass tank-track bracelet. *Courtesy of Roseann Ettinger (Remember When ...).* $75-$100.

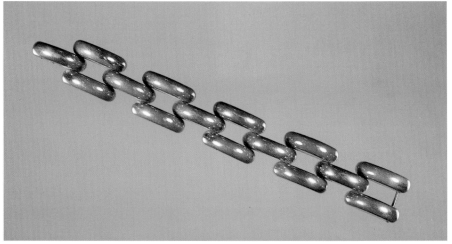

# MATERIALS

## Marcasite

Marcasite is a mineral known as iron pyrite. It was first used during the 18th century as an inexpensive substitute for diamonds. It is opaque and, therefore, relies on the light reflected from its facets for its sparkle. Quality marcasite was "nick" or "gouge" set (not glued) into sterling-silver jewelry. It was often combined with onyx, moon stone, chrysoprase, amazonite, coral, smoky quartz, lapis, chalcedony, or carnelian for striking dress clips, pendants, necklaces, earrings, bracelets, rings, clasps, and hair and hat ornaments.

Inexpensive *faux* marcasite was produced by silver plating faceted glass stones. However, the silver plate often wears off, a condition which is visible through a jeweler's loupe.

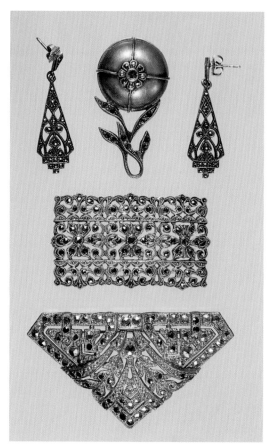

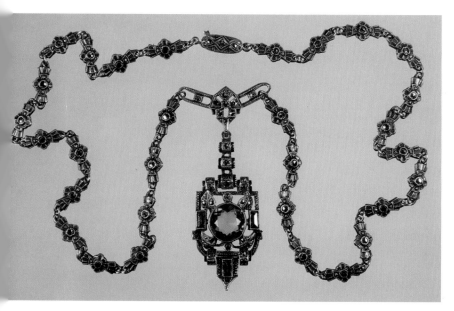

Art Deco-style silver necklace containing a round faceted citrine and marcasites. Marked: sterling, Germany. *Courtesy of Mary Anne Faust (Yesterday's Delights).* $275-$325.

*Top:* Delicate silver filigree pendant earrings set with marcasite. Marked: 925. $60. / Silver and marcasite orb dress clip. Marked: sterling, PAT 1852188 (1932). *Courtesy of Mary Anne Faust (Yesterday's Delights).* $100. *Center:* Sterling and marcasite plaque brooch Marked: 925. $150. *Courtesy of Rose Jamieson. Bottom:* Triangular silver-plated plaque brooch set with marcasite. $75.

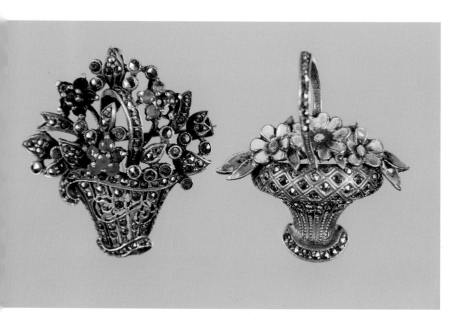

*Left:* Sterling flower-basket brooch/pendant containing sapphires, emeralds, rubies, and marcasites. Marked: 925. *Right:* Silver-plated flower basket brooch with enameled flowers and marcasite ornamentation. *Courtesy of Mary Anne Faust (Yesterday's Delights).* $120-$150.

## Pearls

Most pearl necklaces of the 1930s were made of graduated pearls in one, two, or three strands. Short 15-18 inch or 18-22 inch strands were the most common.

Natural Oriental pearl necklaces were the most costly and usually featured filigree clasps made of platinum or 14k gold, accented with pavé-set diamonds. In 1915, a Japanese man by the name of Mikimoto perfected the process of growing less expensive "cultured" pearls by placing a grain of sand inside each oyster shell. Inexpensive but high-quality imitation pearls were also produced by the Richelieu, Deltah, Técla, and de La Mer (of the sea) companies. Richelieu reproduction pearls were guaranteed not to peel or discolor. In addition to creamy white, imitation pearls were available in rose, aquamarine blue, green, gray, and brown. Sterling or rhodium-plated base metal clasps, often accented with semiprecious stones, were used for less expensive pearls.

## Silver

The sterling silver jewelry produced by Danish silversmith Georg Jensen commanded world attention at the Exhibition of Decorative Arts in Paris in 1925 and the Stockholm exhibit in 1930. Typical Jensen designs included stylized birds, animals, fruit, flowers, and foliage. The company's embossed and chased silver jewelry was widely copied and many of the old designs are still produced by the Jensen company today. Silver pieces set with semi-precious stones are generally more valuable. Sterling silver brooches and segmented bracelets were also produced by costume jewelry firms such as Beau, Danecraft, Trifari, Hobé, Napier, and Coro.

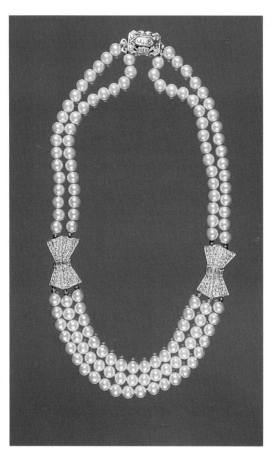

Pearl necklace in the late '20s-early '30s configuration, three strands above and two below connected by bow-knot shaped rhinestone ornaments. $25-$50. *Courtesy of Rose Jamieson.*

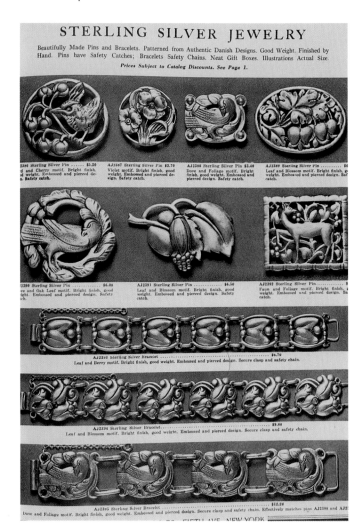

A page from the L.& C. Mayers jewelry catalog (1939) devoted to sterling-silver jewelry "patterned after authentic Danish designs."

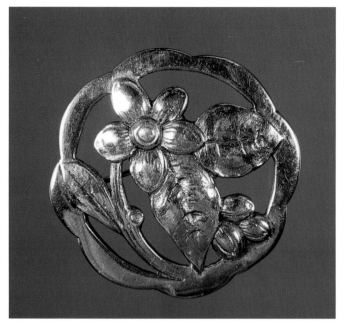

Sterling-silver brooch given to the author's mother by the author's father on their wedding day, April 8, 1939. Marked: Genova, sterling. *Courtesy of Elizabeth Pascoe Whitfield.* $100-$150.

## Celluloid

Celluloid was introduced in the late 19th century and was originally used as an inexpensive substitute for natural substances such as ivory, amber, coral, and tortoise shell. Celluloid is a mixture of cellulose (plant fiber), nitric acid, and camphor. It is a thermoplastic, which means it becomes soft with the application of heat. Care must be taken with celluloid as it is extremely flammable. It can also craze (crack) or crystalize if it is subjected to moisture, heat, or corroded metals. When in this disintegrating state, it "off-gasses" a corrosive gas which is contagious and can infect other celluloid pieces with which it comes in contact. Infected celluloid pieces should be quarantined in a sealed container.

Although on the decline after the introduction of Bakelite, celluloid remained in use during the 1930s for pins, dress clips, buttons, and hair and hat ornaments. (For examples of celluloid hat ornaments, see Hair and Headgear, Chapter 8.) Celluloid was also used for the lightweight chains on which Bakelite charms were suspended.

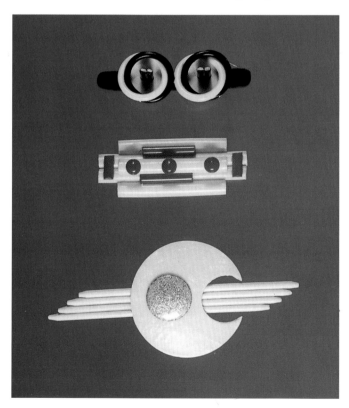

Art Deco-style celluloid pins. *Courtesy of Carl Faust.* $10-$50.

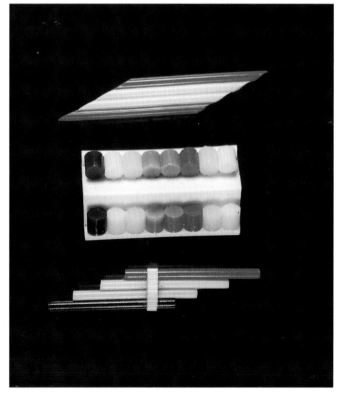

Colorful Art Deco-style celluloid pins. *Courtesy of Carl Faust.* $10-$50.

## Bakelite

Bakelite jewelry was all the rage from the late 1920s into the 1940s. Its cheerful colors, whimsical motifs, and affordable prices made it an ideal antidote for the doldrums of the depression. During its height of popularity, it was not only sold in five and ten cent stores and mail-order catalogs but in better department stores and high-class boutiques in New York, London, and Paris.

Bakelite was the brand name for a phenolic resin invented in 1907 by Belgian chemist, Dr. Leo Hendrik Baekeland. It was the first manmade thermoset plastic, which means that once it has hardened it can not be softened again by the application of heat. Bakelite was also lightweight, non-flammable, moisture resistant, and durable.

Like celluloid, Bakelite was initially used as an affordable substitute for more expensive natural materials such as ivory, bone, onyx, coral, jade, tortoise shell, cinnabar, and amber. With the advent of Art Deco design, however, people began to appreciate synthetic materials for their own merits and the new and unusual effects they could produce.

Bakelite was poured into molds or extruded to form long rods, sheets, and blocks. (For examples of Bakelite rods see the section on buttons under Accessories and Related Items, Chapter 12.) After hardening in an oven, the rods were cut into pieces of the desired thickness. Flat sheets of Bakelite were cut into the desired shapes by the use of a jigsaw. These pieces were then ready to be sanded, carved, engraved, back carved, inlaid, or laminated (two or more colored layers bonded together with glue). They were then polished to a high sheen by tumbling them in a large drum with a fine grit silica or saw dust. Some were given a touch of paint, while others were set with rhinestones, or clad with metal. Bakelite jewelry was not only produced by artisans in factories, it was created by hand crafters in homes as well.

In the early '30s, the Catalin Corporation began producing a phenolic resin substance (similar to Bakelite) which it called "Catalin." In 1937, this company introduced a new clear phenolic resin called "Prystal," an acronym of the words plastic and crystal. This substance was often used for "bracelet" handles and zipper pulls on crocheted purses in the late '30s and '40s.

Martha Sleeper, ended her acting career to become a celebrated Bakelite jewelry designer. Her sense of humor and innovative ideas are evident in her spunky cats on picket fences, tulips with comical faces, and necklaces with champagne bottles and swizzle sticks (a reflection of the repeal of prohibition.) Since she is one of the few Bakelite jewelry designers to sign her work, her pieces are now very valuable.

*Colors.* Bakelite could have an opaque, translucent, transparent, pearlized, or marbleized appearance. The latter was called "variegated" or "end-of-the-day" bakelite as it was produced by mixing the residue of the various colors used on that particular day. Bakelite was produced in a wide spectrum of colors including pure white and pastels. An advertisement from the Butler Brothers Dry Goods catalog (1934) promotes Bakelite jewelry in white and "summer pastels" including willow green, light blue, pink, and yellow. These colors are extremely rare and quite valuable today, as the surface of Bakelite oxidizes with exposure to light, creating a yellowish patina. For this reason, Bakelite is now found in a far narrower range of warm or autumn shades. Over time blue has aged to black, violet to brown, pink or peach to orange, and turquoise to green. What had been patriotic red, white, and blue is now red, custard, and black. The easiest way to describe these aged colors is in terms of the following foods: catsup, tangerine, mustard, butterscotch, caramel, custard, apple juice (once clear), avocado, spinach, chocolate, and licorice.

Like most collectibles, the styles which were produced in limited quantities are the most highly sought after and consequently the most expensive. There was an endless variety of Bakelite jewelry produced during this period. I will touch on just a few of the most popular techniques, forms, and designs.

*Techniques.* Two-toned laminated Bakelite was made with a base layer of one color and a top layer of a contrasting color. When this jewelry was beveled on the edges or deeply carved, the color beneath was revealed, highlighting the design.

As with textile designs of the 1930s, playful polka dots were all the rage. Perky bangle bracelets, necklaces, rings, clips, earrings, and buttons contained colorful dots called "gum drops" which are now very collectible.

Another technique involved clear (now apple juice) Bakelite which was "reverse-carved" or "under-carved" (carved on the reverse side), usually in floral motifs. These carved areas were then painted in multicolored enamels which appeared three-dimensional from the front. (For examples of reverse-carved Bakelite buttons see Accessories and Related Items, Chapter 12.) Particularly amusing are the bangle bracelets with tiny reverse-carved fish which appear to be swimming around the wearer's wrist.

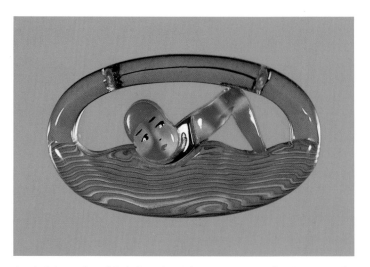

Apple juice colored Bakelite pin with reverse-painted swimmer and reverse-carved waves. *Courtesy of Mary Anne Faust (Yesterday's Delights).* $800-$1,000.

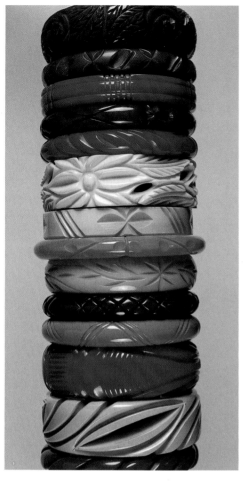

A tower of carved Bakelite bangle bracelets. Note: two pierced models. From center down - *Courtesy of Nancy Moyer*. $75-$500.

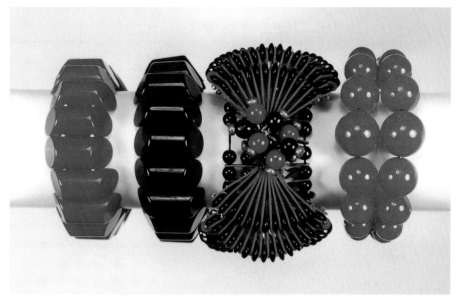

Bakelite bracelets in the desirable Art Deco colors - red and black. *Left:* Three elastic stretchy bracelets. $250-$300. *Right:* One red beaded wrap bracelet. $150-$200. *Courtesy of Mary Anne Faust (Yesterday's Delights).*

*Bracelets.* Bracelets were produced in a variety of styles. The most common was the bangle bracelet which could be plain, carved, laminated, metal clad, back carved, or hinged. Bangles with intricate, deeply-carved tropical flowers and foliage are very collectible today.

Other styles included "stretchy" bracelets (segments strung on elastic), charm bracelets, "wrap" bracelets (strung on coiled wire), and broad cuff-style bracelets. Wide tank-track bracelets with rows of large, overlapping links were inspired by machine-age technology.

Diana Vreeland owned several Chanel cuff bracelets made of Bakelite and embellished with multicolored faceted rhinestones. These bracelets sold at Sotheby's in 1987 for nearly $1,800 each.

*Necklaces.* German costume jewelry designers, influenced by the Bauhaus school of design, preferred to design sleek modernistic jewelry. They alternated smooth geometric-shaped Bakelite pieces with chrome, silver, or nickel-plated brass elements to form necklaces and bracelets with a stark "Machine Age" appearance. At times only one or two pieces of colored Bakelite were used as an accent for an all metal necklace. These accents were usually black, red, or green, common Art Deco colors.

In sharp contrast, American jewelry designers, preferred to let Bakelite stand on its own. They concentrated their talents on carving, laminating, painting, and setting Bakelite with glass stones. American Bakelite was gay and fanciful in nature. Thematic necklaces and bracelets contained charms which were all related to a particular subject such as fruits, vegetables, sporting goods, school supplies, tropical marine life, nautical motifs, south of the border (Mexican), patriotic symbols (late '30s, early '40s), and smoking paraphernalia. (Cigarette smoking, a habit which became popular during the 1920s, was very much a part of everyday life in the 1930s. It was considered so sophisticated that models and movie stars were often photographed nonchalantly holding a cigarette.)

*Clips and Pins.* Popular motifs for pins of the 1930s were Scottie dogs, horses, and whimsical animals with roly-poly eyes. Pins resembling ladies' wide-brim hats, hands, and shoes were also popular. Three-dimensional pins contained clusters of charms, suspended on a celluloid chain or plastic-coated string from a small placque or bar pin. The plaques often took on the shape of something relating to the charms, i.e. a globe, a pen nib, and a book suspended from a miniature ruler. Factory-made Bakelite brooches produced during the 1930s have a metal pin on the back which was either riveted on or the barbs on the back of the pin were pressed into the Bakelite before it hardened.

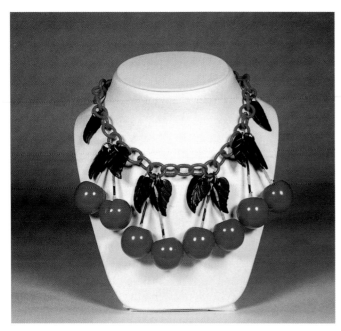

Necklace containing red Bakelite cherries and celluloid leaves on a celluloid chain. *Courtesy of Mary Anne Faust (Yesterday's Delights).* $225-$250.

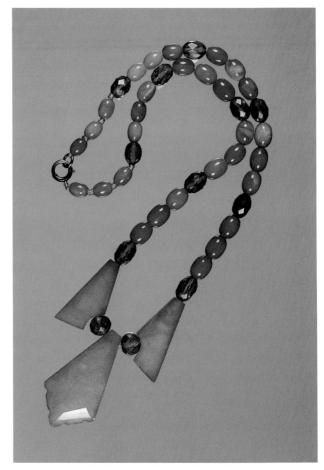

Art Deco-style necklace made of faceted amber and butterscotch-color Bakelite beads. *Courtesy of Margaret Place.* $200-$250.

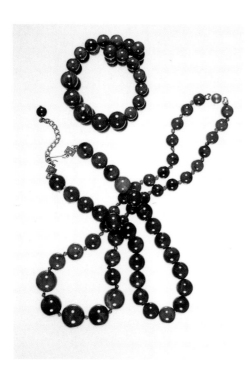

Two beaded necklaces and a wrap bracelet made of dark green Bakelite beads. *Courtesy of Mary Anne Faust (Yesterday's Delights).* $80.00 ea.

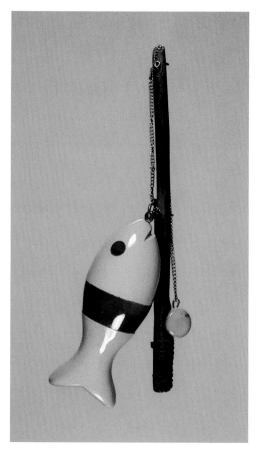

Pin containing a Bakelite fish and reel chained to a wooden fishing pole. *Courtesy of Carl Faust.* $150-$200.

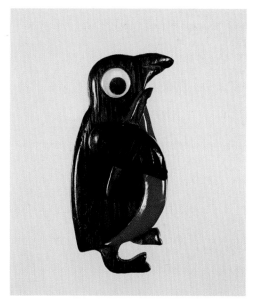

Wood and Bakelite penguin pin with googley eyes and an articulated arm. *Courtesy of Mary Anne Faust (Yesterday's Delights).* $200-$250.

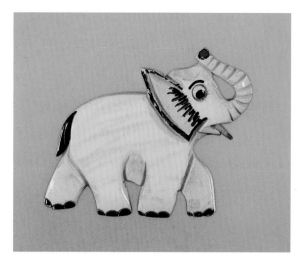

Yellow Bakelite and enamel elephant pin. *Courtesy of Mary Anne Faust (Yesterday's Delights).* $350-$400.

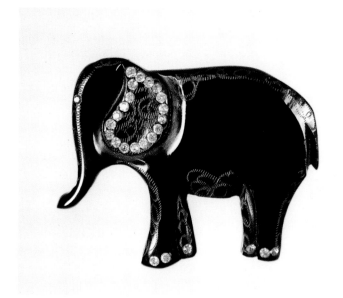

Black Bakelite elephant accented with rhinestones and engraving. *Courtesy of Ina Stoudt (Antique Treasures).* $350-$400.

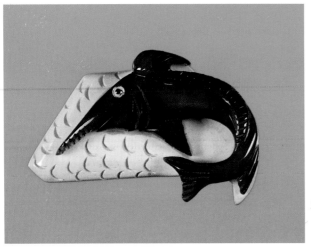

Green Bakelite swordfish dress clip accented with carvings and a glass eye. *Courtesy of Suzanne M. Checksfield.* $250-$300.

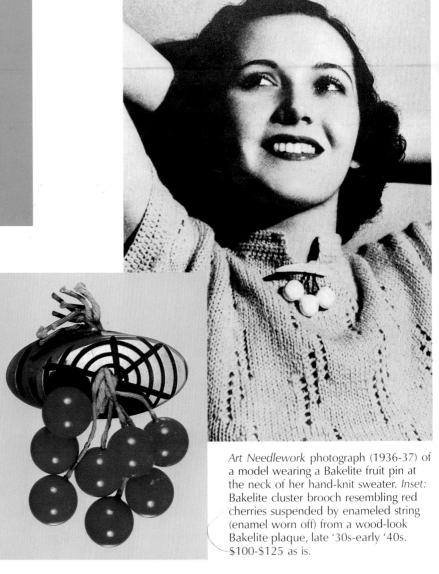

*Art Needlework* photograph (1936-37) of a model wearing a Bakelite fruit pin at the neck of her hand-knit sweater. *Inset:* Bakelite cluster brooch resembling red cherries suspended by enameled string (enamel worn off) from a wood-look Bakelite plaque, late '30s-early '40s. $100-$125 as is.

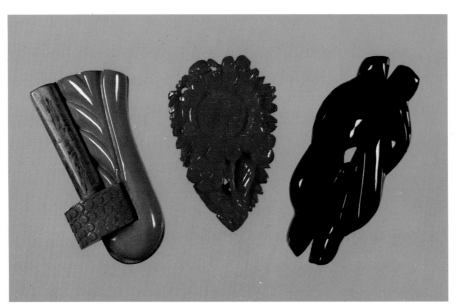

Carved Bakelite dress clips. *Left:* Orange Bakelite and wood clip. *Courtesy of Mary Anne Faust (Yesterday's Delights). Center:* Red floral clip. *Right:* Black square-knot clip. Marked: PAT 1852188 (1932). *Courtesy of Anna Shwak.* $100-$150 ea.

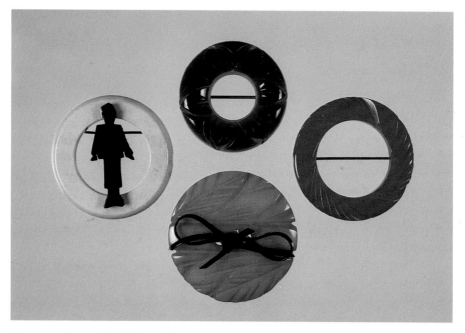

A quartet of carved Bakelite circle pins. Bottom pin is a converted button. *Courtesy of Mary Whitehouse.* $25-$50 ea.

***Earrings.*** Bakelite earrings were made in the dangle, hoop, or button style and contained screwback or clip-back findings.

# TECHNIQUES / STYLES

## Filigree

Filigree jewelry was extremely popular from the turn of the 20th century into the 1940s. It was used for pendants, bracelets, bar pins, earrings, rings, and circle pins. Filigree was originally fashioned by hand by twisting white gold or platinum wire into delicate openwork similar to lace. After the First World War, filigree was die-cast from white gold, sterling silver, brass, nickel, and base metal. Within this lacy framework stones were set in round, square, rectangular, hexagonal, octagonal, and marquise-shaped settings.

Inexpensive filigree jewelry set with *cabochons* and faceted glass stones was produced in Gablonz, Czechoslovakia, during the 1920s and 1930s. (At the end of World War I, the area known as Bohemia became part of Czechoslovakia. Production of jewelry was curtailed after the German invasion in 1939; therefore, jewelry marked Czechoslovakia can be dated between the two world wars.)

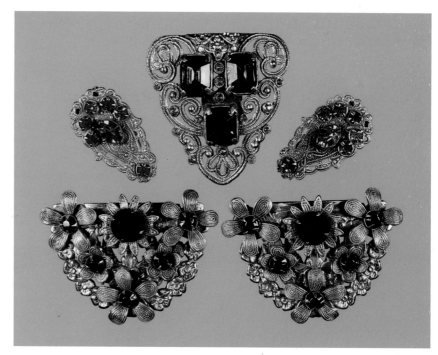

Five gold-plated Czechoslovakian Victorian-Revival filigree dress clips containing blue and black rhinestones. (Small pair) *Courtesy of Mary Anne Faust (Yesterday's Delights).* Small $50-$75. Large $100-$150.

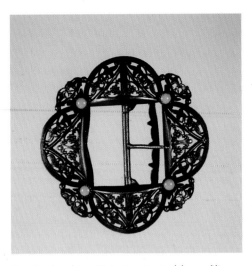

Czechoslovakian Victorian-Revival brass filigree buckle containing prong-set *faux* turquoise and mauve rhinestones. *Courtesy of Rose Jamieson.* $100-$125.

## Star-Cut Crystal

Jewelry made from "star-cut crystal" or crystal with the "star-burst cut" was extremely popular. The star-burst motif was originally etched into the reverse side of a thin piece of frosted rock crystal using a cutting tool. A diamond was set in the center of the star and the crystal was placed in a 14k white gold or gold-filled filigree setting. Star-cut crystal was made into pendants, pins, rings, earrings, bangle bracelets, and even men's tie clasps. Necklaces and bracelets were created by linking the crystal segments together or alternating them with plain filigree segments. Inexpensive imitation star-cut crystal was created from frosted glass (called "camphor glass") which was etched with acid to form the star burst. It was then set with a small diamond chip or clear rhinestone and placed in a rhodium or silver-plated setting.

## Pavé Settings

Pavé is the technique for setting small gems or rhinestones so close together that they cover the piece with continuous sparkle. Pavé means paved in French, implying that this jewelry is paved like a cobblestone street. Fine jewelers used this method for setting diamonds and precious gems in platinum and white gold. It was imitated by costume jewelers who pavé-set marcasite in sterling or rhinestones in base metal. Many of the Art Deco and Retro Modern clips, brooches, bracelets, and rings of the 1930s were embellished with pavé-set rhinestones.

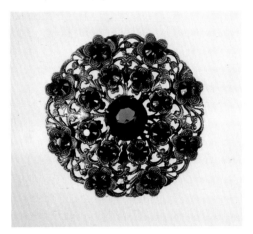

Czechoslovakian Victorian-Revival gold-plated filigree brooch set with blue rhinestones. $75-$100.

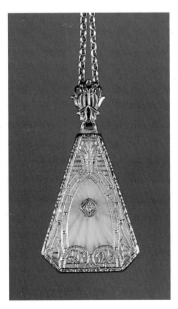

Star-cut crystal pendant set in silver-plated filigree frame with diamond center. *Courtesy of Jan Landis.* $50-$75.

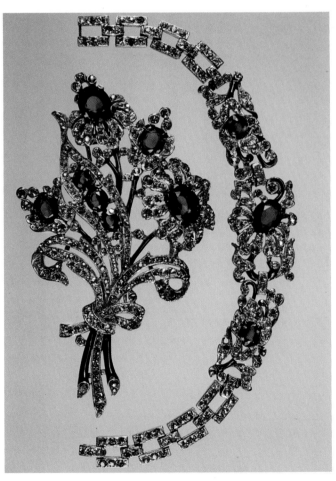

Rhodium-plated fur clip and matching bracelet accented with green oval and pavé-set clear round rhinestones. Marked: Trifari, DES PAT 123,173 (1940). $150-$200 ea.

The "all white" look of the early 1930s was exemplified by movie star Jean Harlow with her platinum-blonde hair and white satin gowns dripping with white fox or marabou. All white jewelry made of platinum and pavé-set diamonds was promoted by Cartier, Fouquet, and many other fine jewelry designers. It was imitated by costume jewelers, at a fraction of the cost, using marcasite and silver or clear rhinestones and base metal.

Rhinestone jewelry should be stored in individual plastic bags so that the prongs from one will not scratch another. Plastic bags are also useful to safeguard any stones which might work their way loose from the settings.

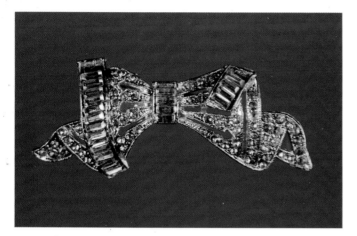

All-white rhodium-plated bow brooch with pavé set round and *baguette* rhinestones. *Courtesy of Rose Jamieson.* $75-$100.

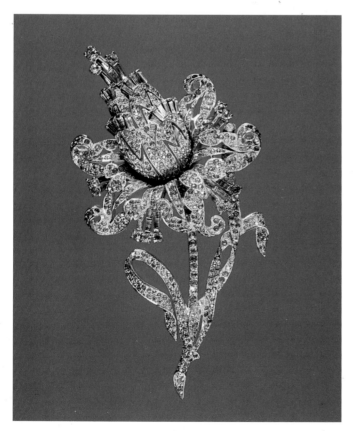

All-white rhodium-plated floral brooch with pavé-set clear rhinestones. Marked: Mazer. *Courtesy of Bonny Yankauer (Menagerie).* $300-$500.

## Cabochons

Smooth, round, dome-shaped *cabochon*-cut stones were frequently used in 1920s and 1930s jewelry. The stones most often cut *en cabochon* were amazonite, moonstone, and star sapphires. Glass *cabochons* for use in costume jewelry were produced in Gablonz, Czechoslovakia, in a variety of colors, shapes, and sizes. Various shapes included round, oval, triangular, diamond, and square cushion-shaped *cabochons*. These stones were either prong or bezel set in gold, silver, or rhodium-plated base metal jewelry, often accented with a common foliate motif consisting of two enameled leaves and a berry.

***Transparent Cabochons.*** Rock crystal or clear glass *cabochons* were used in the production of sports jewelry, discussed later in this chapter.

***Satin Glass Cabochons.*** Cabochons made of colored glass with a slight matte finish were called satin glass. These cabochons could be found in many costume jewelry pieces of the 1930s.

***Mottled Cabochons.*** Glass *cabochons* could have a mottled appearance by introducing tiny glass chips of one shade into glass of a slightly lighter shade of the same color.

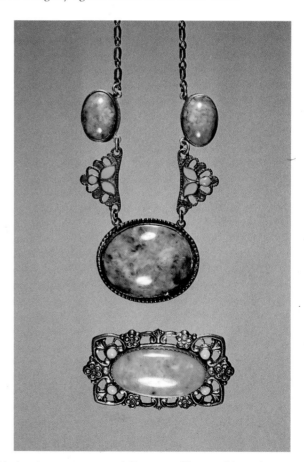

Gold-plated Victorian-Revival filigree necklace and brooch containing green mottled glass cabochons. The enameled leaf and berry design on the green and accompanying yellow cabochon necklace was a common motif used in Czechoslovakian jewelry of the late '20s-early '30s. *Courtesy of Roseann Ettinger (Remember When....)* Necklace $70-$80. Brooch $50-$75.

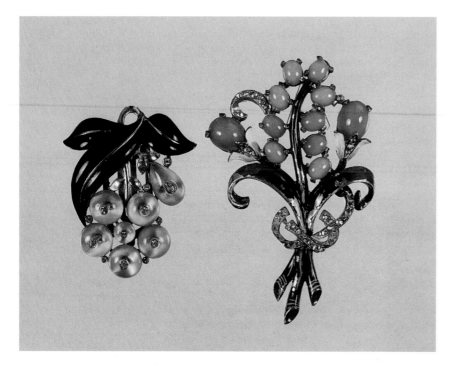

Victorian-Revival cabochon brooches. *Left:* Gold-plated, blue simulated moonstone cabochons with rhinestone centers, enamel. *Right:* Silver-plated, pink glass cabochons, enamel. *Courtesy of Roxanne Stuart.* $75-$150 ea.

***Moonstone Cabochons****.* Moonstone is a pale blue-gray translucent gemstone with an inner opaline luster, which is usually cut *en cabochon.* Imitation glass moonstones were produced by combining a bottom layer of opaque colored glass with a top layer of clear glass. By viewing the *cabochon* from the side, one can see the two layers. It was produced in a variety of colors (including yellow, pink, blue, and green) which were described in mail-order catalogs as "yellow moonstone" or "pink moonstone." (Plastic opaline *cabochons* of the 1940s do not have the discernible layers and the surface has a different feel then glass.)

***Star Cabochons****.* A six-pointed star of reflected light, called an asterism, is a phenomenon found in *cabochon*-cut star sapphires. This star-effect was imitated by glass makers, using not only the blue of sapphires, but other colors such as yellow and pink.

## Cluster Jewelry

***Wired Clusters****.* The queen of "cluster jewelry" was Miriam Haskell, a jewelry designer who began her career in the early '20s. Inspired by Victorian jewelry, she created a unique style which is easy to recognize. When making cluster jewelry, Haskell began with a perforated metal or flexible mesh base to which she painstakingly hand wired Czechoslovakian glass beads, rhinestones, molded-glass leaves, and of course scores of her tiny signature pearls. She arranged these elements into complicated three-dimensional abstract designs or clusters of flowers resembling miniature Hawaiian leis. The technique of wiring jewelry elements into necklaces, wrap bracelets, and earrings was soon imitated by other costume jewelry manufacturers using such materials as glass, wood, celluloid, bakelite, and metal.

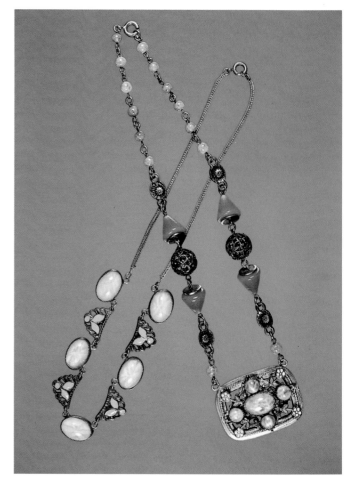

*Left:* Yellow-glass star cabochons alternate with enameled leaf and berry segments. *Right:* Mottled blue glass cabochons set in openwork silver-plated brass plaque. Both made in Czechoslovakia, late '20s-early '30s. $75-$100.

166

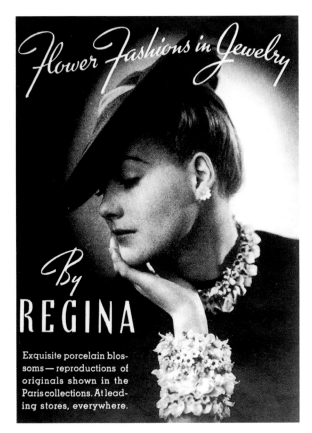

This ad for cluster jewelry by Regina appeared in *Harper's Bazaar* (3/15/38). It features porcelain trumpet flowers and leaves.

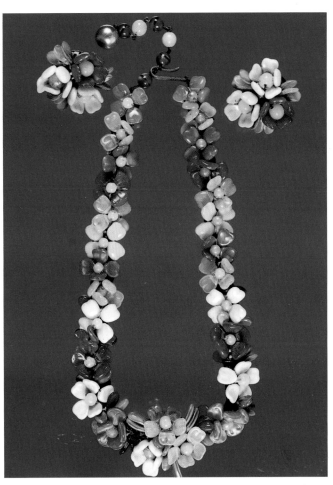

Miriam Haskell-style miniature-lei necklace and earrings of multicolored glass petals with *faux*-pearl centers and pressed-glass leaves, all wired to mesh backing. Marked: Germany. $75-$100.

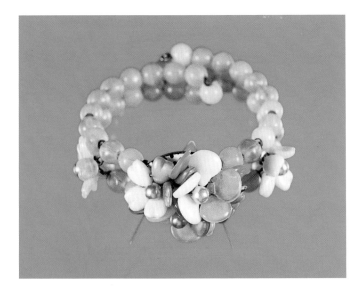

Floral-cluster wrap bracelet made of glass beads and petals with *faux*-pearl centers. *Courtesy of Mary Anne Faust (Yesterday's Delights).* $60-$75.

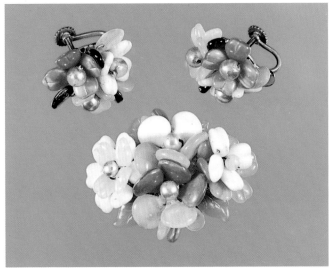

Floral-cluster brooch $50, earrings $40. *Courtesy of Mary Anne Faust (Yesterday's Delights).*

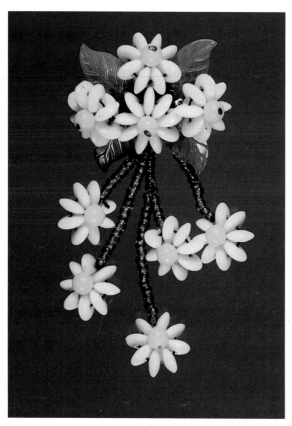

**Suspended Clusters.** Cluster jewelry was also made by suspending elements from silk cord or chains made of celluloid or metal. These elements included tiny Czechoslovakian lampworked-glass flowers, fruits, bells, balls, and birds. Green molded-glass leaves were very common in cluster jewelry. A fine wire was embedded in each leaf, which was used to secure it to the jewelry. These leaves were very fragile and it is common to find cluster jewelry with a few or all of the leaves missing. Sometimes all that remains are the tiny wires still wrapped around the chain links.

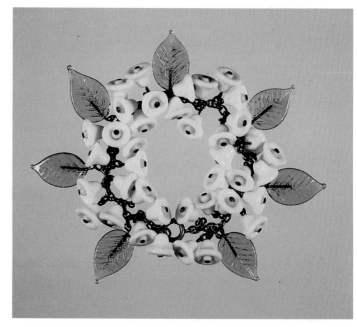

Daisy cluster pin made from white rondells with yellow bead centers, pressed-glass leaves, and seed bead stems. $60-$75.

Cluster bracelet made of white Czechoslovakian-glass bell flowers and green pressed-glass leaves. $45-$60.

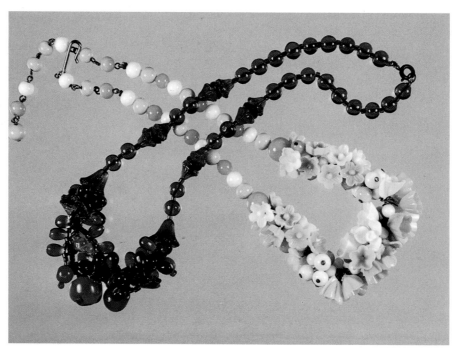

Czechoslovakian cluster necklaces. *Left:* Purple glass beads with lampworked fruit beads. *Right:* Pastel beads with lampworked flower-head beads. $100-$125.

168

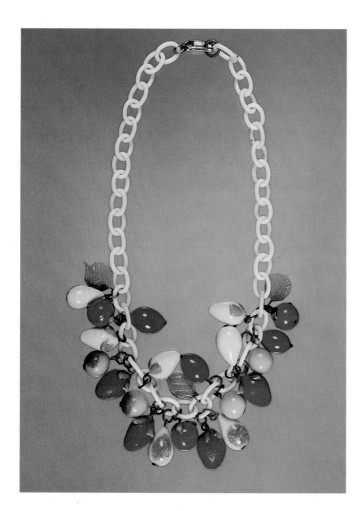

Cluster necklace containing colorful glass fruit and pressed-glass leaves suspended from celluloid chain. *Courtesy of F. Paul Laubner.*

Cluster necklace and matching bracelet containing large gold-plated brass buds. $25-$50.

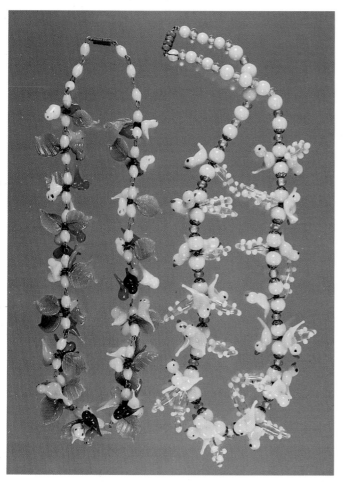

Two cluster necklaces made with tiny lampworked glass birds, leaves, and berries. $100-$150.

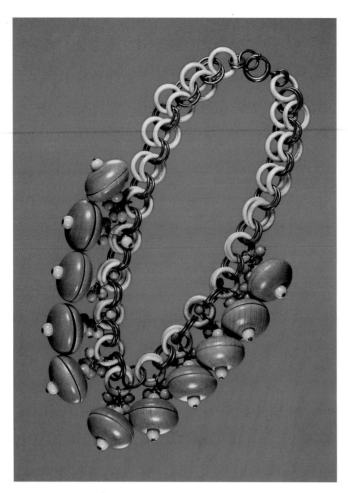

Necklace made of wooden baubles suspended from a celluloid and brass chain. *Courtesy of Mary Anne Faust (Yesterday's Delights).* $75-$100.

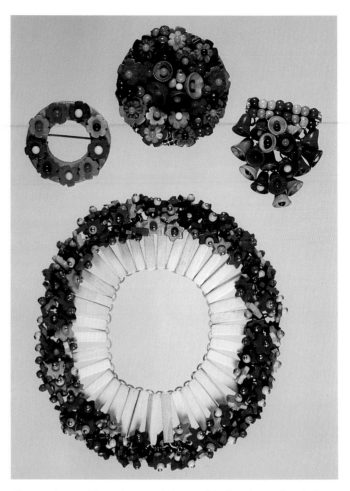

Cluster pins and bracelet containing multicolored wood and glass beads from Czechoslovakia. $60-$70.

Miriam Haskell also created "bubble" necklaces and bracelets featuring hollow-glass bubbles fastened to a silk cord or metal chain. This technique was imitated by other jewelry manufacturers who also suspended glass bubbles from brooches or placed them on the tips of hat ornaments. They were made of colored or enameled glass as well as clear glass filled with colorful chenille yarn or shiny tinsel.

Unfortunately the wires on cluster jewelry are susceptible to corrosion and jewelry in an advanced stage often falls apart.

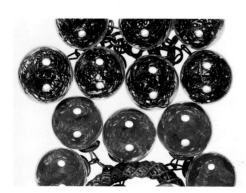

Close-up of glass bubbles containing blue tinsel and orange chenille.

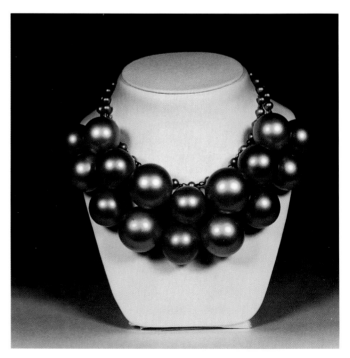

Necklace containing large pink pearlized-glass bubbles fastened to a metal chain containing small pink pearls. *Courtesy of Mary Anne Faust (Yesterday's Delights).* $175-$225.

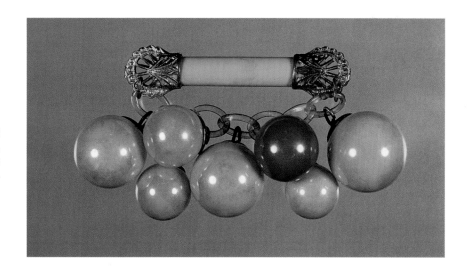

Pearlized-glass bubbles suspended on a celluloid chain from brass filigree and enamel bar pin. *Courtesy of Mary Anne Faust (Yesterday's Delights)*. $75-$100.

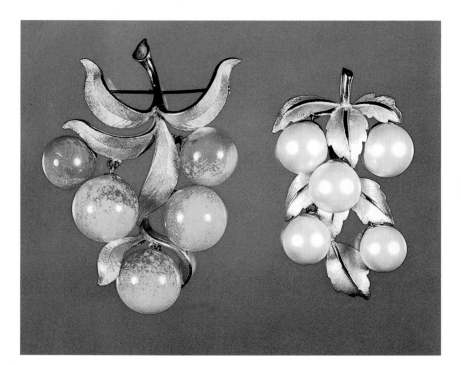

Gold and silver-plated bubble brooches. *Courtesy of Mary Anne Faust (Yesterday's Delights)*.

# MOTIFS

## Monogram and Name Jewelry

Art Deco geometric-shaped monogram pins were created in round, oval, rectangular, diamond, or marquise shapes. They usually featured three cut-out block-style or script initials. Monogram pins were made of sterling or rhodium-plated base metal decorated with pavé-set marcasites or rhinestones. For greater contrast, the letters were often set against a black or green background which could be onyx, Bakelite, or enamel. Some pins were custom made by piercing the initials by hand. Less expensive versions contained grooves, channels, dovetails, or prongs under which the desired interchangeable, pre-formed letters were inserted. A style which surfaced towards the end of the decade featured a plain, modernistic bar pin from which three individual initials were suspended on chains.

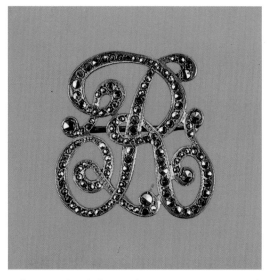

The initial "R" made of silver and pavé-set marcasite. Marked: sterling. *Courtesy of Rose Jamieson*. $70-$80.

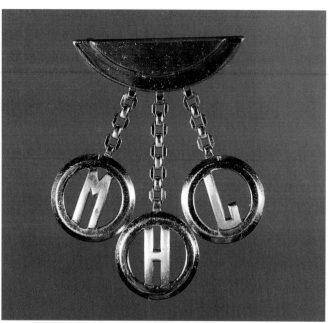

Chrome-plated modernistic bar pin containing the initials MHL suspended by square open-link chains. A similar pin appeared in the 1936-37 Sears, Roebuck and Co. catalog. Marked: Monocraft. $40-$50.

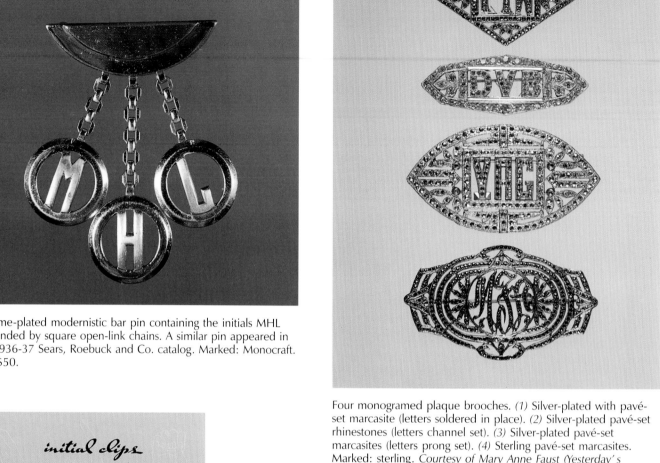

Four monogramed plaque brooches. *(1)* Silver-plated with pavé-set marcasite (letters soldered in place). *(2)* Silver-plated pavé-set rhinestones (letters channel set). *(3)* Silver-plated pavé-set marcasites (letters prong set). *(4)* Sterling pavé-set marcasites. Marked: sterling. *Courtesy of Mary Anne Faust (Yesterday's Delights).* Top 3: $30-$50. Bottom: $75-$100.

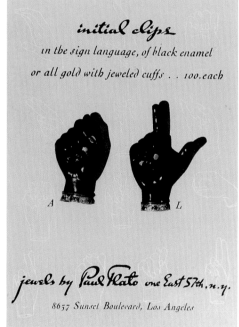

These clever monogram clips by Paul Flato appeared in *Harper's Bazaar* (1/38). Each black-enameled hand with jeweled cuff represented a letter of the alphabet in sign language.

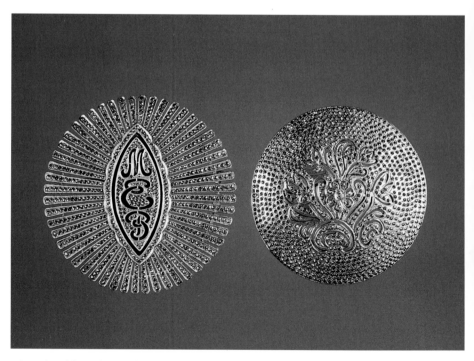

Silver-plated brooches with pavé-set marcasite. *Left:* Sunburst with pierced monogram over black celluloid underlay. A similar brooch appeared in the L.&C. Mayers jewelry catalog (1939). Marked: sterling. $50-$75. *Right:* Plaque brooch with pierced foliate design. Marked: Sterling. *Courtesy of Rose Jamieson.* $100-$125.

172

Fine jewelry designer, Paul Flato, took the initial pin concept one step further. He designed clever "sign-language" brooches and cuff links each resembling a human hand signing a particular letter of the alphabet.

## Sports Jewelry

Sports jewelry was introduced in the 1930s to complement the tailored suits, coats, blazers, and sweaters worn by sports enthusiasts. The ubiquitous Scottie dog, inspired by FDR's dog "Fala," was a special favorite, along with the wire-haired terrier, popularized by the 1930s *Thin Man* movies staring William Powell and Myrna Loy. Sail boats, horses, trout, foxes, and stop-action figures engaged in sports activities were also popular. These motifs were incorporated in pins and segmented bracelets. Each segment was stamped with a cutout silhouette of one of these motifs or they were reverse painted on the underside of small round, square, or rectangular clear-glass *cabochons*. Slender bar pins were made to resemble the accoutrements of various sports such as golf clubs, riding crops, horse bits, polo mallets, tennis rackets, and fishing poles. (See examples of sports tie clips in Men's Wear, Chapter 13).

Bakelite cluster pins, charm bracelets, and necklaces contained charms associated with a particular sport. Popular sports themes and associated charms included riding (horseshoes, nails, stirrups, bits, hurdles, hunting horns), golf (clubs, balls, tees), tennis (rackets, balls, sneakers), archery (bows, arrows, targets), football (helmets, megaphones, footballs, shoes), baseball (bats, mitts, and balls), and nautical (sailboats, ship's wheels, anchors, life preservers, signal flags). Bakelite was also used for horse head and sailboat pins.

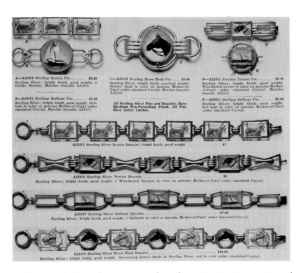

This sterling sports jewelry appeared in the L. & C. Mayers jewelry catalog (1939). It features sailboats, horse heads, Scotties, and wire-haired terriers either in silhouette or enameled under simulated-crystal cabochons.

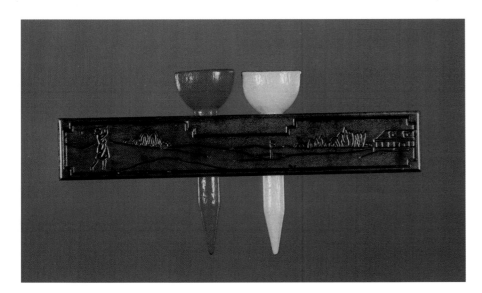

Gold-plated bar pin with an engraved woman golfer. Reverse side contains brackets for golf tees. Marked: Tee Addle, Herff-Jones Co., Indianapolis. $40-$50.

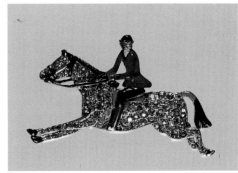

Rhodium-plated horse and rider pin embellished with pavé-set rhinestones and enamel. Marked: Trifari. *Courtesy of Bonny Yankauer (Menagerie).* $100-$200.

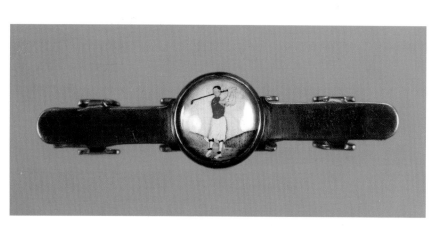

Silver bar pin containing a golfer painted on the reverse side of a clear-glass cabochon. Marked: sterling. *Courtesy of Mary Anne Faust (Yesterday's Delights).* $40-$50.

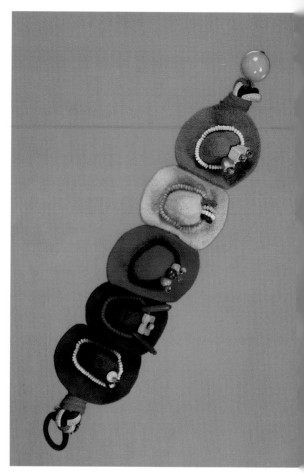

Novelty bracelet made of tiny multicolored-felt Tyrolean hats decorated with glass and wooden beads. $35-$45.

## Figural Jewelry

Figural jewelry was made in the likeness of living creatures including humans, animals, birds, and fish. These were made of metal, celluloid, Bakelite, and wood in the form of brooches and fur clips. Scottie pins were extremely popular and are known as "cross-over" collectibles which are sought after by jewelry collectors as well as Scottie enthusiasts.

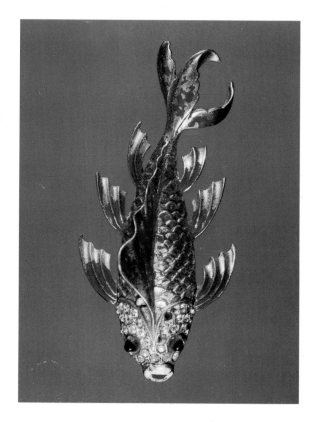

Gold-plated and enameled fish brooch featuring pair of articulated fins, set with rhinestones and glass eyes. Marked: MB (Marcel Boucher original prototype.) *Courtesy of Mary Anne Faust (Yesterday's Delights).* $200-$250.

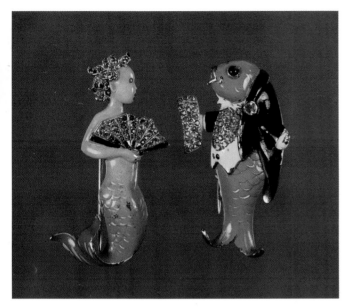

Mermaid and fish fur clips decorated with pavé-set rhinestones and enamel. *Courtesy of Roxanne Stuart*. Rare.

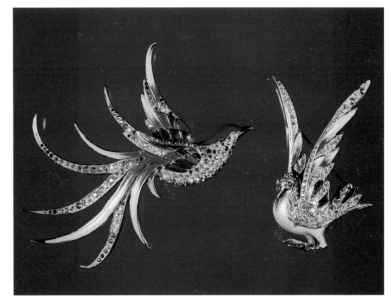

Rhodium-plated bird brooches decorated with pavé-set rhinestones and enamel. Marked: MB. (Marcel Boucher original prototypes.) *Courtesy of Mary Anne Faust (Yesterday's Delights)*. $275-$325 ea.

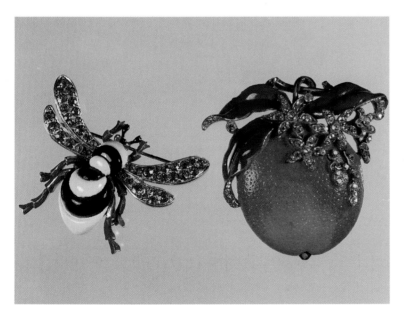

Rhodium-plated bee pin and orange clip embellished with enamel and pavé-set rhinestones. Both marked: Trifari. *Courtesy of Bonny Yankauer (Menagerie)*. Bee $100-$200. / Orange $400-$600.

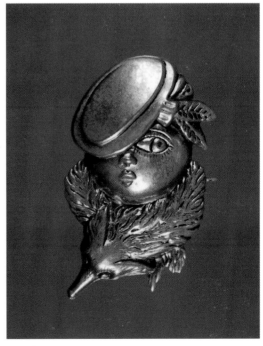

Gold-plated brass brooch, woman wearing early 1930s hat and fox-fur piece. *Courtesy of Mary Anne Faust (Yesterday's Delights)*. $40-$50.

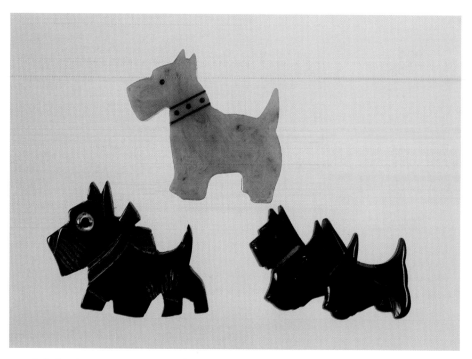

Bakelite Scottie pins. *Top:* Mottled butterscotch with black enamel. *Courtesy of Anna Shwak. Left:* Green, carved with glass eye. *Courtesy of Roxanne Stuart. Right:* Green twins, gold enamel. $40-$80.

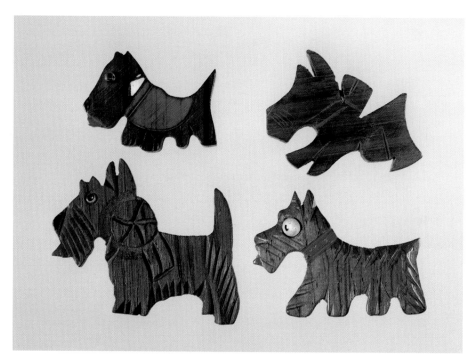

Wooden Scottie pins. Several decorated with enamel and glass eyes. Lower left - *Courtesy of Rose Jamieson.* $10-$60.

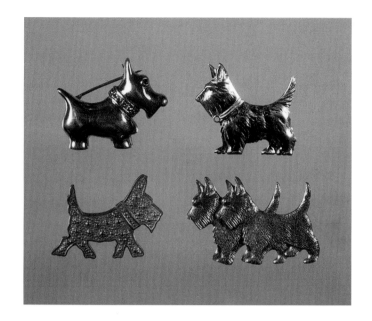

Metal Scottie pins. *Top left:* Sterling with marcasite collar and green glass eye. Marked: 825. *Top right:* Missing opposing Scottie and connecting chain. Marked: sterling. *Bottom left:* Brass. *Bottom right:* Marked - Beau sterling. $25-$80 ea.

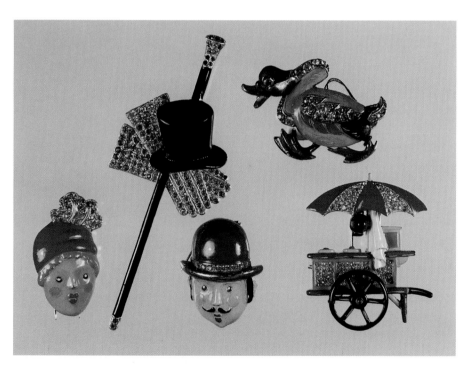

Whimsical rhodium-plated pins all decorated with enamel and pavé-set rhinestones. All marked: Trifari. *Courtesy of Bonny Yankauer (Menagerie).* $100-$350.

Other popular motifs of the 1930s were the Maltese cross (favored by Chanel) and the scimitar (a curved Arabian sword).

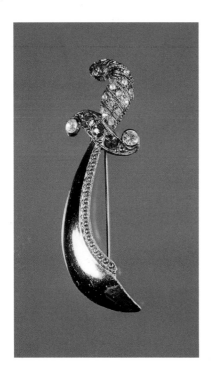

Gold-plated scimitar brooch set with blue and clear rhinestones. $25-$45.

# JEWELRY FORMS

## Clips and Double-Clip Brooches

In lieu of the extravagant beadwork so typical of 1920s evening wear, elegant, understated gowns of the 1930s were accented with glittering dress clips, brooches, buckles, and clasps. They were produced in platinum and gem stones, silver and marcasite, or base metal and rhinestones.

*Dress Clips.* The most popular form of jewelry, during the first half of the decade, was the dress clip which was usually produced in Art Deco-style geometric designs. Dress clips may be recognized by the flat hinged clamp on the back of the clip, which contains sharp barbs to grip the fabric. Sold singly or in pairs, they could be clipped to the edge of a lapel, the base of the popular V-shaped neckline, or at the corners of the square, boat, or sweetheart necklines. They could also be fastened to either side of the draped cowl neckline to create a squared-off look. Clips added interest to the shoulders or accented the deep back openings so popular during the late '20s and early '30s. They were even used to accent hats, belts, or evening bags.

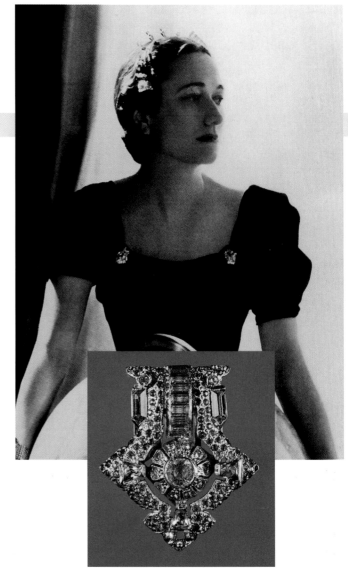

*Harper's Bazaar* published this photograph (7/37) of the Duchess of Windsor wearing dress clips in the popular arrow motif. *Insert:* Similar Art Deco all-white arrow dress clip in base metal and rhinestones. $50-$75.

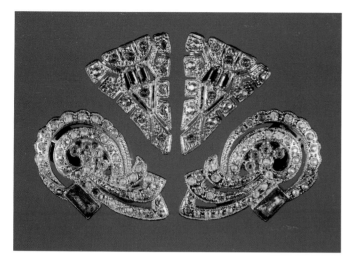

Dress clips of base metal and pavé-set rhinestones and yellow *baguettes*. Top - *Courtesy of Mary Anne Faust (Yesterday's Delights)*. $30-$60. pair.

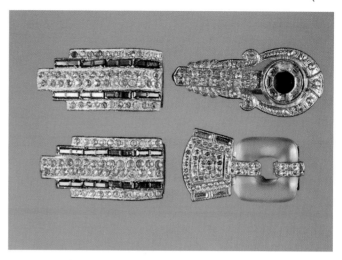

Art Deco-style dress clips made of base metal with pavé-set rhinestones, colored *baguettes*, and frosted glass. *Courtesy of Mary Anne Faust (Yesterday's Delights)*. $40-$50 ea.

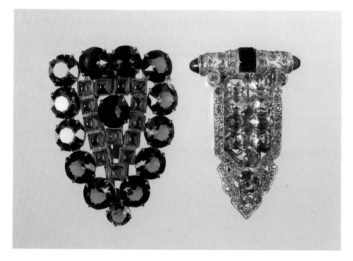

Art Deco-style dress clips decorated with multicolored faceted and cabochon-cut stones. *Courtesy of Roxanne Stuart*. $75-$100 ea.

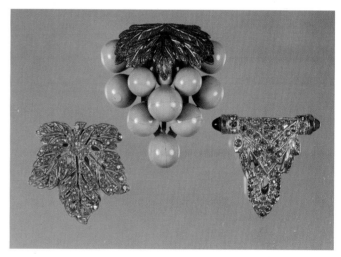

A trio of dress clips. *Top:* Simulated grapes of green plastic, leaf of gold-plated brass. *Left:* Gold-plated base-metal leaf with pavé set clear rhinestones. *Right:* Rhodium-plated base metal accented with green glass cabochons and pavé-set clear rhinestones. *Courtesy of Betsey Pacini*. $40-$50 ea.

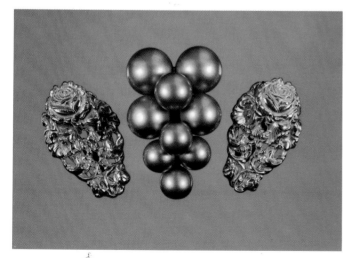

*Left & Right:* Pair of gold-plated base-metal dress clips. *Center:* Dress clip made of gold-plated glass bubbles. *Courtesy of Rose Jamieson*. $40-$50 ea.

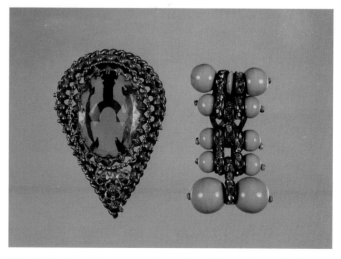

*Left:* Gold-plated base-metal dress clip with large faceted yellow rhinestone. *Right:* Dress clip of turquoise glass beads and rhinestones. $40-$50.

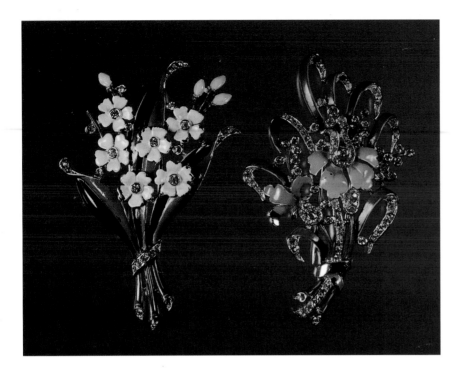

Retro Modern rhodium plated floral-bouquet fur clips accented with enamel and clear rhinestones. Both marked: Trifari. $75-$110 ea.

***Fur Clips***. Dress clips were replace by fur clips during the second half of the decade. They can be recognized by the two sharp needle-like prongs hinged to the reverse side of the clip. Fur clips were attached to fur coats and capes or woolen suits and coats by pushing the prongs into, then out of the fur or fabric. A third tiny curved prong on the underside of the clip also gripped the fabric and held the clip closed. This mechanism allowed the wearer to place the clip in the middle of the fabric rather than at the edge, like a dress clip. Fur clips were also fastened to muffs and crocheted handbags.

While dress clips had a hard-edged geometric look, fur clips were more open and three-dimensional with the soft, fluid lines of Retro Modern. Asymmetrical floral bouquets or figurals were the most common motifs for fur clips. They were generally made of rhodium-plated base metal accented with rhinestones and enamel. Many fur clips were marked with the maker's name and/or a patent number.

***Double-clip Brooches***. In 1927 Cartier patented the versatile "double-clip" brooch. This unique piece of jewelry consisted of two dress clips or fur clips which could be fastened together, by the use of a metal frame, to form a brooch. Art Deco-style double-dress-clip brooches from the first half of the decade were generally "mirror image," while the halves of double-fur-clip brooches from the mid-to-late '30s could be quite different from one another, creating an asymmetrical brooch when joined together. The double-clip brooch was widely imitated by costume jewelry firms such as Trifari and Coro. In 1931, Coro patented its version of the double-clip brooch using the trade name "Coro Duette." The maker and the patent number were often marked on the piece. (It should be noted that some double-clip brooches have two patent numbers, one on the frame and one on the clips. The invention patent for the frame mechanism may have been issued in the early '30s, while the design patent for the clips themselves could be from a later date.) Double-clip brooches remained popular into the 1940s and are quite collectible today.

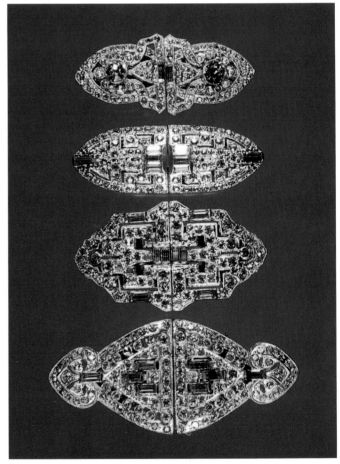

Four Art Deco all-white double dress-clip brooches containing pavé-set rhinestones. (1) Rhodium-plated. Marked: PAT. 1798867 (1931) *Mary Anne Faust.* (2) Rhodium-plated. Marked: PAT. 1798867 (1931) on frame and PAT. 1852188 (1932) on clip. (3) Rhodium-plated. Marked: PAT. 2044225 (1936) *Elizabeth Whitfield.* (4) Silver-plated. Marked: PAT. 2044225 (1936). *Mildred Kelly.* $75-$110 ea.

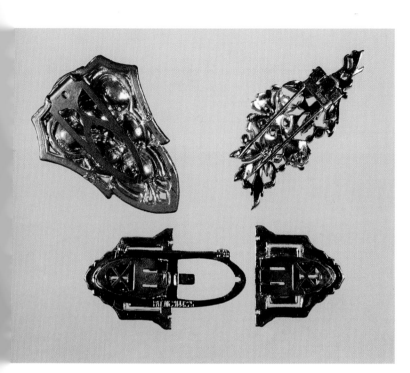

The reverse side of clips and a double-clip brooch. *Left:* Dress clip with flat hinged clamp. *Right:* Fur clip with two hinged prongs. *Bottom:* Double-clip brooch showing one dress clip removed from the oval frame which holds the two clips together to form a brooch.

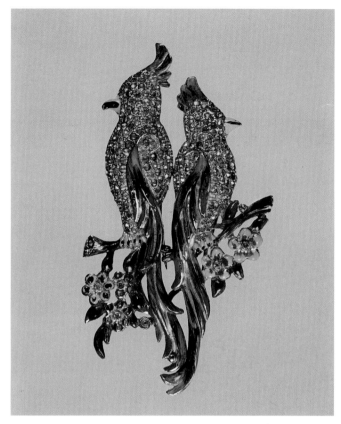

Asymmetrical Retro-Modern rhodium-plated bird-of-paradise double fur-clip brooch embellished with rhinestones and enamel. Marked: Coro Duette, PAT. 1798867 (1931) on the frame and PAT. 1164?? [illegible] (1939) on clip. $200-$375.

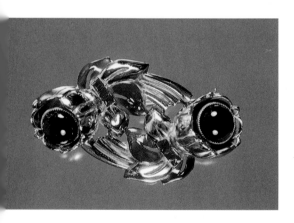

Asymmetrical gold-plated double fur-clip brooch, red cabochons and square glass stones, green enameled leaves. Marked: Coro Duette, PAT 1798867 (1931) on the frame. $125-$150.

## Brooches/Pins

Rectangular, oval, round, or lozenge-shaped "plaque" brooches were pavé-set with precious or semi-precious stones, rhinestones, or marcasites. Many 1930s brooches had a geometric-shaped frame which encompassed an intricate openwork central design.

Retro-Modern brooches were characterized by light, airy, asymmetrical floral sprays and figurals embellished with rhinestones and colorful enamels.

The novel *tremblant* brooch featured one (or more) elements fastened to it by the use of a tiny spring(s). The spring caused the elements to quiver as the wearer moved about. Typical motifs were animals with bobbing heads and flowers with trembling blossoms. This technique was introduced during the 18th century and is also know by the names "trembler," "nodder," "bobbler," and "springer."

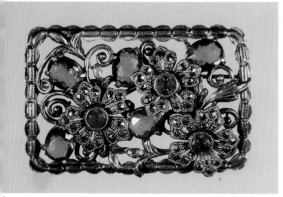

Silver-plated base-metal plaque brooch with rectangular frame and openwork floral design decorated with marcasite, and blue and purple glass stones. *Courtesy of Margaret Place.* $30-$40.

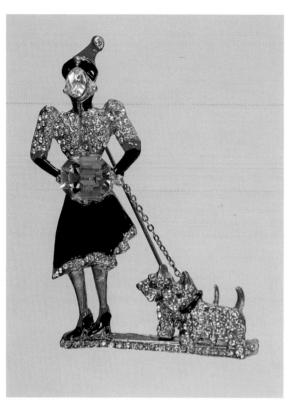

Woman walking *tremblant* Scotties. Rhodium-plated and enameled base metal with pavé-set rhinestones, larger faceted stones for face and muff, late '30s. *Courtesy of Roxanne Stuart.* $200-$250.

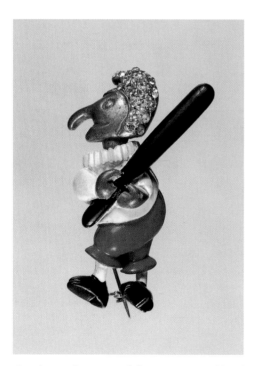

Rhodium-plated "Punch" pin (English puppet), *tremblant* head, pavé-set rhinestones and enamel. Marked: Chanel (script). *Courtesy of Bonny Yankauer (Menagerie).* $2,500-$3,500.

## Necklaces

Short, beaded necklaces were made of semi-precious materials such as rock crystal, rose quartz, carnelian, chrysoprase, jade, topaz, amethyst and amber. Beads imitating semi-precious stones were made of glass or Bakelite. The beads were cut in a variety of geometric shapes including the sphere, cube, prism, cylinder, pear, and lantern (diamond). A majority of these necklaces were made of graduated stones which were either smooth, frosted, carved, or faceted. The beads were often alternated with tiny gold-filled spacers or smaller beads in a contrasting color. The most popular lengths were 15 to 18 inches. Beaded necklaces were strung on a fine chrome-plated chain or waxed silk cord and were fastened with screw-barrel, spring-ring, or fish-hook findings.

Pearls and other beads were often strung in interesting configurations imitating necklaces designed by Cartier. A necklace might have three strands on the top (around the neck) and five strands on the bottom (over the bust) joined together on either side by pavé-set rhinestone ornaments. Unusual "back drop" necklaces featured two or three dangling beaded ends suspended

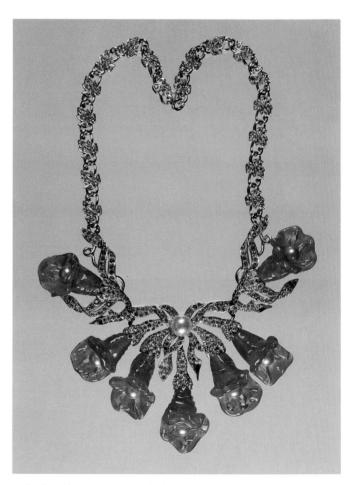

Pink glass lilies accented with *faux* pearls suspended from a rhodium-plated necklace covered with pavé-set clear rhinestones. Marked: MB (Marcel Boucher). *Courtesy of Bonny Yankauer (Menagerie).* Rare.

from the clasp at the back of the neck. They were designed to accent the deep, plunging necklines at the backs of dresses during the late 1920s and early '30s.

For Schiaparelli's Zodiac Collection, Jean Clément designed a necklace containing bright enameled-metal links resembling various star signs. Schiaparelli's Pagan Collection of 1938 included an outrageous necklace made from a clear-perspex (plastic) collar embedded with enameled metal insects. At first glance the wearer appeared to be crawling with bugs! Designs of this type were characteristic of Schiaparelli's playful nature.

## Bracelets

It was considered quite stylish to wear several glittering bracelets on each wrist. Whether made of diamonds or rhinestones, they generally contained numerous flexible segments with geometric or oriental-style links. Diamonds or clear rhinestones were pavé-set in even rows or in abstract openwork designs, often accented with colored stones.

Chanel often wore her famous twin bangle bracelets designed for her by the Duke of Verdura. They were made of white enameled metal and decorated with large colored stones in the form of Maltese crosses, a motif revived by Kenneth Jay Lane in the 1960s.

## Earrings

Long pendant earrings, worn by flappers of the previous decade, were still worn for the evening, while button earrings became the accepted style for day wear. Mercury wings and hoops were popular motifs. The new "clip-on" style findings (patented in 1934) began to replace pierced and screw-back styles. Art Deco-style earrings often incorporated a variety of geometric shapes and cuts.

## Rings

Due to the poor economy, smaller diamonds and gemstones were used in the creation of rings. They were mounted in "illusion" settings to give the appearance of a larger stone.

Large semi-precious stones such as aquamarine, topaz, citrine, zircons, and carnelian were in demand as substitutes for more expensive gemstones. They were cut into a variety of bold geometric shapes and were often accented with marcasites.

The reversible Romany ring provided the wearer with two rings in one. The top surface of the ring flipped over to reveal a different head on the reverse side. The customer could chose from two of the following heads: a cameo, birthstone, onyx with a diamond center, or a star-cut crystal.

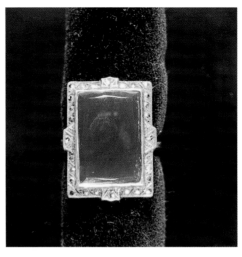

Sterling-silver Art Deco-style ring with large rectangular sardonyx stone surrounded by marcasite. Marked: sterling. *Courtesy of Jan Landis.* $60-$80.

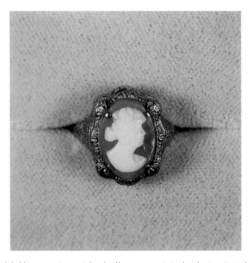

White-gold filigree ring with shell cameo. Marked: A&S 10k. *Courtesy of Margaret Place.* $90-$110.

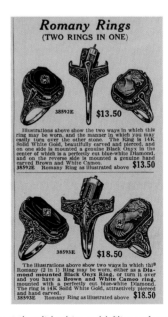

Romany rings in 14k solid white-gold filigree from the Baird-North jewelry catalog (1930). These rings can either be worn on the black onyx and diamond side or the hand-carved cameo side, 1930.

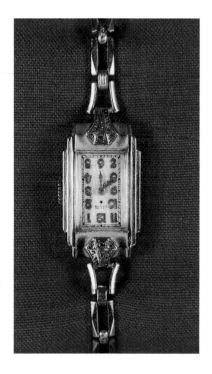

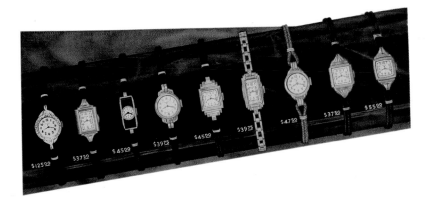

Left: Rectangular Art Deco-style watch by Elgin incorporating the popular step design, band of rectangular open links. Marked: Simmons, PAT 1,966,063 (1934). *Courtesy of Elizabeth Pascoe Whitfield.* $175-$200.

Below: Watches by Elgin. Note: geometric-shapes, step design, and bands of black-silk cord or square open links.

## Watches

Watches were produced in a variety of geometric shapes, including the rectangle, square, circle, hexagon, or variations of these shapes. They were made of platinum, 14k white gold, or gold filled and were often engraved with mini-border designs. The 1939 L.& C. Mayers Co. wholesale catalog offered platinum watches and bands set with diamonds. Women's watch bands were made of filigree, tiny brick-work links (like the Ludo bracelet), woven mesh, black grosgrain ribbon, black silk cord, gold mouse-tail chain, or square, rectangular, or circular open links.

# FINE JEWELRY DESIGNERS

Large French jewelry firms such as Cartier, Van Cleef & Arpels, and Boucheron were in the forefront of jewelry design and an inspiration to other smaller firms such as Jean Fouquet, Raymond Templier, and Jean Després. Tiffany was the largest producer of fine jewelry in the United States.

# COSTUME JEWELRY MANUFACTURERS

**Coro** - The name Coro was created from the first two letters of the founders' last names, Emanuel Cohn and Karl Rosenberger. The company opened its doors in 1927, in Providence, Rhode Island, and became one of the largest manufacturers of costume jewelry in the world. Over the years, the company used various trademarks including "Coro," "Coro Craft," and "Coro-Duette."

**Theodor Fahrner** - Fahrner founded a jewelry company in Pforzheim, Germany, which became famous for Art Deco-style jewelry during the 1920s and 1930s. This company mass produced art jewelry for the middle-class market using silver, low-carat gold, and semi-precious stones such as amazonite accented with marcasites. Fahrner jewelry is highly sought-after by collectors for its dramatic Art Deco and oriental styling. It was marked with "TF" in a circle.

**Trifari** - In 1918, Gustavo Trifari and Leo F. Krussman joined forces and founded the Trifari and Krussman Company in New York. Carl Fishel joined the firm in 1925. Trifari established a reputation for using only the finest rhinestones from the renowned Austrian rhinestone manufacturer, Daniel Swarovski. The high lead content of Swarovski stones created an extraordinary sparkle without the need for foil backings. The company's wide-spread use of these brilliant stones earned Trifari and his associates the nickname "rhinestone kings." After the stock market crash, Trifari hired Alfred Philippe, a talented young designer whose fine jewelry had been sold by Van Cleef & Arpel and Cartier. Under Philippe's direction, each stone was set by hand, as it was done in fine jewelry houses. Philippe was responsible for the Cartier-style "carved" (pressed glass) jewelry produced by Trifari during the 1930s and '40s. Trifari was inspired by Van Cleef & Arpels to make jewelry with "invisible settings" using square stones. Stones were placed edge to edge on metal rods, producing a solid unbroken surface. Trifari became one of the leading manufacturers of costume jewelry during the 1930s. Trifari jewelry was signed with the initials "TKF" until 1937, when it was replaced by the name "Trifari" with a crown over the "T."

**Eisenberg** - Jonas Eisenberg established an exclusive ladies' apparel shop in Chicago in 1914. He accented many of his dresses with sparkling rhinestone clips and brooches. Eisenberg's all-white pieces were made of large, clear Swarovski rhinestones imported from Austria. These dazzling pieces made such a hit that many were removed from the dresses and stolen by eager costumers. Eisenberg then decided to develop a line of *couture* jewelry to sell separate and apart from his clothing and he eventually discontinued his clothing line altogether. His jewelry, during the first half of the decade, was geometric in design, influenced by the Art Deco movement. As the decade progressed, his lines became more fluid with the sweeping curves of ribbons and gently bending flowers. During the 1930s this jewelry was marked "Eisenberg ORIGINAL."

**Napier -** The Napier Company was established in North Attleboro, Massachusetts, in 1875. During the 1920s, the company's president, James Napier, built a reputation on copying jewelry designs of the famous French *couture* houses of Chanel, Schiaparelli, Patou, Lelong, and Premet. This jewelry was marked "Napier."

**Boucher** - Marcel Boucher, a former jewelry designer for Cartier, started his own costume jewelry business in New York during the 1930s. He produced fine quality geometric pieces and enameled figurals. His designs were marked: "Boucher" or "MB" (with a bird).

**Hobé** - This French family-owned costume-jewelry firm was managed by several generations of Hobés. Robert Hobé had a keen interest in period costume and was often commissioned by movie moguls to design historic costumes and jewelry for period movies. His Victorian-revival jewelry often featured three-dimensional roses and ribbons. This jewelry is marked "Hobé."

**Joseph of Hollywood** - Eugene Joseph became a costume jewelry designer for Hollywood movies during the late 1920s. He rented his glamorous originals to the studios, primarily for period movies. They were usually larger in scale than ordinary jewelry to enhance their visibility on screen. They were often finished in matte-gold to prevent glare under the powerful studio lights. In 1937, Joseph launched a line of jewelry which he sold to the exclusive shops and department stores in Hollywood. These pieces are marked "Joseff Hollywood" or "Joseff."

**Barclay** - McClelland Barclay was a successful artist who's illustrations appeared on the cover of *Pictorial Review* magazines during the 1930s. He is known for his gold and rhodium-plated Art Deco-style geometric brooches, embellished with large *faux* gemstones and pavé-set clear rhinestones. He also produced necklaces and pins in the form of maple leaves pavé-set with clear rhinestones. His unique style is easy to recognize but his pieces are difficult to find. Barclay was killed in action during World War II.

# Chapter 12

# Accessories & Related Items

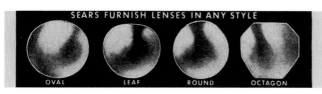

The Sears, Roebuck and Co. catalog (1936-37) offered lenses inthese four shapes.

## EYE WEAR

There were four main lens shapes produced during the 1930s. The oval lens was a carry-over from the Victorian era, while round lenses were introduced in the late teens. Octagonal lenses appeared in the late '20s and the leaf-shaped lens was a product of the 1930s.

The popular 10k white gold-filled rims were often engraved or chased with a border design. Most glasses had soft cable temples which adjusted to the contours of the individual ear. Self-adjustable swivel nosepads were covered with pearlized-celluloid for comfort.

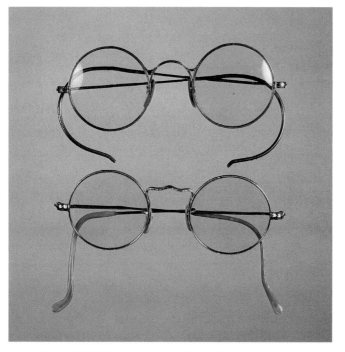

White gold-filled eyeglasses with round engraved rims. *Top:* Flexible cable temples, rocking nose pads. *Bottom:* "Spoon-tip" temples with Pearl-Zylo tips. *Courtesy of Margaretha J. Laubner.* $25-$35.

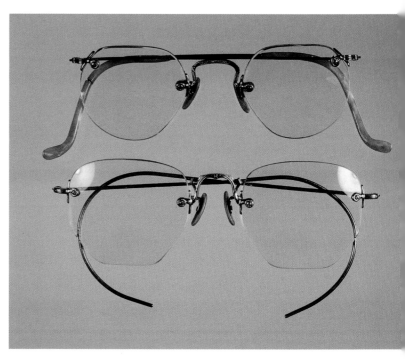

Rimless eyeglasses. *Top:* Leaf-shaped lenses, spoon-tip temples with Pearl Zylo tips Marked: SHURON. *Courtesy of F. Paul Laubner.* Bottom: Modified octagonal-shaped lenses Marked: SHURON 1-10 12k GF. *Courtesy of Margaretha J. Laubner.* $25-$35.

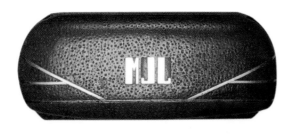

Brown frog-mouth style eyeglass case with Art Deco-style monogram and linear design. *Courtesy of Margaretha J. Laubner.* $30-$40.

## Oxford *Pince-nez*

The oxford *pince-nez* (pinch nose) style eyeglasses were worn by the older generation. They required a more sedate, dignified carriage as they were held precariously on the nose by the bow-bar spring bridge. For this reason a grosgrain ribbon, automatic chain reel, or safety chain was often attached. Folding oxfords had a spring bridge which could be bent so that one lens lay directly over the other. They were held in this position by a decorative clasp. Eyeglass cases were made to fit oxford glasses in both the open and folded positions.

Folding oxford *pince-nez* glasses, round rims. *Left:* (Folded) yellow gold-filled filigree clasp with Art Deco-style sunburst motif. Marked: 1/10 12k. *Right:* (Open) white gold-filled filigree clasp. Marked: 1/10 12k SPG LEMAY. $20-$40.

## Lorgnette/dress clip

The most unique spectacles of the 1930s were the *lorgnette*/dress clips. They were made in three hinged sections. The first two sections consisted of rectangular rims which were hinged to the bridge, allowing them to fold together, one on top of the other. The third section consisted of a short decorative handle embellished with marcasites. This handle clamped against the lenses by the use of a spring, thus converting the *lorgnette* into a fancy dress clip. When clamped over the edge of a pocket, lapel, or neckline, the lenses remained behind the fabric and only the decorative handle was visible. This style of eyeglass is rather rare and consequently quite expensive.

Silver *lorgnette*/dress clip with magnifying lenses. (Open) - *lorgnette* with rectangular rims, ornate open-work handle accented with marcasites. (Closed) - When handle is folded against the lenses it becomes a dress clip. Marked: 835. $150-$200.

# BELTS

When the waist returned to its normal position in the 1930s, it signaled the return of belts in a wide variety of styles. The most common materials for belts were calf, suede, kid, imitation leather, simulated alligator, and patent leather. They were usually 1 to 3-inches wide. Common decorations for belts were perforations, inlay, metal studs, and contrasting piping. Suede sport belts were top-stitched, woven, or braided. As the decade progressed, 3-inch-wide crushable-suede belts were introduced. The soft suede was gathered or crushed into its narrow buckle.

"Monk-cord girdles" with tasseled ends appeared mid-decade, possibly to accompany the popular monk shoes. They were available in a variety of colors plus silver and gold.

Novelty belts were assembled from links made of gold and silver coins, hammered metal, Bakelite, and wooden beads. Belts were also made of interconnecting leather links similar to leather-link handbags. Schiaparelli instructed her accessories designer, Jean Clément, to design belts of aluminum, lacquered string, and cellophane. The 1939 Sears, Roebuck and Co. catalog featured a braided cellophane belt with a leaf-shaped gold-toned buckle. Another belt called the "corselette," which appeared in the same catalog, was 3 1/2-inches wide in front where it laced up like a corset. This may have been influenced by the interest in Victorian fashions.

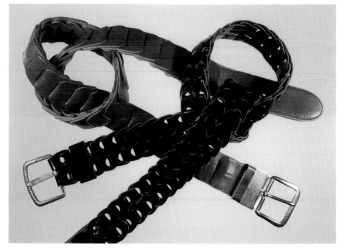

Two belts made of interlocking leather links. (This technique was also used in the production of leather-link purses.) *Courtesy of Rose Jamieson.* $25-$35.

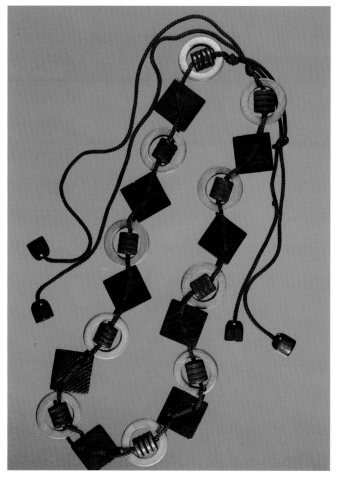

Art Deco-style wooden bead and cord belt. *Courtesy of Mary Anne Faust (Yesterday's Delights).* $30-$40.

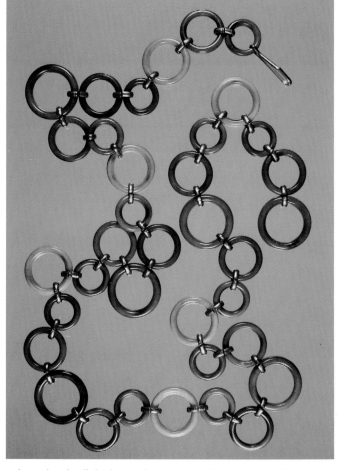

Belt made of celluloid rings fastened together with metal links. *Courtesy of Mary Anne Faust (Yesterday's Delights).* $35-$45.

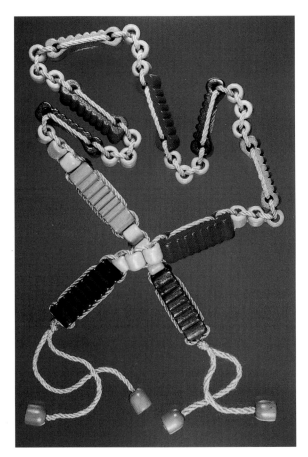

Belt made of colorful wooden beads and cord.
*Courtesy of Rose Jamieson.* $30-$40.

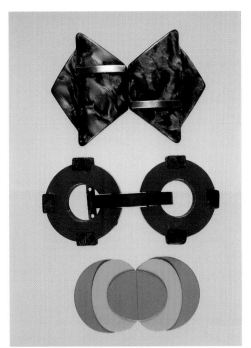

Art Deco-style mirror-image belt clasps. *(1)* Marbleized Bakelite and metal. *(2)* Bakelite and wood. *(3)* Plastic. *Courtesy of Mary Anne Faust (Yesterday's Delights).* $10-$40 ea.

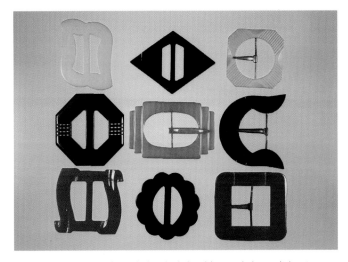

Typical Art Deco-style Bakelite belt buckles and dress slides in a variety of geometric shapes. *Courtesy of Mary Anne Faust (Yesterday's Delights).* $10-$50 ea.

Belt colors echoed those of shoes and hats of the period. During the first half of the decade, they were produced in standard black, brown, navy, gray, tan, beige, red, and white for summer. By 1936-37, Sears, Roebuck and Co. had added the new shades of wine, russet (rust), winter green (olive), and royal blue to coordinate with the latest styles.

## Belt Buckles, Slides, and Clasps

Dresses of the 1930s were often made with "self" belts. They were fastened with geometric-style buckles, belt slides (buckle without a hasp), or mirror-image clasps which were made of celluloid, bakelite, wood, metal, or combinations of these materials. Sets including buckles or clasps and matching buttons were also popular. Nothing escaped the monogramming craze of the 1930s, not even belt buckles! Precut block-style letters were applied to the buckle at the time of purchase. Buckles covered in self fabric were also worn.

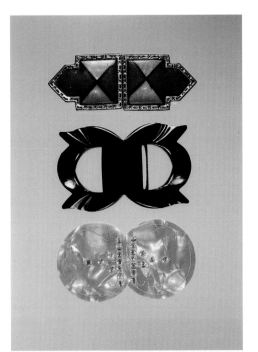

Art Deco-style mirror-image belt clasps. *(1)* Gold-plate with celluloid overlay. *(2)* Black Bakelite. *(3)* Pink marbleized celluloid with rhinestones. *Courtesy of Ina Stoudt (Antique Treasures).* Top and bottom $25-$30 ea. Middle $50-$60.

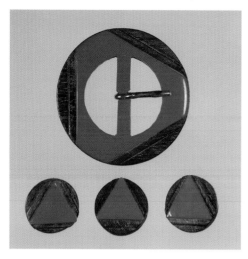

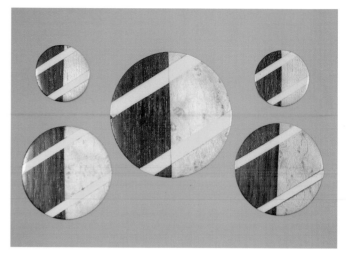

Art Deco-style Bakelite and wood belt buckle and buttons. *Courtesy of Mary Anne Faust (Yesterday's Delights)*. $50-$75 set.

Art Deco-style celluloid and wood belt clasp and buttons. *Courtesy of Mary Anne Faust (Yesterday's Delights)*. $40-$50 set.

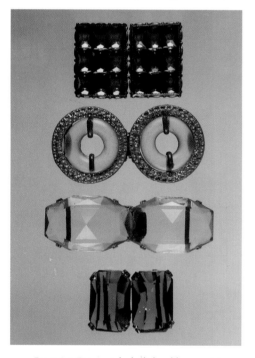

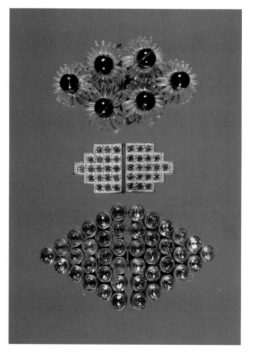

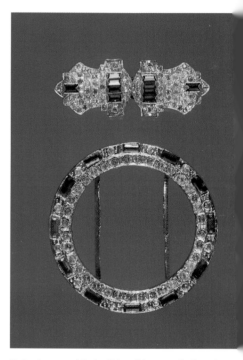

Four Art Deco style belt buckles containing green, frosted, pink, and blue glass stones. $20-$40 ea.

Art Deco style belt buckles. *(1)* Base metal and glass. *(2)* Base metal and rhinestones. *(3)* Gold-plated brass and blue rhinestones. *Courtesy of Mary Anne Faust (Yesterday's Delights)*. $10-$50.

Belt clasp and belt slide of base metal and pavé-set clear rhinestones and colored *baguettes*. *Courtesy of Mary Anne Faust (Yesterday's Delights)*. $25-$40 ea.

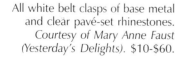

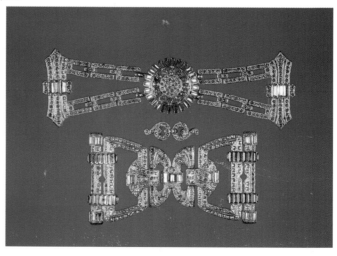

All white belt clasps of base metal and clear pavé-set rhinestones. *Courtesy of Mary Anne Faust (Yesterday's Delights)*. $10-$60.

# BUTTONS

The 1930s was the heyday for novelty buttons. Bright whimsical buttons were ideally suited to the 1930s; they were an inexpensive antidote to the doldrums of the depression. For many women, the failed economy meant making do with last year's frocks. What better way to liven up an old dress (or a new dress for that matter) then by adding a few cheerful buttons —perhaps ones that looked like flowers, dogs, fish, or even insects.

This "button-mania" was sparked by French designer, Elsa Schiaparelli, whose witty innovative buttons are now legendary. She accented her garments with "realistic" buttons resembling lollipops, spinning tops, padlocks, spoons, candlesticks, mermaids, crayfish, lobsters, cicadas, butterflies, swans, lips, hands, fish hooks, paper clips, safety pins, Christmas tree balls, spoons, peanuts, assorted fruits and vegetables, and the list goes on. Items in her "Music Collection" of 1937 contained buttons resembling musical notes. In 1938, she trimmed the garments in her "Circus Collection" with buttons that resembled clowns, prancing horses, and trapeze artists.

Schiaparelli's clever buttons were designed by Jean Clément, a graduate of the *École des Beau-Arts* with a degree in painting. He also had a degree in chemistry from the University of Paris. His previous training served him well as he devoted his life (from 1927 until his untimely death in 1949) to the creation of original and highly imaginative buttons, costume jewelry, and accessories for Schiaparelli. The majority of these items were made of Bakelite, which he baked in a small electric oven.

Buttons of the 1930s were produced in every color, size, shape, and style imaginable. They were made of a wide variety of materials including amber, crystal, glass, china, metal, wood, wood pulp composition, porcelain, celluloid, Bakelite, and other plastics. (For further information on Bakelite, see Jewelry, Chapter 11.) The following are but a few of the popular button styles produced during the 1930s.

*Realistics*. Buttons which resembled familiar objects such as flowers, household objects, plates of food, faces, hats, shoes, birds, fish, and animals are called realistics. President Roosevelt's Scottish terrier "Fala" was the inspiration for many a Scottie button. Realistics were often produced in sets which included types of fruits, vegetables, musical instruments, gardening tools, circus performers, under-sea life, sporting goods, cigarette packs, and cocktails (a reflection of the repeal of prohibition). Realistics were usually molded or carved from Bakelite or other forms of plastic.

The 1937 Sears, Roebuck and Co. catalog advertised a dress decorated with "good luck" buttons which included a four leaf clover, the number seven, a horseshoe, and dice. Their 1939-40 catalog featured a dress with alphabet buttons which spelled the wearer's name down the bodice.

*Cookies*. Flat sew-through buttons in various shapes were made by cutting slices from a long Bakelite "cane." When the cane contained two colors, the result was buttons that resembled cookies made from sliced rolls of dough, thus the name "cookies". Since the two colors ran the entire length of the rod, a cookie button looked the same on both sides.

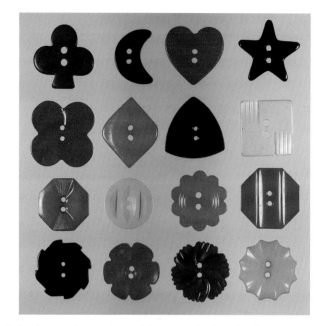

Bakelite buttons in a variety of shapes and colors. $5-$10 ea.

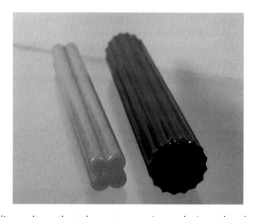

Two Bakelite rods ready to be cut crosswise and pierced to form buttons. *Courtesy of Nancy Moyer*. $20-$50 ea.

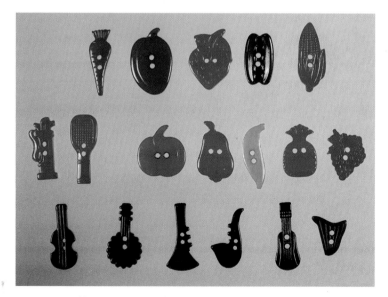

Four series of buttons: vegetables, sporting goods, fruits, and musical instruments. *Courtesy of Nancy Moyer*. $30-$100. per set.

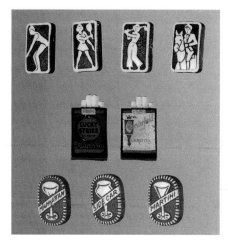

Three series of buttons: celluloid sports buttons, plastic cigarette buttons, and celluloid cocktail buttons (a reflection of the repeal of Prohibition. *Courtesy of Nancy Moyer.* $50-$125. per set.

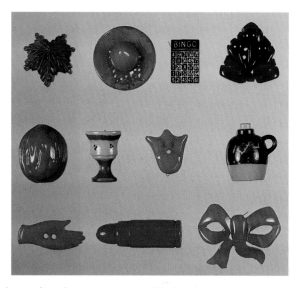

Bakelite realistic buttons. *Center*: tulip-face button attributed to renowned costume jewelry and button designer Martha Sleeper. *Courtesy of Nancy Moyer.* $10-$50 ea.

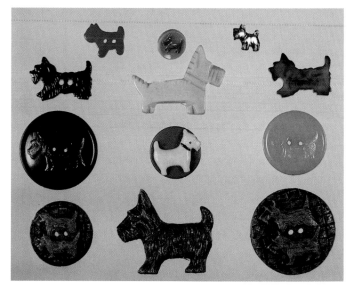

Popular Scottie buttons made of Bakelite, plastic, glass, celluloid, and wood composition. *Courtesy of Nancy Moyer.* $5-$50.00 ea.

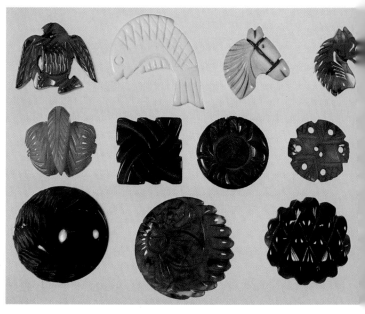

A variety of carved Bakelite buttons. (Row 1) Realistics. $40.00 - $75.00 ea. (Rows 2 and 3) Foliate and abstract designs. $10-$25 ea. *Courtesy of Nancy Moyer.*

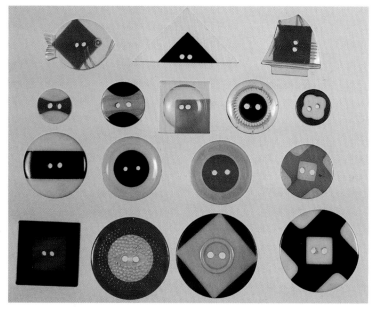

A sampling of Bakelite cookie buttons. Note: the fish and sailboat in the top row. *Courtesy of Nancy Moyer* $5-$40.

**Clear Glass-Dome Buttons.** Buttons often paralleled costume jewelry of the 1930s, sharing many of the same materials and techniques. Clear *cabochon* (glass-dome) buttons were first cousins to the domed cuff links, tie bars, sports pins, and bracelets so popular during this period. Common motifs for this type of button were horses, Scottish terriers, sailboats, and sports figures, which were reverse painted on the underside of the dome.

**Reverse-Carved Buttons.** Clear Bakelite (now the color of apple juice) was used to create reverse-carved buttons. A design was carved into the reverse side of a transparent button which was visible from the front. These indentations were either enhanced by the use of colored enamels or left untouched. Florals were the most popular motif for this type of button. The same technique was also used in the production of Bakelite jewelry.

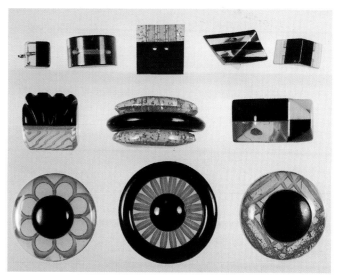

These laminated buttons were made of black and clear (now apple juice color) Bakelite . *Courtesy of Nancy Moyer.* $5-$40.

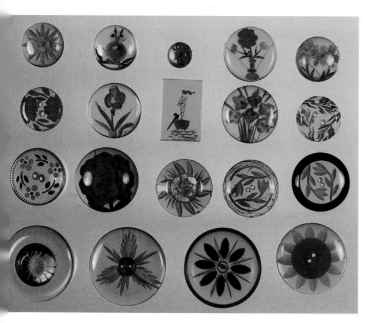

Various reverse-carved buttons made of apple juice (once clear) Bakelite and enamel. *Courtesy of Nancy Moyer.* $10-$50 ea.

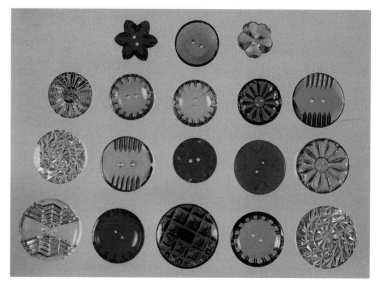

Pressed or depression glass buttons. *Courtesy of Nancy Moyer.* $1-$5 ea.

**Laminated Buttons.** Black and clear (now apple juice) Bakelite were laminated (glued) together to form striking geometric Art Deco-style buttons.

**Depression Glass Buttons.** Transparent and translucent depression glass buttons were made in sew-through and shank style in a variety of colors. Opaque Art Deco-style buttons were embellished with sleek modernistic ornamentation.

**Commemorative Buttons.** Buttons were also produced to commemorate such events as the 1939 World's Fair, which featured the stylized Trylon and Perisphere motif. World's Fair buttons are "cross-over" collectibles which are sought after by button collectors, World's Fair enthusiasts, and vintage clothing collectors alike.

**Platter Buttons.** Coats of the 1930s were fastened with large platter buttons measuring a whopping 2 to 2 1/2 inches in diameter. They were made of celluloid, Bakelite, metal, and wood in interesting colors, shapes, and textures.

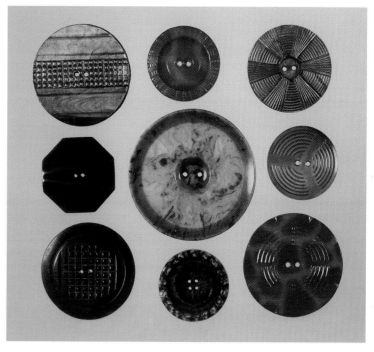

Large Bakelite platter buttons used on coats. Celluloid, Bakelite, and metal in interesting textures. *Courtesy of Sue Irons (Irons Antiques).*

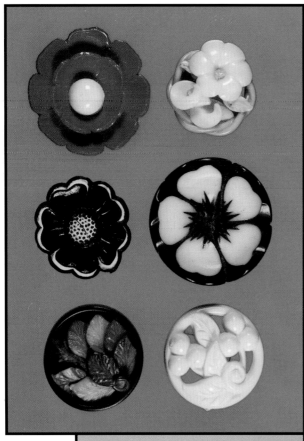

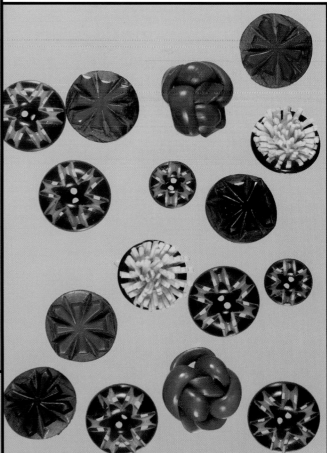

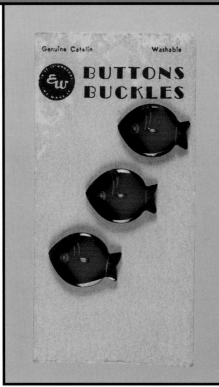

Genuine Catalin          Washable

**BUTTONS
BUCKLES**

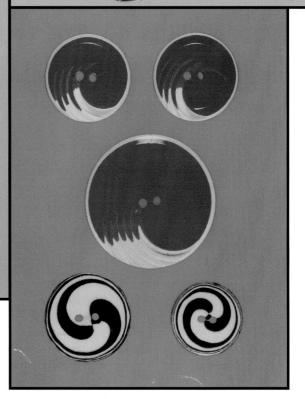

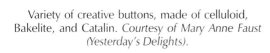
Variety of creative buttons, made of celluloid,
Bakelite, and Catalin. *Courtesy of Mary Anne Faust
(Yesterday's Delights).*

# UMBRELLAS

Umbrellas were still made in the short "stub" length, a carry-over from the 1920s. The silk and linen close-weave, water-proof cover was usually striped, although solids and woven borders did exist. In 1939, the Sears, Roebuck and Co. catalog featured the new clear Pliofilm umbrella made of transparent rubber composition for better visibility.

The handles of umbrellas were made of carved wood, amber-colored celluloid, Bakelite, and (at the end of the decade) clear carved Prystal.

# GLOVES

The glove continued to be an important accessory throughout the 1930s. The rather ambiguous terms *gauntlet* and *mousquetaire* are explained in the following passages.

Gloves of the first few years of the decade were a continuation of the styles worn during the 1920s. These wrist-length gloves had short, dainty, turn-back cuffs which were saddle stitched, embroidered, or appliquéd with Art Deco designs. In lieu of a cuff, pleated or gathered ruffles were attached at the wrist and could be worn over the forearm or turned back over the glove. By 1931 the cuff began to disappear and triangular gores were inserted into the hem of gloves for a slight flare. In 1932-33, the lower edge of the hem began to droop to a point or a large sagging curve.

***Gauntlets***. By 1934-35, the area over the wrist and forearm grew to an enormous funnel-shaped extension, reminiscent of the *gauntlets* worn by 17th century French *mousquetaires* (musketeers). The flared portion of the glove, also called a *gauntlet*, was usually made of stiffer fabric than the hand to give it body. Typical fabric combinations were a cotton mesh hand - organdy tiered *gauntlet*, cotton chamois hand - cotton pique *gauntlet*, rayon hand - taffeta *gauntlet*, Bemberg mesh hand - organdy *gauntlet* with ruffled edge, rayon mesh hand - corded rib rayon bengaline *gauntlet*, kid hand - quilted *gauntlet*. *Gauntlet* were often piped with a contrasting color which accentuated the design. They often featured a buckled wrist strap or buttoned tab. In winter, the funnel-shaped *gauntlet* area was worn up over the edge of the coat sleeve.

Once the *gauntlet* had reached such exaggerated proportions, there was nowhere to go but to recede. In 1937, the wrist seam disappeared and by 1939 the flare was minimal.

***Mousquetaires***. *Mousquetaires* were long, usually white, lambskin gloves with a buttoned slit at the wrist. They were used with formal afternoon or evening wear and could be worn smooth or crushed down casually below the elbow.

***Fingerless mitts***. Also worn for evening were long or short fingerless gloves called mitts, yet another example of Victorian revival fashions influenced by period movies.

Gloves were not only made of the *usual* silk, lambskin, *glacé* kid, pigskin, and doeskin, but of the *unusual* washable chamoisuede, cotton piqué, organdy, cotton *matelassé*, and Lastex. Printed woven fabrics were also made into gloves to match a particular garment. Typical colors for gloves were beige, brown black, gunmetal gray, coco, sand, and eggshell. In 1939, Sears, Roebuck and Co. added the new shades of wine, grape (purple), russet (rust), winter green (olive), and royal blue to coordinate with their latest styles.

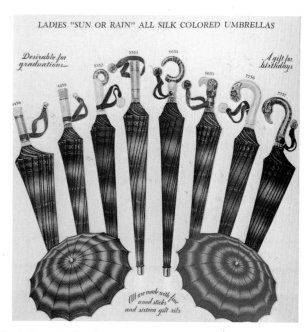

Ladies' silk umbrellas, from E.L. Rice & Co. (1931), made of fine wood sticks, moonglow or tortoise-shell colored Pyralin (plastic) handles, and silk cord. Note: the two hand-carved bird-head handles.

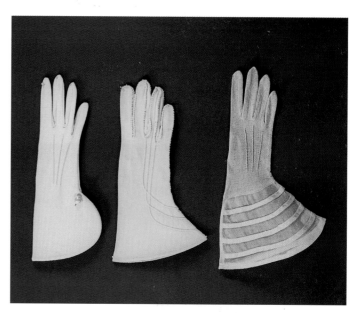

*Gauntlet*-style gloves. *(1)* Pale yellow rib-knit rayon. Label: Van Raalte. *(2)* Yellow cotton with parallel tucks. *(3)* Light blue rayon knit, wide organdy *gauntlets* trimmed with rows of bias tape. Label: Made in Germany. $25-$40.

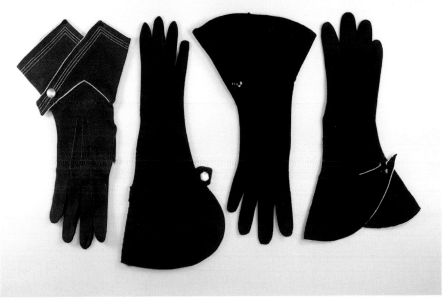

*Gauntlet*-style gloves. *(1)* Brown cotton, white piping, railroad stitching. *(2)* Navy rayon with stiff textured cotton *gauntlet*. *(3)* Black ribbed cotton, textured cotton *gauntlet*. *(4)* Black cotton, textured cotton *gauntlet*, white piping. All made in Czechoslovakia. $40-$70

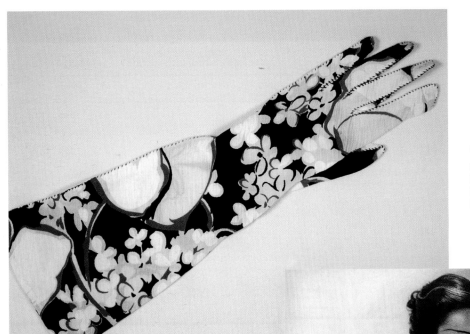

*Vogue* photograph featuring a black and white satin dress, matching gloves, and ostrich cape. Bergdorf Goodman. *Vogue*, 5/34. / Gloves handmade from printed-rayon fabric which may have matched a dress or hat band. $30-$40.

In typical fashion, Schiaparelli created shocking pink gloves that ballooned out into enormous puffed sleeves at the top. She also designed gloves with appliquéd fingernails.

Van Raalte, Aris, and Daniel Hays were three of the major glove manufacturers. Gloves were also imported from Czechoslovakia and Germany during this period.

## NAILS

There were two techniques for polishing fingernails during the 1930s. The first was polishing the entire nail. The second involved polishing all but the white areas located along the cuticle and the tips of the nails.

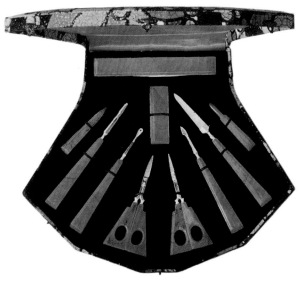

This striking Art Deco-style manicure set by Premier contains implements with geometric-shaped Premalite handles. Velvet lined presentation box, 1931.

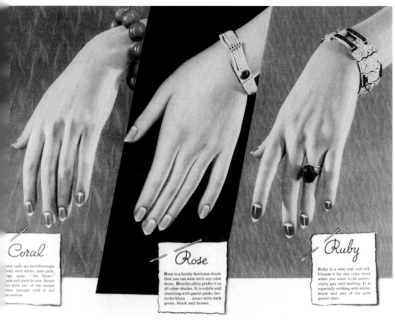

Cutex nail polish advertisement from *Ladies' Home Journal* (8/38) illustrating a popular method of coating all but the white areas of the nails.

## BUREAU SETS

Bureau sets were sold in most jewelry and department stores. They contained from three to twenty matching items which could include a brush, comb, mirror, cuticle scissors, shoe button hook, nail file, nail buffer, shoe horn, hair receiver, atomizer, salve boxes, corn knife, cloth brush, puff box, and a tray.

Some sets were made of sterling silver with embossed or engine-turned designs and often featured a *cartouche* for monogramming. Other sets were gold, silver, or chrome-plated and decorated with *guilloché* enameling. Pearlized du Pont Lucite or Pyralin was also used in such pastel colors as peach, rose, orchid, maize, buff, and jade. They were decorated with delicate floral sprays, garlands, and wreaths, or Deco-style geometric shapes.

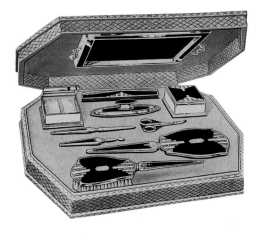

Elgin American Manufacturing Company advertisement for a ten-piece chrome-plated boudoir set with black enameled Art Deco step motif. Set contains: brush, mirror, nail cleaner, nail file, cuticle scissors, nail buffer, comb, powder box, cigarette humidor, and tray in velvet-lined presentation box, 1931.

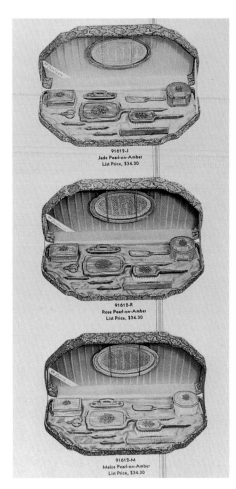

Twelve-piece boudoir sets by Madelon made from du Pont Pyralin in three popular pearlized colors - jade, rose, and maize, 1930-1931.

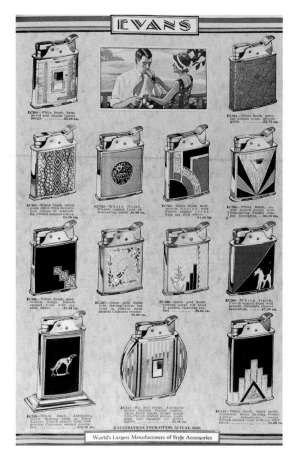

Evans advertisement for colorful cigarette lighters, 1931.

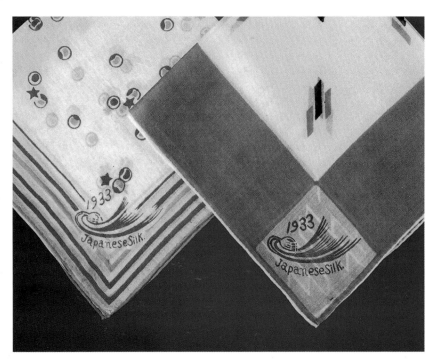

Two Japanese silk handkerchiefs decorated with the 1933 World's Fair logo and Art Deco-style geometric designs. $10-$15.

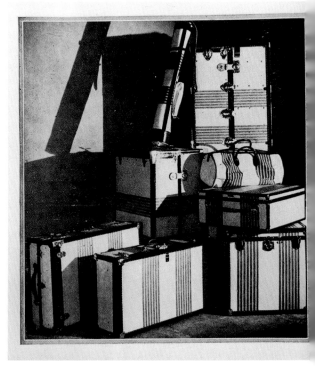

Advertisement for Oshkosh "Chief" luggage which appeared in *House and Garden* (7/30). "The name Chief means permanence in style. People who bought Chiefs ten years ago can match them today. And those who buy Chiefs now can do the same thing ten years from now." The most distinguishing characteristics were "the red and yellow stripes woven into the duck which covers it [the luggage]."

# Chapter 13

# Men's Wear

Men's wear manufacturers around the world looked to the English tailor for inspiration in the same way the women's wear industry looked to the Paris *couturier*. The Prince of Wales (later the Duke of Windsor) gained a reputation as a connoisseur of men's fashion. When he emerged in something new and innovative, it quickly set an international trend. During the 1920s and '30s he popularized such items as the double-breasted dinner jacket, the Fair Isle sweater, "plus fours," Scottish *gillie* oxfords, Argyle socks, glen plaid suits, the wide Windsor knot (for tying ties) and shirts with collars designed to accommodate this wide knot.

The ideal male now had a more rugged athletic appearance, with broad shoulders, and a narrow waist and hips. Hollywood was now featuring male stars like Clark Gable and James Cagney with a more assertive, commanding presence.

## UNDERGARMENTS

With the trend towards central heating, long knitted union suits were not the necessity they had once been. "Long johns" were still worn, however, by those men who worked in cold weather conditions or participated in winter sports. One-piece undergarments were being replaced by rib-knit tank-top-style undershirts and striped cotton boxer shorts. Brief-style knitted underpants became available towards the middle of the decade.

Clark Gable dealt the men's undergarment industry a blow when he removed his shirt in the movie "It Happened One Night" and viewers noticed that he was not wearing an undershirt.

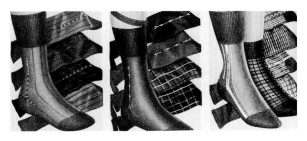

Montgomery Ward catalog illustrations (1937) featuring silk and rayon socks with vertical stripes, knit-in clocks, and grid patterns. Note: built-in garters on center pair. Montgomery Ward, 1937.

Socks were made in solid colors plus plaids, grids, Argyles, and stripes. Solids were often decorated with clocks (vertical arrows embroidered above the ankles). Common fibers used in the production of socks were silk, glossy rayon, cotton *lisle*, wool, or combinations of these fibers. Standard colors were black, navy, brown, tan, gray, and white. Garters were still a necessity until the late '30s, when Lastex was added to the rib-knit bands at the tops of socks.

## SLEEPWEAR AND LOUNGE WEAR

### Pajamas

Pajamas were available in both the button-front cardigan and the pull-over style tops. Collarless cardigan tops often featured Oriental frog fasteners, a carry-over from the preceding

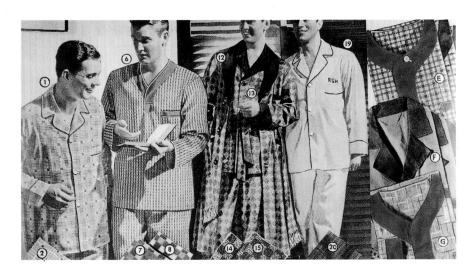

Montgomery Ward catalog illustration (1937) offering pajamas in the notched-collar open-front and placket pullover styles with contrasting trim and piping, cotton batiste and broadcloth. Note: matching bath robe.

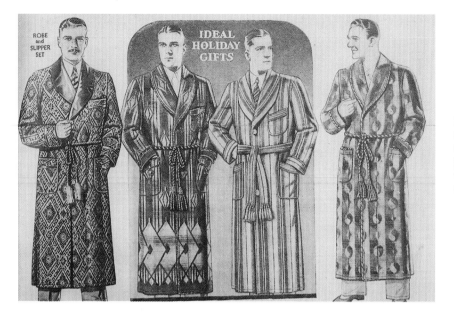

decades. Notched collars became more common for cardigan-style tops as the decade progressed. When pajamas were made of solid-color fabric, the collar, pocket, and cuffs were often made of a contrasting color or a coordinating stripe or plaid. The neckline placket on pull-over tops was often made of a coordinating fabric. Contrasting piping was also used as a decorative trim. Broadcloth, muslin, flannelette, rayon, and silk were the common fabrics in stripes and solids.

## Robes

Genuine Beacon robes were made of fluffy cotton blanket cloth in geometric *ombré* patterns. Silk cord was used for the tasseled girdle and trim along the shawl collar and front edges. Robes were also made of wool, rayon brocade, flannel, seersucker, and terry cloth. They featured a shawl or notched collar and patch pockets.

## Slippers

Men's slippers came in a variety of styles. The kidskin "Romeo" style had a long pull tab in back and elastic gores in the sides for a snug fit. The "opera" slipper resembled a woman's *d'Orsay* model with a closed toe and heel and cut-away sides, forming a broad "V". Natural-color tan sheepskin slippers were also popular. The fuzzy fleece side of the skin was used on the inside of the slipper creating a thick soft lining. The edge of the skin was turned down to form a fuzzy wool collar. Slippers made of felt and terry cloth were also available.

# EVENING WEAR

*Tails.* Formal occasions called for a black or midnight-blue tailcoat with matching pleated cuffless trousers. The wide peaked lapels, trouser stripes, and covered buttons were made of lustrous satin or matte-finish silk faille. A white dress shirt with a stiff bosom and detachable wing collar was worn with a white piqué single-breasted waistcoat (vest) with a shawl or "wide-angled" collar, and a white piqué bow tie. The shirt and waistcoat were fastened with gold studs and cuff links set with mother-of-pearl or onyx. A black silk-faille top hat, black patent leather oxfords or dance pumps trimmed with black grosgrain *faux* bows, and white kid gloves completed the ensemble. A white pocket

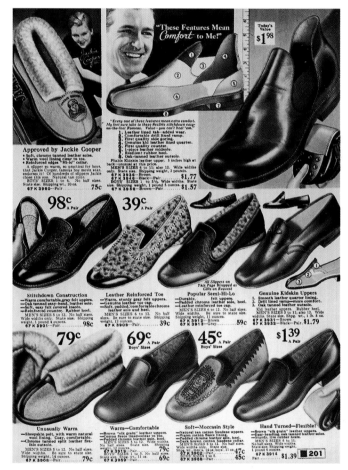

Sears, Roebuck and Co. catalog page (1935-36) devoted to men's and boy's slippers. *(Top left)* "Jackie Cooper" sheepskins. *(Top right)* Kidskin "Romeo". *(Rows 2 and 3)* Felt, kid, and sheepskin.

handkerchief and *boutonnière* were icing on the cake. White spats were worn for only the dressiest of occasions.

*Tuxedo*. Semiformal occasions called for a black or midnight-blue tuxedo or dinner jacket. The emphasis was shifting from single to double-breasted jackets with peaked lapels or shawl collar. Lapels, trouser stripes, and covered buttons were made of satin or silk faille. White dinner jackets made of rayon gabardine were an option for summer. The single-breasted dinner jacket was worn over a black or white piqué single or double-breasted waistcoat or a cummerbund. (No waistcoat or cummerbund was required under the double-breasted dinner jacket.) Those men who preferred a cummerbund could choose from conservative black satin or a variety of colors and subdued patterns. The white dress shirt with starched bosom and detachable wing collar was giving way to soft shirts with attached turned-down collars. Shirts were fastened with gold studs and cuff links set with mother-of-pearl, onyx, or colored stones (often matching the cummerbund.) A black bow tie, black patent leather oxfords or pumps, a white pocket handkerchief and *boutonnière* completed the ensemble.

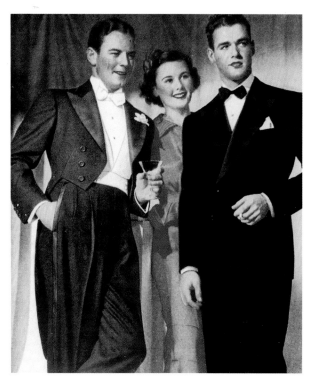

Howard Clothes advertisement (1937) for tails and double-breasted tuxedo (dinner suit) available in midnight blue and black with grosgrain or satin peaked lapels and trouser stripes.

# DAY WEAR

## Suits

*Morning Suit*. For formal afternoon weddings, a morning suit was required. It featured a black "cutaway" coat with a long, knee-length skirt which was cut away on an angle from the center of the waist in front diagonally down to the knees at the sides. It was worn with black and gray striped or checked trousers and a black, gray, or lavender waistcoat. This ensemble required a wing-collar shirt and a solid or striped four-in-hand tie or ascot held in place by a decorative stickpin. A black top hat, black patent leather oxfords, white spats, and white pocket handkerchief and *boutonnière* completed the outfit.

*Classic Suit*. During the first few years of the decade, men wore conservative snug-fitting three-piece suits. Two and three button jackets were available with straight-leg trousers.

*English Drape Suit*. The English drape-suit made its debut circa the mid-1930s and was made in both double and single-breasted models. It had broad shoulders, wide lapels, a semi-fitted waist, and snug-fitting hips. What set this suit apart from previous styles, however, was the fullness over the chest and shoulders which caused a slight wrinkle or indentation in the fabric between the collar and the sleeves. (The contrast between the broad shoulders and the nipped-in waist was more exaggerated on collegiate-style suits designed for young men.) The matching high-waisted trousers had two pleats on each side of the waist and wide 19-inch cuffs at the bottom (22-inch cuffs on young men's suits.) Circa 1934, manufacturers began to substitute slide fasteners (zippers) for buttons in fly-front closings. Many suits had a pleated "action back" which allowed for more freedom of movement. This style often had a stitched-down "half belt" in back, a last vestige of the Norfolk jacket.

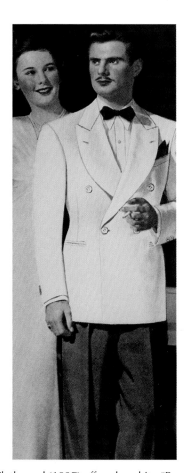

This Howard Clothes ad (1937) offered a white "Breeze Cloth" double-breasted dinner jacket with unusual peaked-shawl lapels, two-button cuffs. Note: black bow tie and handkerchief. .

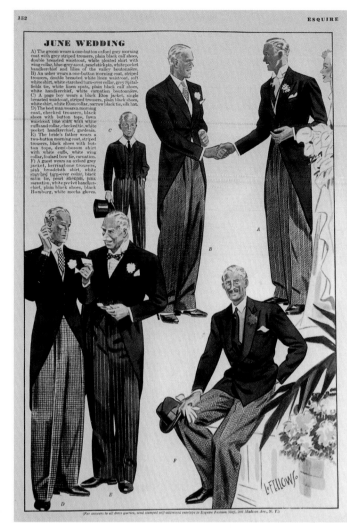

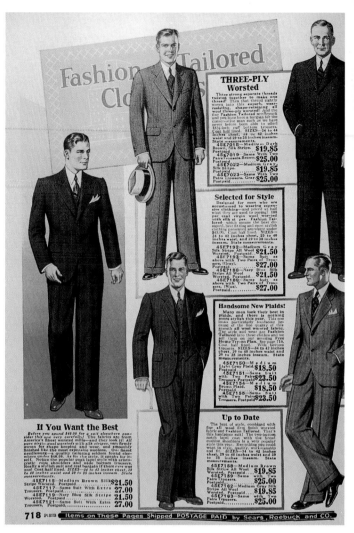

*Esquire* illustration (6/38) for formal day-time attire. Morning coats (cutaways) and striped trousers for *(A)* groom, *(B)* best man, and *(E)* father of the bride. Checked pants for *(D)* usher. Eton jacket, vest, shirt with Eton collar, striped trousers for *(C)* ring bearer. Oxford gray jacket, herringbone trousers, homburg for *(F)* guest. *Esquire*, 6/38.

Catalog page from Sears, Roebuck and Co. (1931) offered classic three-piece single-breasted wool-worsted suits featuring two and three button jackets with notched collars or peaked lapels, vests, and straight-leg pants with cuffs.

Suits were made of worsted, flannel, gabardine, cheviot, and sharkskin in solids, tweeds, herringbones, and fine checks. Double-breasted dark-blue pin-stripe suits were commonly worn for business. The Prince of Wales created a fad for suits made of glen plaid. Named for Glen Urquhart, a valley in Invernessshire, Scotland, this plaid was also referred to as the "Prince of Wales check." Since more fabric and time were required to carefully match this plaid both horizontally and vertically, well-made glen plaid suits were more expensive and, consequently, quite desirable.

In 1936, light-weight summer suits in pale colors were introduced. They were made of tropical wool worsted, rayon, cotton, linen, silk, and blends of these fibers. Popular Palm Beach suits were made of cotton and mohair in white, oatmeal, or light gray. Seersucker was another cool, lightweight fabric used for suits.

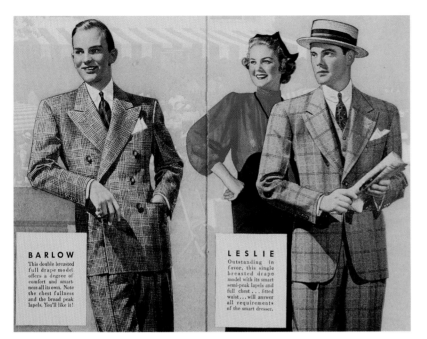

Howard Clothes advertisement (1937). *Left:* English-style glen-plaid drape suit with double-breasted jacket featuring peaked lapels and slight indentations over the chest. *Right:* Plaid suit with two-button single-breasted jacket, wide peaked lapels. Matching vest and trousers.

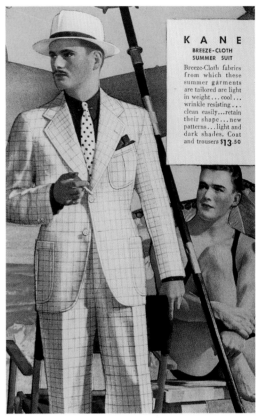

Howard Clothes advertisement (1937) for men's single-breasted summer suits, white with blue windowpane pattern, notched collar, pleated pockets. Note: Panama straw hat, navy shirt, and white tie.

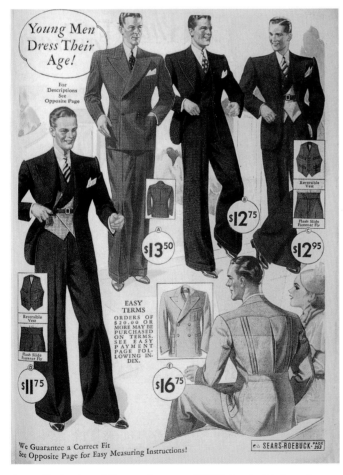

Sears, Roebuck and Co. catalog page (1935) devoted to broad-shouldered suit jackets with fitted waists. High-waisted pleated trousers with wide 22-inch bottoms. Reversible vests (check or solid). Note: pleated pockets and pleated action back with half belt.

## Trousers

*Oxford Bags*. In 1925, the undergraduates at Oxford University began to wear trousers with wide baggy legs. These pants measured a whopping 25-30 inches around the knee, thus the name "Oxford bags." Legend has it that the Oxford rowing team wore these wide-leg pants over their rowing knickers, which were unacceptable attire for class.

*Wide-legs.* Trousers with full-cut legs became popular for American college men during the late 1920s and 1930s. This influenced older men's trousers as well. The standard cuff bottoms for young men's trousers was 22 inches around the bottom. More conservative men's trousers were 19 inches. Trousers were high waisted with wide waistbands and two pleats on each side in front. Zippers replaced buttons in fly-front closings circa 1934. Many styles also featured adjustable side buckle straps attached below the waistband.

Trousers were made of gabardine, wool flannel, worsted, linen, cashmere, corduroy, and cotton whipcord. They were available in solids, tweeds, plaids, stripes, herringbones, and checks in various shades of gray, brown, and navy. Towards the end of the decade, dark green and marine blue were added. Trousers made of white and light-colored summer fabrics were introduced circa 1936. These fabrics included cotton duck, cotton crash, linen, wool flannel, and tropical worsted.

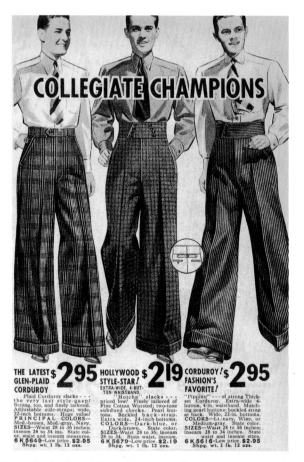

This Sears, Roebuck and Co. ad (1936-37) features young men's high-waisted slacks with 2-4 inch wide waist bands and wide 22-24 inch bottoms. *(1)* Glen-plaid corduroy. *(2)* Checked worsted. *(3)* Corduroy.

## Shirts

Dress shirts were made of pre-shrunk cotton broadcloth or oxford cloth with soft attached collars. Dress shirts were produced not only in white but light shades of blue, green, tan, yellow and gray. Towards the middle of the decade, "deep tones" like marine blue, navy, brown, dark green, maroon, metal gray, and burgundy were worn with contrasting light ties. Patterned shirts were popular in pin stripes, checks, and tattersalls (window panes). Shirts were made of jacquard weaves featuring a pastel pattern on a white ground and cotton fabric with a shiny rayon stripe. Shirts in the "Duke of Kent" button-down-collar style were another alternative. It was considered stylish to wear patterned ties with patterned shirts. Shirts with French cuffs suitable for cuff links were also available.

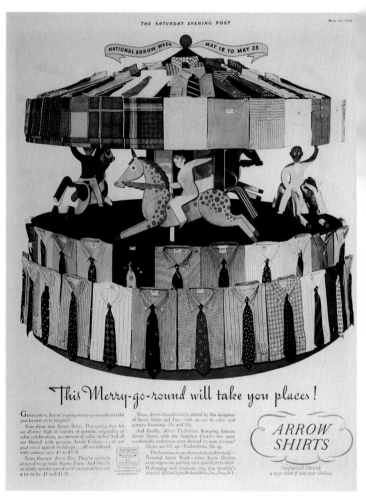

Arrow men's wear (5/23/36) including assorted patterned shirts, and coordinating ties, plaid handkerchiefs, and under shorts.

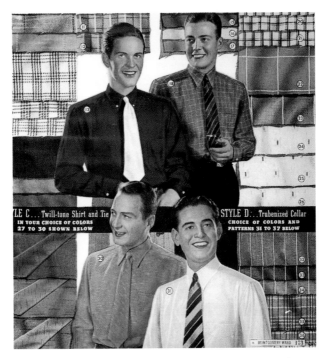

Montgomery Ward catalog page (1937) featuring men's shirts and ties. Note: Dark-maroon shirt with white tie and shirts with matching ties.

## Neckwear

*Four-in-Hand Ties*. From 1930 through 1936, men's four-in-hand neckties were primarily conservative featuring solids, diagonal stripes, window panes, plaids, Argyles, and small dots or geometric shapes (randomly spaced or in even rows). From 1936 on, larger, bolder designs began to appear, a trend which would continue into the 1940s. Blurred *chiné* fabrics in which the warp yarn was printed before the weft yarn was woven in, were also used. Ties were made of silk and rayon or combinations of these fibers. Popular tie fabrics included wide-wale twill, jacquard, bouclé, moiré, and flat crepe with a satin over design. College men preferred knitted or crocheted ties.

*Windsor Knot.* The Windsor knot, named for the Duke of Windsor, was a more complicated method of tying the standard four-in-hand tie which produced a larger knot. This knot required a special shirt with a collar which was spread far enough apart to accommodate the wide knot.

*Bow ties.* Bow ties were available in both the "self-tie" and the "made-up" versions which featured an adjustable neckband. They appeared in solids and conservative mini prints in the same colors as four-in-hand ties.

Standard colors for ties were navy, black, gray, brown, maroon, green, and purple. Ties were generally interlined with wool to minimize wrinkles and retain their shape. The ends were then lined with silk. A line of less expensive ties without a lining were offered in Sears, Roebuck and Co. catalogs during the early years of the depression (1931).

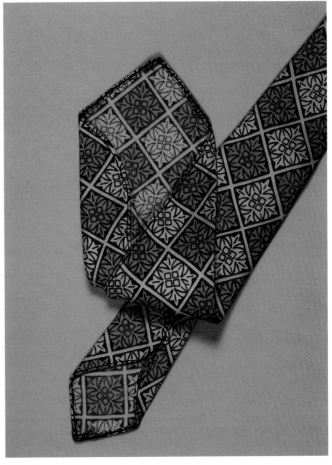

During the depression, ties were often made without linings in an effort to make them more affordable. Reverse side of unlined rayon neck tie. $25-$30.

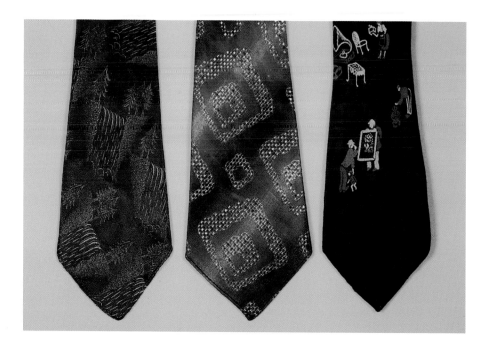

Three rayon neckties, two in the popular rust color. *Courtesy of Mary Anne Faust (Yesterday's Delights).* $30-$50.

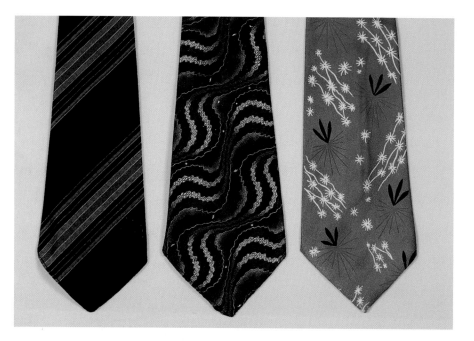

Three rayon neckties, one conservative, two more flamboyant. *Courtesy of Mary Anne Faust (Yesterday's Delights).* $30-$50.

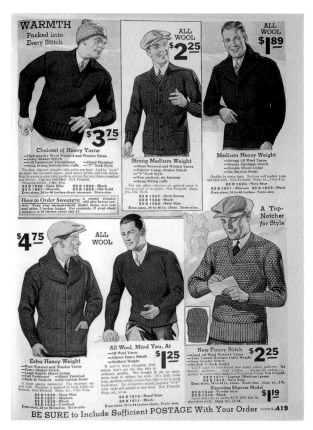

An assortment of men's sweaters from the Sears, Roebuck and Co. catalog (1933-34). V-neck pull-over sweaters. / Collarless and shawl-collar cardigans.

## Sweaters

*Pullovers.* Sweaters were offered in figure-hugging pullover styles with crew, boat, turtle, and V-necklines. They were produced in plain, rib, or heavy shaker knits with slash or patch pockets.

*Cardigans.* Button-front V-neck cardigans were also available and some retained the high shawl collar of the 1910s and '20s. Many pullover and cardigan styles featured a "rustless zip" (zipper) closing. Some sweaters also featured a zippered pocket. Common colors were navy, brown, tan, rust, gray, maroon, green, fawn, and heather mixtures produced primarily in solids; however, a few striped sweaters were also offered. Towards the end of the decade, the chest area of some sweaters were fashioned of a color or texture to contrast with the raglan sleeves and waistband. Knitted sleeveless vests in pullover and cardigan styles were also available.

# ACTIVE SPORTSWEAR

## Swimming

Swimwear for men was influenced by the bathing suits worn by Olympic Champions like Johnny Weissmuller and Buster Crabbe. In 1932, Weissmuller starred in his first Hollywood film *Tarzan the Ape Man* and began modeling bathing suits for BVD.

*Crab-back Suits.* Men's bathing suits were becoming more and move revealing. The trend for suntanned skin led to the "crab-back" wool-knit suit of the late '20s and early '30s which featured large cut-outs stretching from the center back to the sides.

*Topper Suit.* Regulations on public beaches of the early '30s required that men cover their chests. On private beaches, however, adventurous young men were basking and bathing

topless. Circa 1934, Jantzen introduced its ingenious "topper" suit which could be worn with or without the top. This suit consisted of dark two-ply woolen trunks (briefs) and a light-colored crab-back-style woolen top fastened together by a zipper. Topless brief-style high-waisted trunks became commonplace by the late 1930s and contained a contrasting white cotton belt with a metal buckle and a narrow white vertical stripe down the side seam. Some suits featured a small zippered pocket.

*Lastex Yarn.* In 1931, the United States Rubber Company introduced a new elastic yarn, called "Lastex." This yarn had a rubber core wrapped with cotton, rayon, wool, or silk fiber. Lastex could be woven or knitted into fabric with high elasticity and two-way stretch which revolutionized the garment industry. Lightweight Lastex swim trunks with a shiny rayon-satin finish dried quicker, held their shape better, and were less itchy than woolen suits. Bathing suits for men were produced in navy, royal blue, maroon, black, and gray with white trim.

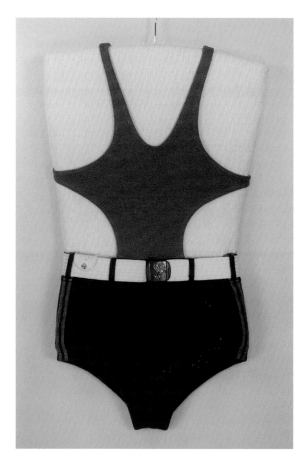

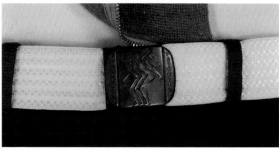

Men's bathing suit featuring a bib top which can be removed by the use of a hidden zipper, white rayon belt with small pocket and copper buckle. $30-$40.

207

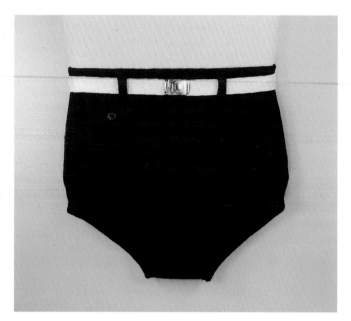

Men's maroon (50% wool, 50% cotton) bathing suit with white rayon belt. $25-$30.

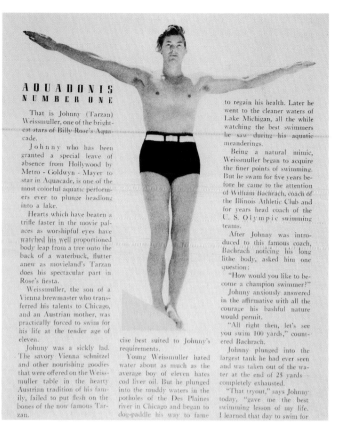

Johnny Weissmuller, two-time Olympic swim champion and star of the movie series *Tarzan* (1932-1948), wearing a typical late '30s wool-knit swimsuit featuring a white belt, 1939.

**Beach Accessories.** Cotton seersucker or terry cloth robes were popular for the beach. Navy and white striped knit shirts resembling those worn by French sailors were a popular cover-up to wear with trunks. Colorful rope-soled espadrilles or woven leather *huaraches* were also worn at the beach.

## Golf

Golfers began the decade by wearing tweed knickers, a carry-over from the 1920s. They were gradually replaced by pleated flannel or gabardine slacks in gray, tan, or white. Khaki-colored shorts with knee-length socks became a third option circa 1936. These pants styles were worn with short-sleeved wool-jersey shirts with pointed collars. Golf caps were still in vogue, although they were receiving competition from linen or wool "porkpie" hats. Brown brogues, brown buckskins, and moccasin-style golf shoes with steel spikes completed the look.

## Tennis

Tennis players of the late 1920s and early 1930s wore short-sleeved light-weight polo shirts, white wool flannel trousers, and white sneakers. In cool weather, off-white cable-stitch sweaters were worn with contrasting navy or maroon bands at the V-neck, cuffs, and waistband.

English tennis player, Bunny Auston, made fashion history in 1932 when he arrived in shorts for the Men's National Tennis Championship at Forest Hills, Long Island. By the end of the decade, tennis shorts were commonplace.

## Skiing

**Ski Suits.** Manufacturers of ski wear looked to the Norwegians, the Swiss, and the Austrians for inspiration. Short double-breasted Tyrolean-style jackets were popular as they were lightweight and waterproof. Single-breasted jackets and jackets with an off-center zipper closing were considered quite fashionable. Towards the end of the decade, hip-length parkas with drawstring waists and detachable hoods were available. Skiers during

the early 1930s continued to wear heavy wool knickers, a carry-over from the 1920s. These were worn with heavy-wool cable-stitch knicker socks. As the decade progressed, knickers began to lose their fullness and were eventually replaced by ski trousers which could be tucked into the ski boots. The most popular fabric for these snow togs was wool or cotton gabardine in navy or other neutral colors such as tan or brown.

**Accessories.** Norwegian peaked ski caps made of navy blue Melton, serge, or gabardine featured flaps which could be pulled down over the ears. Three-inch wide wool-knit headbands covering the forehead and ears were another popular head covering. Tyrolean-style hats with cord bands were a third option. Snow goggles were a must for the serious skier. Leather mittens were often worn over wool-knit gloves for added warmth.

## Horseback Riding

Horseback riding was steeped in English tradition and a strict code of dress developed which has changed very little over the years. Informal riding required a tweed single-breasted hacking jacket with high, short lapels and three or four leather buttons. Under the jacket was a white flannel or wool shirt with an attached collar. A silk, piqué, or linen stock was fastened around the neck with a stickpin. Either breeches or *jodhpurs* were appropriate for informal riding. They were both cut full over the hips and fitted from the knee to the ankle. *Jodhpurs* (originally from Jodhpur, India) had a cuff at the ankle and were worn over ankle-high *jodhpur* boots. Breeches (brE- chez), on the other hand, had buttons from the knee down with no cuffs and were worn inside of knee-high riding boots. Breeches and *jodhpurs* were held down with stirrup straps which passed either under the foot or under the shank of the *jodhpur* boot. *Jodhpurs* and breeches were made of sturdy cotton cavalry twill, cotton whipcord, or gabardine and the insides of the knees were reinforced with leather knee guards. Common colors were tan, brown, stone, navy, dark green, and black. Boots were made of black or brown calfskin. Either a hard bowler or a Tyrolean-style hat completed the habit.

# OUTERWEAR

## Coats

*Guardsman Coat.* The dark-blue double-breasted guardsman coat was patterned after the greatcoats worn by English Grenadier guards. It had broad shoulders, wide lapels, and a half belt in back.

*Polo Coat.* Single-breasted camel's hair polo coats were also popular. They featured narrow notched lapels, slashed pockets, and either a full or a half belt. The dashing wraparound coat, of

1934, was also made of camel's hair. This style was loose and roomy with no buttons—only a belt/sash to keep it closed.

*Prince of Wales Coat.* The single-breasted Prince of Wales top coat, introduced in 1936, was made of Glen Urquhart plaid. It was a loose-fitting coat with broad shoulders, raglan sleeves, wide lapels with blunt points, and a fly-front closing with hidden buttons.

*Loden Coat.* The dark olive-green Loden coat, originally from Austria, became popular in the late '30s along with other Tyrolean-inspired fashions. It was made from the soft wool of mountain sheep and featured a military collar, set-in sleeves, and slash pockets. It was also popular in a mid-thigh-length jacket with raglan sleeves.

## Jackets

*Field Jacket.* The fingertip-length gabardine field jacket was popular with college men. It had raglan sleeves, a military collar, and side vents.

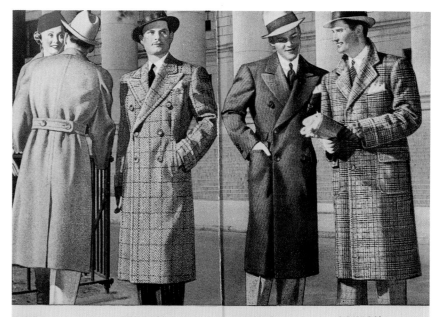

Howard Clothes advertisement (1937) featuring top coats. *(1)* Raglan-sleeved camel's hair coat. *(2)* Double-breasted drape coat, peaked lapels, slash pockets. *(3)* Double-breasted drape coat of covert cloth, peaked lapels. *(4)* Three-button plaid box coat, notched collar, patch pockets.

**KENT...**
Here we show one of the most beautiful 100% Camel's Hair Raglan Topcoats we have yet produced. It is a three button, single breasted, notch lapel garment.

**KENDALL...**
Indicative of the vital present-day trends, this double breasted drape coat with its convenient slash pockets is bound to wend its way into the wardrobe of every well dressed man.

**SPENCER...**
All evidence indicates that this double breasted drape coat with its smart dignified lines will be a spotlight fashion this season. Shown here in the much preferred Covert Cloth.

**BOXTON...**
One of the most important contributions to the spring style showing is this new three button, single breasted box coat. Developed with a straight back with center vent.

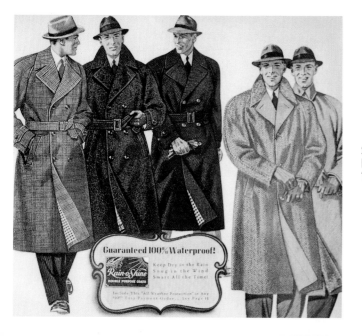

Sears, Roebuck and Co. ad (1939). *Left:* Men's waterproof belted topcoats in Glen plaid, herringbone, and twill. *Right:* Two-in-one reversible gabardine and herringbone top coats.

209

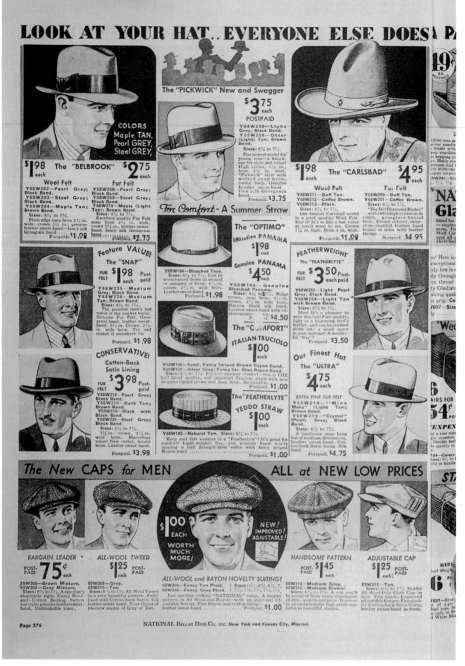

Bellas Hess (1931) offered a variety of men's hat styles including the felt snap-brims, felt Homburg, straw Panama, Italian-straw pork-pie, straw boater, Carlsbad (cowboy), and wool caps.

# HAIR AND HATS

## Hair

Men's hair was worn fairly short with a side part. Wavy hair was considered an asset. A thin, straight moustache was worn by mature men over the upper lip.

## Hats

*Homburg.* This large firm-felt hat appealed to older established gentleman. It could be worn with a dinner jacket (tuxedo) as well as a business suit. It contained a high crown with a crease running from front to back and a brim which was turned up all around.

*Snap Brim.* The crown of this felt hat had a teardrop-shaped creased on top and an indentation on either side. The brim was worn up in back and snapped down "swagger style" in front. The wide, contrasting grosgrain band featured a *faux* bow on one side. Snap brims were offered in shades of gray with a black band and shades of brown or tan with a dark brown band. During the late 1930s, a small feather was tucked into the band behind the bow.

*Tyrolean Hat.* This sport hat originated in the Alpine Tyrol region of Austria and Bavaria and was popular for football games and outings in the country. It had a high tapered crown with a center crease, a medium-sized brim (worn down in front and up in back). It was accented with a cord band and a bristle or barnyard-feather. Common colors were green, rust, black, and brown.

*Panama Hat.* This summer hat was actually made in Ecuador from the reed of the South American *jipijapa* plant. It got its name after President Theodore Roosevelt wore it for his visit to the Panama Canal in 1906. The fine, light-weight straw was shaped into an oval crown with a raised ridge running front to back. It featured a solid or striped silk band and was unlined which made it a cool choice for summer. Panama hats were worn until the Second World War.

*Porkpie.* This casual sport hat was introduced in the 1930s. It featured a snap brim and a circular crease running around the edge of its flat crown. This hat was made of felt, fabric, or straw with a solid or striped band. Summer straw porkpies were beginning to replace the boater.

*Cap.* This popular sport hat was worn for golf, motoring, and informal country wear. It was also a popular all around hat for blue collar workers. It was made with a flat one piece or "eight-quarter" piece top (eight pie pieces). Wool tweeds, checks, and herringbones were popular for winter, while cotton, linen, and corduroy were used for spring and fall. Common colors were tan, gray, and brown. Some models had a fur-lined inband which could be turned down over the ears for warmth in cold weather.

# FOOTWEAR

It was not uncommon to see holes in the soles of men's shoes during these hard times. Yet, those who could afford new shoes had a wide variety of sporty new styles to choose from. Men's shoes were evolving from the square toes of the 1920s

toward the more rounded toes of the late '30s and early '40s. Shoes were made predominantly of kidskin (from young goats), calfskin (from young cattle), or "reverse calfskin" which was the rougher flesh side of the leather used on the outside of the shoe and the grain side the inside. Also popular was buckskin, made from deer or elk hide which was given a suede finish. Common colors for men's shoes were black, brown, tan, gray, and white. Crepe rubber soles, introduced in the teens, were still used for sport shoes.

*Brogue.* The most common shoe, worn during the 1930s, was the brogue. It was made in black or brown calfskin or brown buckskin and was decorated with broguings (small perforations). These perforations were placed along the edges of the leather and either straight across the toe or in a wing-tip formation.

*Spectator.* Known as a co-respondent in the U.K., the spectator was a popular two-toned sport oxford. It consisted of a white shoe with a brown or black calfskin wing tip and quarter (brown being the most popular.) During the second half of the decade, another dark calfskin section was added over the instep. The dark sections were decorated with broguings along the outer edges. Calfskin with an embossed alligator grain was occasionally substituted for the dark leather.

*Trouser-Creased Oxford.* This sport shoe featured a raised seam running from the bottom of the lacing down the center of the vamp to the tip of the toe.

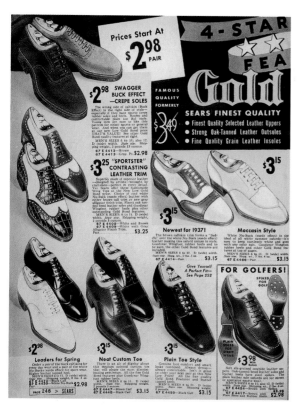

Sears, Roebuck and Co. catalog page (1937) promoting men's shoe styles including bucks with crepe soles, spectators in brown calf or gray alligator wing-tips, straight-tip, blucher, moccasin-style golf shoe, variation of spectator, white buck with moccasin toe.

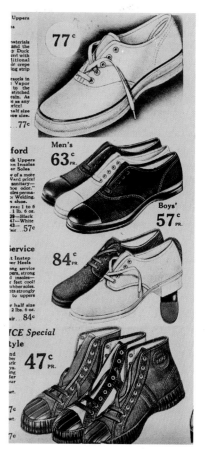

Montgomery Ward illustrations (1935) featuring men's sport oxfords. *(1,2,3)* Duck uppers, crepe rubber soles. *(4)* "Laced-to-toe" style, duck uppers, rubber soles and toe caps.

**Buck and Saddle Shoe.** These two shoe styles were made of deer or elk suede. They were available in white, brown, and tan with red rubber soles. The saddle shoe, introduced for men and women during the 1920s, was still worn in white or tan with a brown saddle and quarter.

**Weejun.** The weejun was originally handmade by Norwegian fishermen. It became a popular sport shoe during the 1930s and a forerunner of the all-American loafer. It contained a U-shaped moccasin-style seam circling the vamp. It was made in brown calf or two-tone brown and white which emphasized this "U" seam. Slip-on models had a strip of leather stitched-down over the instep with a slit through which a penny could be inserted. Oxford-style weejuns were also available.

**Monk Shoe.** Also introduced during the 1930s was the monk shoe. It featured a strap which crossed over the instep and buckled on the side of the shoe. It was available in polished and reverse-calf.

**Huarache and Espadrille.** In 1936, new styles in men's summer shoes began to reflect seasonal changes. The *huarache*, worn by Mexican peasants, was a sandal made of woven strips of leather which allowed for ventilation. Also popular were Spanish *espadrilles* with colorful canvas tops and rope or rubber soles. Beige or white canvas shoes were also popular.

# JEWELRY

**Tie Clasps.** Tie clasps were generally made of sturdy curved wire similar to a paper clip. They were decorated with sports motifs such as tennis rackets, guns, horses, sailboats, polo mallets, and dogs. Commemorative motifs such as the symbols of the 1932 summer Olympics in Los Angeles and the 1933 and 1939 world's fairs were also popular. These motifs were either executed in metal or reverse painted on dome or cushion-shape clear-crystal *cabochons*. An ornament was often suspended on a chain from the clasp. This ornament could be decorated with engine turnings (machine engravings), pavé-set marcasites, or a *cartouche* for monogramming.

**Collar Bars.** Gold-plated collar bars were used to hold the collar in place. They were attached to the collar points under the knot of the tie.

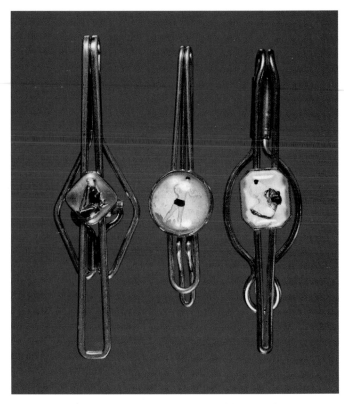

Silver-plated tie bars with horse-head, prizefighter, and terrier motifs under clear-glass cabochons. *Courtesy of Anna Shwak.* Marked: NU-LOK. $25-$35.

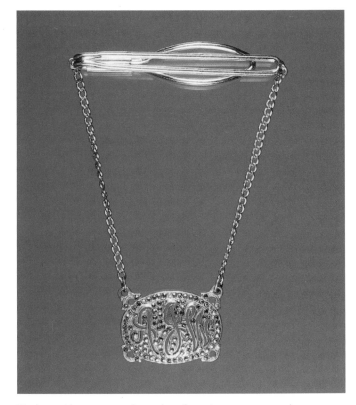

Tie bar with ornamental pendant featuring an openwork monogram and pavé-set marcasites. Marked: sterling, Manleigh. $75-$100.

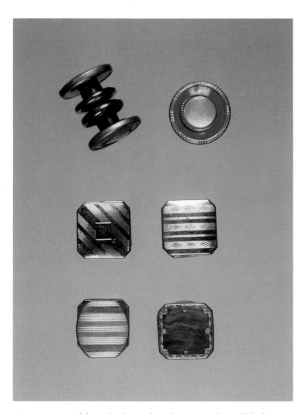

**Cuff Links**. Cuff links were a form of decorative jewelry used to fasten French- style shirt cuffs together. They were produced in a multitude of geometric shapes and materials. Many were hand engraved, engine-turned, chased, or brocaded. Others were set with precious or semi-precious stones, mother-of-pearl, onyx, moonstone, ribbed or star-cut crystal, sports crystal, or colored rhinestones. Cufflinks were produced with various findings. KUM-A-PART brand cuff links featured two sections which pulled apart like a snap. Other types included the "link button" and the "swivel bar." "Dress sets" containing two matching cuff links and four shirt studs were designed to fasten the formal dress shirt. Nine piece sets contained three additional vest studs.

**Watches**. Chains for pocket watches with a belt sleeve were still offered in sets with matching belt buckles. Wrist watches were becoming more and more popular and would eventually replace pocket watches. They were made in a variety of geometric shapes including rectangle, square, circle, hexagon, and variations of these shapes. Watch bands were made of tan or black leather or metal in parallel bar links, square or rectangular open links, tiny brick work links, or woven mesh.

Five men's gold and silver-plated snap-style cuff links. *(Row 1)* Red celluloid with mother-of-pearl center. Side view revealing the indentations for shirt cuffs. *(Row 2 and 3)* Engine turnings. $25-$40.

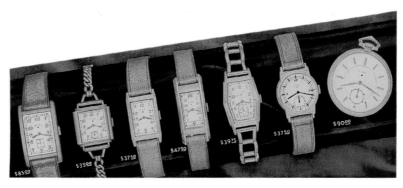

Watches by Elgin. Note: geometric-shapes, step design, and bands of black-silk cord or square open links.

# Chapter 14
# Uniforms

## WORK UNIFORMS

### Nurse

Nurses' uniforms resembled a tailored shirtwaist-style dress and were usually made of white cotton poplin. They opened all the way down the front with removable mother-of-pearl buttons and cuff links for easy laundering. Zipper front closings appeared in the late thirties. These uniforms featured notched, pointed, or Peter Pan collars, a buttoned-band waist, and three patch pockets (one breast, two hip).

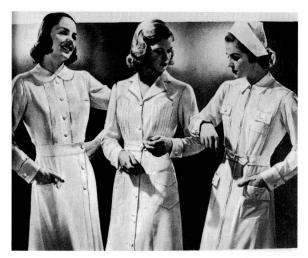

Advertisement from the Sears, Roebuck and Co. catalog (1939) for white cotton shirtwaist-style poplin nurses' uniforms (third style contains zipper front) and white cloth nurses cap.

### Maid

The maid's uniform included a dress in black, burgundy, navy, or dark green with white pointed collar and cuffs. A white headpiece and apron completed the ensemble.

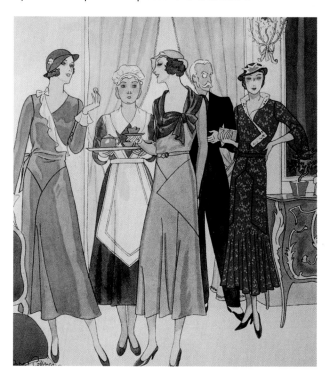

*McCall's* fashion illustration (1931), featuring a typical maid's uniform containing a black mid-calf dress with white collar and cuffs, white apron with pointed panel and wide straps which converge at the center waist.

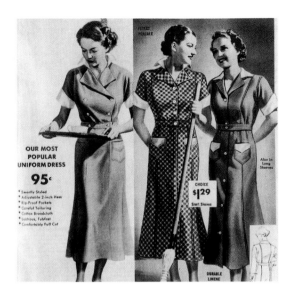

The Montgomery Ward catalog (1937) offered these single and double-breasted cotton-broadcloth waitress uniforms in solid colors (blue, green, rose, and lavender) and checks (black, red, medium green, copen blue with white). They were accented with white collar, cuffs, and pocket trim.

## Waitress or Beautician

This shirtwaist-style uniform was open to the waist or to the hem with removable buttons. During the second half of the decade, zipper closures were used. Bodices were either single or double breasted with a notched, pointed, or Bermuda collar. The most common fabric was cotton broadcloth in white, copen blue, green, rose, lavender, and burgundy with a white collar, cuffs, and trim on the patch pockets. Stripes and checks using vat-died yarns were also available. Also part of the uniform was a small apron with at least one patch pocket to hold an order tablet.

## Theater Usher

Large swanky theaters required that their ushers wear a short waist-length double-breasted jacket with brass buttons and peaked lapels. The collar and cuffs were made in a darker color to match the trousers. A winged-collar dress shirt and dark bow tie completed the uniform.

## Soda Jerk

The local soda shop was a popular place for teenagers to go after school. Here they could choose from such delectable treats as milk shakes, ice cream sodas, or sundaes. Creating these frosty concoctions was the soda jerk. He was typically clad in a white washable blazer-style jacket topped by a white overseas-style cap. Both were trimmed along the edge with dark binding or piping. In smaller shops a white apron might be substituted for the jacket.

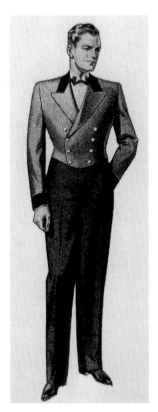

Theater usher's uniform. Short double-breasted jacket, peaked lapel with contrasting collar and cuffs, tailored pants. 1939. *Courtesy of Suzanne Checksfield.*

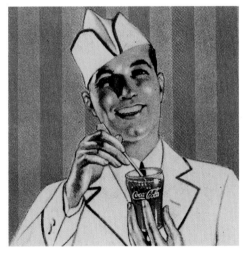

Soda jerk's uniform. White over-seas style cap and jacket with contrasting binding, 1935.

# SCHOOL UNIFORMS

The following descriptions were taken from the Powers Athletic Wear catalog of 1936.

## Cheerleader Uniforms

The male cheerleader's uniform consisted of a wool worsted or rayon pullover sweater with a high shawl collar. The collar front facing, and rib-knit cuffs and waistband were made in a contrasting color. The trousers were made of gabardine, duck, twill, corduroy, or flannel and featured a silk braid stripe down the sides. A skull cap made of six pie-shaped pieces of wool, felt, or corduroy completed the uniform. The female uniform was similar to the men's but with a V-neck sweater. These garments could be made in the school's colors.

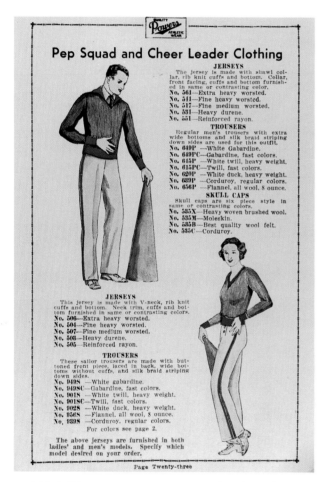

Powers Athletic Wear (1936): men's Pep Squad uniform - long-sleeved sweater with contrasting shawl collar, cuffs, waistband, and silk braid stripe on trousers. / Cheer Leader's uniform - V-neck sweater in contrasting colors and trousers with silk braid stripe.

## Band Cape and Cap

The typical band cape was made of flannel or rayon twill and lined with satin, sateen, or rayon twill. The overseas-style cap was made of flannel or rayon twill and trimmed in a contrasting color.

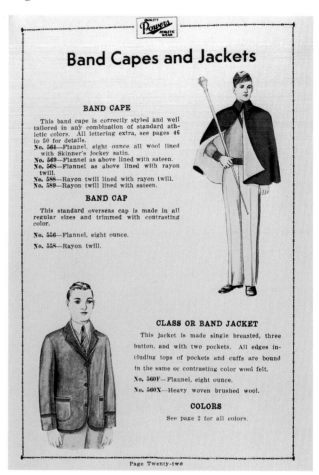

Powers Athletic Wear (1936): band uniform - cape in standard athletic colors, overseas cap. / Class jacket - single-breasted jacket, three buttons, bound in contrasting color.

## Class or Band Jacket

The single-breasted flannel class blazer featured three buttons, two patch pockets. All edges including the tops of the pockets and cuffs are bound in the same or contrasting color wool felt.

## Gym Suit

Girls' one-piece gym suits were notoriously homely. Those of the '30s were usually sleeveless with a V-neck, buttoned self belt, and bloomer-style pants with elasticized hems.

## Hockey Tunic

The sleeveless hockey tunic featured a shoulder yoke with a square neckline. The fabric below the yoke was arranged in three box pleats front and back, which allowed for freedom of movement. A button or tie self belt completed the uniform.

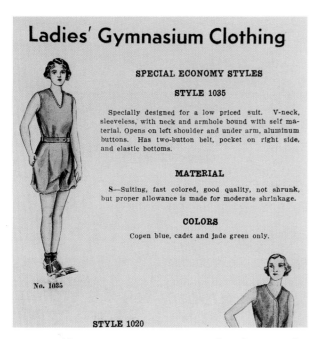

Powers Athletic Wear (1936): gym suit - sleeveless, V-neck, self belt, opens on left shoulder and under arm, elastic bottoms.

## Basketball Uniform

The button-front basketball shirt contained short sleeves and a shawl collar. It was available in sateen, broadcloth, poplin, rayon twill, and satin. The shirt was worn with bloomerettes, abbreviated bloomers with elastic bottom. They could be ordered in flannel, satin, rayon twill, corduroy, poplin, or gabardine.

The preceding athletic uniforms were available in the following standard colors: maroon, scarlet, royal, navy, kelly, black, white, gray, light gold, old gold, light orange, dark orange, dark green, and purple.

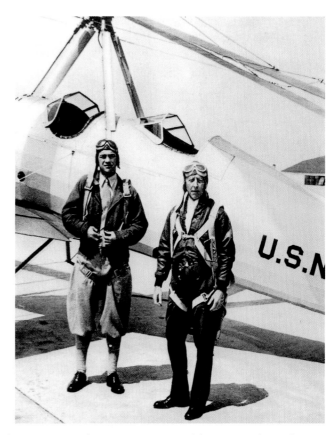

The Secretary and Assistant Secretary of the Navy in front of a Pitcairn Autogiro. Both men wear leather aviator helmets with goggles, leather aviator-style jackets, and parachutes, 1931. (Aviator-style helmets were very popular for young boys.)

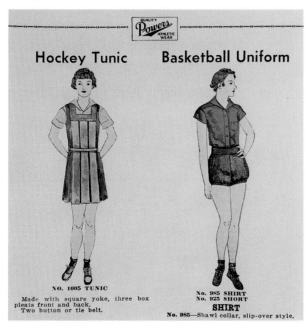

Powers Athletic Wear (1936): girl's hockey tunic - shoulder yoke, three box pleats, belt. / Girl's basketball uniform - Shirt with shawl collar and cap sleeves, bloomerettes with rib knit at bottom. Powers Athletic Wear, 1936.

217

Chapter 15

# Children's Wear

## INFANTS' WEAR

Most clothing for infants was made in pastel colors, the most common of which were pink for girls and blue for boys.

### Day Wear

*Dresses*. Dainty white nainsook or batiste dresses with delicate hand-embroidery were imported from the Philippines. Clusters of vertical pleats or pin tucks emanating from the shoulders or the neckline created a gentle fullness. They were produced with short sleeves in both knee and past-the-toe lengths. Long fancy white dresses with matching hats were traditionally worn as christening outfits.

*Rompers.* Summer cotton "rompers" or "creepers" were all-in-one garments with short sleeves and short pants. They usually featured a Peter Pan or Bermuda collar and a snap crotch. They were made of seersucker, crinkle crepe, and broadcloth and were decorated with lace, embroidery, smocking, or appliqué work.

### Night Wear

*Nightgowns.* Also called "sleeping bags," nightgowns were made of flannelette and contained a buttoned front placket, with or without a small round collar. The hem of the nightgown contained a drawstring which could be drawn to enclose the baby's feet.

*Sleepers.* Dr. Denton sleepers for infants came in two pieces which buttoned together at the waist. They were made of warm double-knit cotton-fleece with long sleeves and legs with feet.

*Wrappers.* Wrappers were simple flannelette garments similar to a kimono. They were fastened with ribbon ties at the neck and were open down the front.

### Outerwear

*Buntings*. Cozy buntings (shaped like grocery bags) had a zipper or button front for convenience and no sleeves or arm holes. They were made of warm Beacon blanket-cloth and were designed to encase the baby, outer clothing and all, like a custom-fitted blanket. They were usually bound along the edges with satin binding and often contained a figural appliqué.

*Sacques.* Loose-fitting cardigan sweaters called *sacques* (also spelled sacks) had long sleeves. A ribbon or tasseled crocheted drawstring was threaded through holes along the neckline, then tied in a bow at the neck. *Sacques* often came in sets with a matching crocheted cap and booties.

*Coats.* Spring and summer coats with matching hats were made of rayon taffeta, silk crepe, or wool flannel. They were embroidered with smocking and other embroidery stitches and their round Peter Pan collars were often trimmed with lace.

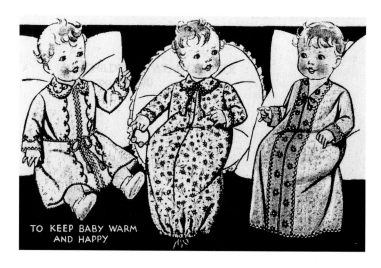

Infant's wear. (1) Blanket cloth bathrobe, embroidery, rayon cord girdle. (2) Printed cotton flannel sleeper, drawstring. (3) Cotton-flannel kimono. Bellas Hess Co., 1930-31.

## Layette

Thirty-four to forty-six piece layette sets were routinely offered in mail-order catalogs of the period. In addition to the items listed above, these sets included cotton flannel vests (undershirts), cotton batiste or cotton flannel gertrudes (slips), white rayon hose (socks), pin-on hose supporters (garters), terry cloth bibs, diapers, diaper pins, terry cloth towels and wash clothes, cotton fleeced blankets, crib sheets, rubber sheets, and quilted mattress pads.

## Accessories

*Bonnets*. Poke-style bonnets had flat or gathered projecting brims which were used to shade the baby's face from the sun. An alternative style had a fussy shirred ruffle which was fastened to the front edge of the hat with the fullness extending back against the sides of the head. Hats were made of organdy, silk crepe, or rayon taffeta and were decorated with picot edging, embroidery, and delicate ribbon rosettes. Winter poke bonnets were made of warm wool flannel.

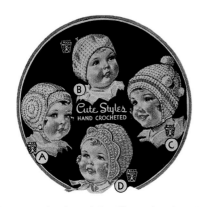

Sears, Roebuck and Co. illustration (1933-34) featuring wool beret, hats, and bonnets.

*Footwear*. Crocheted cotton or rayon booties with tasseled drawstrings were worn by both boys and girls. Silk-crepe moccasin-style shoes decorated with pastel embroidery were popular for dressy occasions.

# GIRLS' CLOTHING AND ACCESSORIES

Young girls' clothing was influenced by the traditional styles worn by the young English princesses, Elizabeth and Margaret and by the perky little dresses worn by child star, Shirley Temple.

## Day Wear

*Dresses.* "Bloomer" or "*sacque*" dresses of the 1920s were still very much in style during the 1930s. These comfortable little frocks hung loosely from the shoulders like a chemise. They often incorporated unstitched pleats which created a slight flare over the matching bloomers. The Peter Pan, Bermuda, or *Pierrot* collars were accented with embroidery or edged with contrasting binding, piping, rickrack, or lace. Baby-doll and ruffled wing sleeves were the most common.

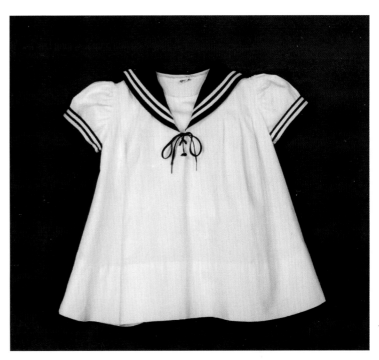

White cotton-twill sailor dress with navy-blue sailor collar, white bias tape trim and navy lacing. Label: DEB.N.HEIR *Courtesy of Janet Senderowitz Loengard.* $25-$45.

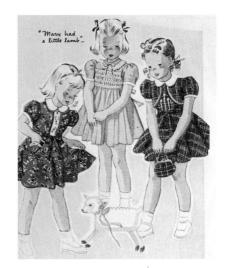

Illustrations from the Sears, Roebuck and Co. catalog (1939) featuring dresses with puffed-sleeves, Peter Pan collars, and high waists. *(1)* Rayon print, full-circle "swing" skirt, red rickrack, embroidery. *(2)* Cotton broadcloth, smocked bodice, full gathered skirt. *(3)* Gingham plaid, bolero effect, white rickrack, full-circle swing skirt.

As the decade progressed, a new high waistline appeared. Dresses consisted of a short bodice stitched to a full-circle "swing" skirt or gathered skirt. They were often trimmed at the waist with a self belt, or a matching sash tied in the back. Bodices were embellished with smocking, a bib front, or a short bolero-jacket effect. Peter Pan collars were the most common followed by the sailor, puritan, and "dog's ear" collars. The classic sailor dress was a perennial favorite with its contrasting tie, braid, and nautical emblems.

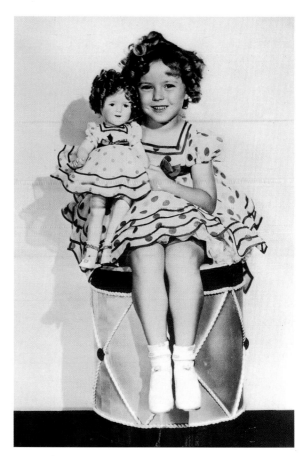

Photograph of Shirley Temple published in *Home Art Needle Craft* (12/36). She is wearing a polka-dot organdy dress trimmed in contrasting binding. She holds a doll in her likeness wearing a miniature version of the same dress.

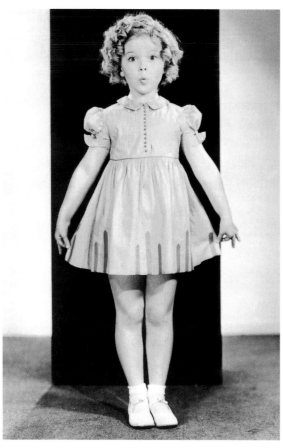

Child star Shirley Temple in typical ringlets, high-waisted dress, and white Mary Jane shoes.

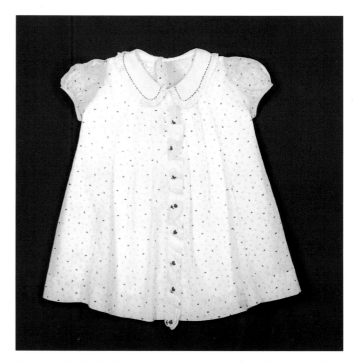

*Sacque*-style Shirley Temple dress made of pale-pink cotton mini-print fabric with baby-doll sleeves. Peter Pan collar is trimmed with a blue running stitch and white lace. Center front trimmed with white ruffle with red embroidered hearts. Label: A Nanette Toddler, Shirley Temple Brand. *Courtesy of Janet Senderowitz Loengard.* $30-$40.

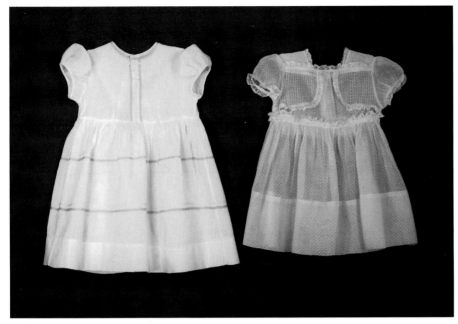

*Left:* White cotton dimity dress with baby-doll sleeves, pink and blue bias-tape trim and tiny mother-of-pearl buttons. Label: Saks Fifth Avenue. *Right:* Dainty dress of pink dotted Swiss with baby doll sleeves, trimmed with tiny tucks and lace. *Courtesy of Kay Senderowitz Breakstone and Janet Senderowitz Loengard.* $25-$35 ea.

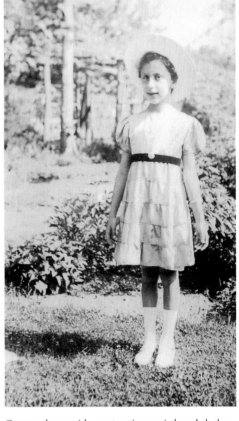

Cotton dress with contrasting waistband, baby-doll sleeves, and tiered skirt, wide-brimmed sailor hat. *Courtesy of Elizabeth Grant.*

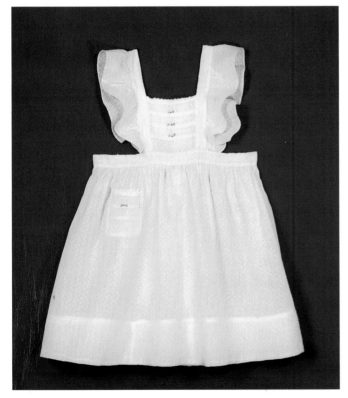

Pink dotted Swiss pinafore, bib and pocket decorated with lace, tucks, and pink embroidered flowers. *Courtesy of Kay Senderowitz Breakstone.*

**Pinafores.** The feminine pinafore was a short skirt with a bib top and shoulder straps, each embellished with a gathered ruffle (like the wing sleeve). Pinafores could be cool and airy when worn alone on hot summer days, or a dainty feminine touch when worn over dresses in cooler weather. They were often made of sheer fabric or white eyelet.

Solid colored fabrics, mini-floral prints, checks, plaids, and stripes were all used for young girl's dresses. Summer dresses were made of cotton piqué, gingham, voile, organdy, batiste, dimity, nainsook, dotted Swiss, crepe, and flocked-dot organdy. Common winter fabrics were wool, corduroy, cotton, and taffeta. Dresses were decorated with lace, ruffles, embroidery, and contrasting piping.

**Sunsuits.** Summer sunsuits consisted of short pants with a bib top and shoulder straps made of cool absorbent cotton. They were designed for toddlers and were worn with or without a blouse or shirt. They were made of seersucker, crinkle crepe, piqué, and broadcloth.

**Overalls.** Overalls were long pants with a bib front and shoulder straps. They were made of corduroy, cotton broadcloth, seersucker, khaki drill, cotton suiting, and chambray.

**Playsuits.** All-in-one play suits (similar to current jumpsuits) were popular for girls as well as for boys. Girls' playsuits, however, were generally more decorative than boys'. They were designed with long pants and either long fitted or puffy baby-doll sleeves and a back-tie sash. The Peter Pan collar, waistband, and patch pockets could be made of a contrasting color or pattern. The bodice was often embroidered or appliquéd with flowers or figurals. They were made of chambray, denim, corduroy, and broad cloth. Lace, rickrack, or braid were typical forms of trim.

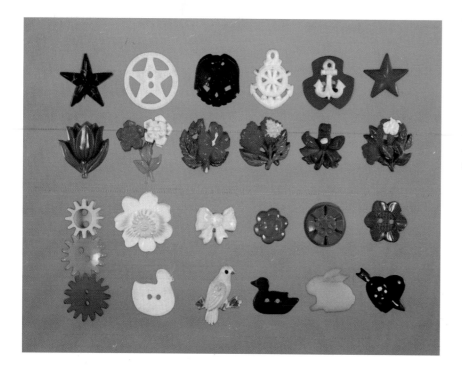

Realistic buttons including nautical, floral, and figural designs. *Courtesy of Mary Anne Faust (Yesterday's Delights).* $1-$10.

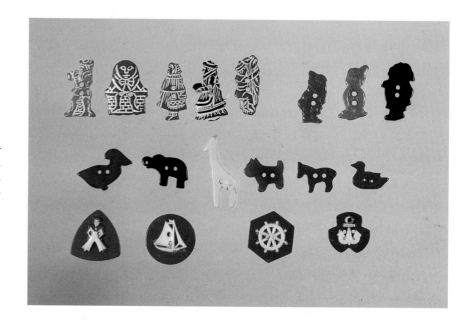

Bakelite and plastic realistic buttons from four different series: nursery rhymes, dwarfs, animals, and nauticals. $35-$150. per set. *Courtesy of Nancy Moyer.*

Brother and sister outfits were offered in mail-order catalogs. They consisted of matching long-sleeved knit shirts with coordinating short pants for the brother and a pleated skirt for the sister. On some styles the colors were reversed (light top and dark bottom for the girl—dark top and light bottom for the boy).

Unisex crew-neck and V-neck pull-over sweaters were offered throughout the decade. Sears mail-order catalogs offered sweaters printed with Mickey Mouse cartoons for boys and girls.

Children's clothing of the 1930s was often accented with cleaver little "realistic" buttons which were sold on cards containing all-of-one kind or a series. (Buttons on their original card are very desirable.) Each series consisted of different buttons with a similar theme such as Snow White and the Seven Dwarfs, nursery rhymes, animal silhouettes, Mickey Mouse and company, and "things that go" (popular for little boys). Button

collectors are always in pursuit of those few illusive buttons to complete a set.

## Sleep Wear

*Sleepers*. Dr. Denton's all-in-one pajamas with feet were the most popular sleep wear. They were made of double-knit cotton fleece or flannel for cold winter nights. The front placket opening was fastened with rubber buttons and the back contained a drop seat.

One-piece summer sleepers were designed with short sleeves, long pants, and a placket front fastened with buttons or Oriental-style frogs (a carry-over from the 1910s and 1920s). They were made of nainsook, cotton crinkle crepe, rayon crepe, cotton pongee, and cotton broadcloth in prints and solids.

*Robes*. The old favorite Beacon cotton blanket-cloth robes (a carry-over from previous decades) featured a shawl or notched collar and rayon cord trim and tie.

## Sportswear

*Bathing Suits*. Little girls wore conventional wool knit tank suits, "crab-back" style knit suits with cut-outs at the sides and back, or bib front bathing suits. Designers began to experiment with Lastex and rayon satin fabrics for quicker-drying figure-hugging suits.

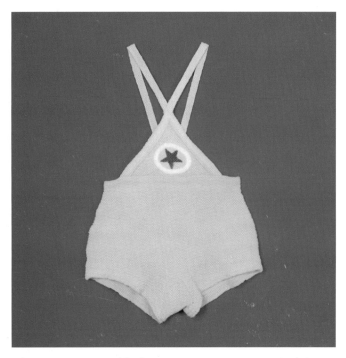

Infant's turquoise wool bathing suit containing a triangular bib front with appliquéd star, circa 1935-36. *Courtesy of Janet Senderowitz Loengard.* $15-$20.

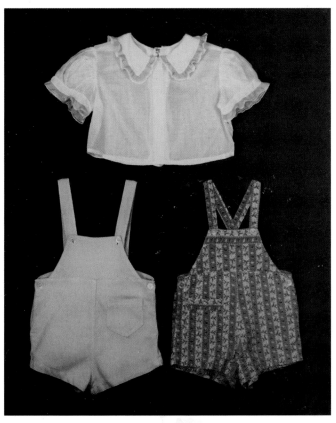

White cotton blouse containing a narrow pink cotton ruffle along edge of collar and sleeves. Two cotton sunsuits. All labeled: Best & Co. *Courtesy of Kay Senderowitz Breakstone.* $15-$20.

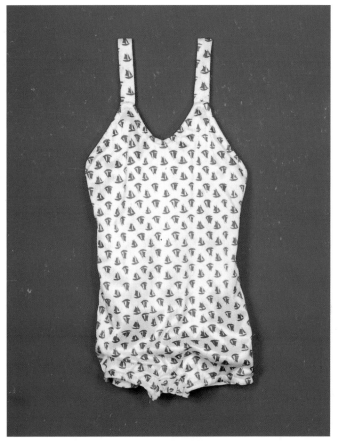

Satin-Lastex bathing suit with all-over sailboat pattern. *Courtesy of Janet Senderowitz Loengard.* $15-$20.

## Outerwear

Dressy double or single-breasted coats with a matching bonnet and zippered leggings were made of warm wool or wool chinchilla cloth. Their little round collars were often trimmed along the edge with a narrow band of fur.

Two-piece or all-in-one snow suits with round or pointed collars and rib knit cuffs were worn for play. These suits came with a matching snug-fitting aviator-style hat, or knitted Alpine-style pointed hat or hood.

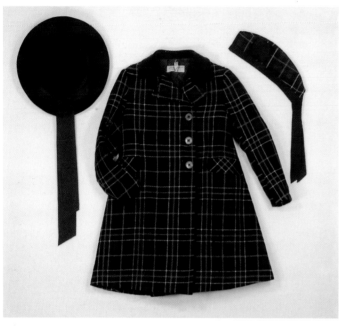

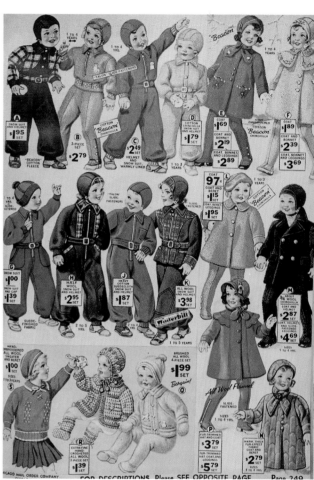

Girl's single-breasted coat of navy, green, and red wool tartan with a green velvet collar. Label: Glenconner, made in England exclusively for Best & Co., New York. / Green fur-felt Breton sailor hat with wide up-turned brim, green grosgrain band and streamers. Label: Best & Company, Lilliputian Bazaar. / Scottish Glengarry cap (to match coat) with navy grosgrain cockade and streamers. Label: same as coat. *Courtesy of Kay Senderowitz Breakstone.* $50-$75 set.

This Sears, Roebuck and Co. catalog page (1936-37) offers / Children's snow suits and matching aviator-style helmets made of Beacon blanket cloth, cotton chinchilla, wool flannel, and suede cloth (some feature zippers). / Coats with matching bonnets and leggings. / Hand-crocheted sweater sets.

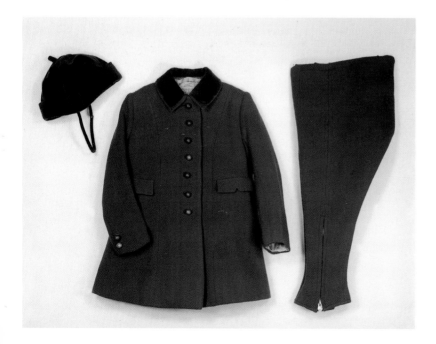

Blue wool herringbone coat and leggings with blue velvet collar and hat. Label: Glenconner, Made in England Exclusively for Best & Co., New York. *Courtesy of Janet Senderowitz Loengard.* $55-$75.

## Hair

Young girls' hair styles included the bob with a side part, the shingle, bouncy Shirley Temple-style corkscrew curls (ringlets), or braids. Hair ribbons to coordinate with a particular outfit were worn under the hair at the back of the neck, then tied in a bow at the top of the head.

## Accessories

*Hats*. *Cloches* were worn for all seasons during the early years of the decade. Spring and summer hats included straw bonnets decorated with delicate flowers and Breton sailor hats. Many hats for young girls had an elastic chin strap or tie to keep the them securely on the head.

Dressy winter hats included the felt or angora beret, feather trimmed Tyrolean hat, felt or wool tartan Glengarry cap, tam-o-shanter, and the wool bonnet (usually part of a matching set including a coat and leggings ). Utilitarian winter hats such as the wool-knit hockey cap, the pointed Alpine hood, and the snug-fitting aviator-style helmet (without a peak) were worn for winter play.

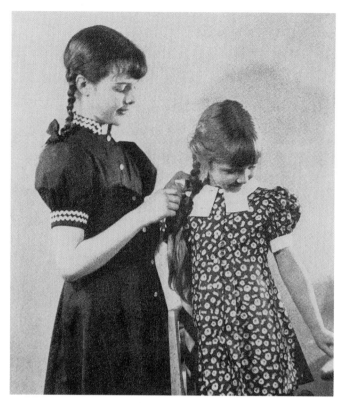

As this *Delineator* photograph (2/37) shows, braids were a popular way of dressing girl's hair, particularly for play as it kept the hair off of the face. *Delineator, 2/37.*

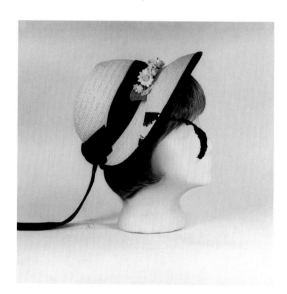

Natural straw bonnet is edged with black velvet, black velvet band embellished with pink and white flowers. Best & Co., Lilliputian Bazaar. *Courtesy of Kay Senderowitz Breakstone.* $20-$30.

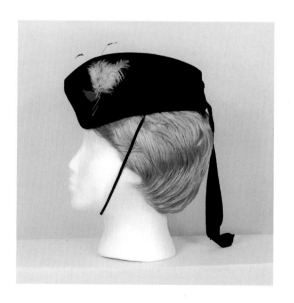

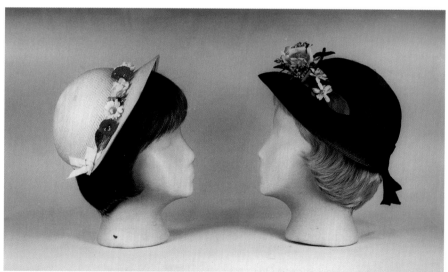

**Above:** Natural-straw bonnet decorated with multicolored flowers. / Navy-blue straw bonnet with grosgrain band accented with multicolored flowers. Label: Saks-Fifth Avenue. *Courtesy of Janet Senderowitz Loengard.* $20-$35 ea.

**Left:** Navy-blue felt Scottish Glengarry cap accented with feathers and grosgrain ribbon. *Courtesy of Kay Senderowitz Breakstone.* $15-$20.

**Handbags.** In most cases, handbags for little girls were smaller, less expensive versions of those carried by their mothers. They included *pochettes* (often of artificial leather), cloth pouch-style bags gathered to metal frames, and suede or velvet muffs with zippered pockets. Bags made of leather links were also popular. Handbags were often accented with some form of appliqué, the Scottie dog being the most common. Miniature *Beauvais* bags, with pastel chain-stitch embroidery surrounded by white seed beads, were used for special occasions.

**Shoes.** Many of the same shoe styles worn by women were offered for little girls as well; however, they had lower heels and broader toes. T-strap sandals with cut-outs and Roman high-top sandals with two to four straps were worn for hot summer days. High-top and low oxfords, kiltie oxfords, tongueless tie oxfords, and oxfords with two-toned moccasin vamps were worn for play. Black or white patent leather Mary Janes were worn for dressier occasions. (This shoe was named after Mary Jane from the Buster Brown comic strips of the early 1900s.)

**Jewelry.** Pearl "anniversary" necklaces were an ideal gift for little girls. A child was given a 14k gold chain and one or two pearls to start. Additional pearls are added on birthdays and special occasions until the necklace was complete.

Dainty white gold-filled lockets were offered in circle, rectangle, hexagon, tear drop, and heart shapes. They were embellished with engine turnings (machine engravings), *guilloché* enameling, engraved initials, or a faceted stone. Engraved 10k gold crosses were another popular gift.

Engraved or filigree bangle bracelets made of white gold were also popular. Charm bracelets featured lucky elephants, Scottie dogs, and nursery rhyme characters. Tiny 10k gold rings were set with simulated birthstones or engraved with a young ladies' initials.

Children's watches offered in the Sears Roebuck and Co. catalog featured Mickey Mouse and Orphan Annie faces. In 1935, both Montgomery Wards and Sears offered enameled silver and gold-tone Mickey Mouse jewelry including rings, pendants, pins, and bracelets.

Less expensive jewelry was made of plated base metal, celluloid, Bakelite, and other forms of plastic.

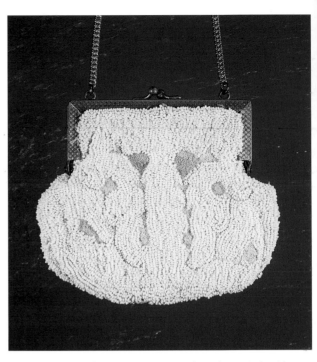

Child's *beauvais* bag containing pastel tambour embroidery surrounded by white seed beads, gold-plated frame and chain handle. $45-$60.

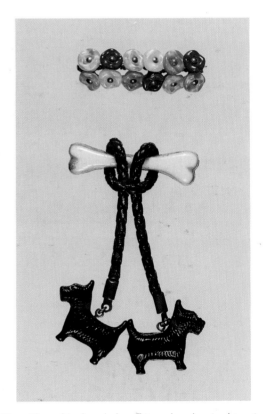

*Top:* Pin with multicolored glass flower heads wired to pin finding. $15-$20. *Bottom:* Pin containing two celluloid Scotties suspended on braided leash from celluloid bone. $35-$40.

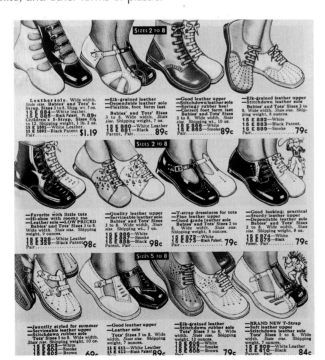

Children's shoes from Sears, Roebuck and Co. (1937). They include Roman (four strap) and T-strap sandals, high-tops, and oxfords with numerous perforations. Not pictured: cowboy boots.

# BOYS' CLOTHING AND ACCESSORIES

## Day Wear

*Suits.* Two-piece suits consisting of short pants which buttoned onto a long-sleeved (in fall and winter) or short-sleeved shirt (in spring and summer) were worn by toddlers. The shirts were made of knitted cotton jersey with a crew neckline or cotton broadcloth with a Peter Pan, Bermuda, or *rever* collar. The pants were made of corduroy, cotton broadcloth, serge, wool jersey, or chambray.

Suits for older boys had single-breasted, double-breasted, or collarless jackets. They were worn with short pants, knickers, or "longies" (long pants) with extra-wide bottoms. A pointed collar shirt and a four-in-hand tie completed the outfit.

Boys' classic sailor suits in white cotton poplin or navy flannel were a perennial favorite. They were trimmed with braid on the collar and cuffs and nautical emblems on the pocket and sleeves. The accompanying "longies" or sailor pants had wide bottoms and a buttoned front fall. A free bosun's whistle was frequently offered as a premium.

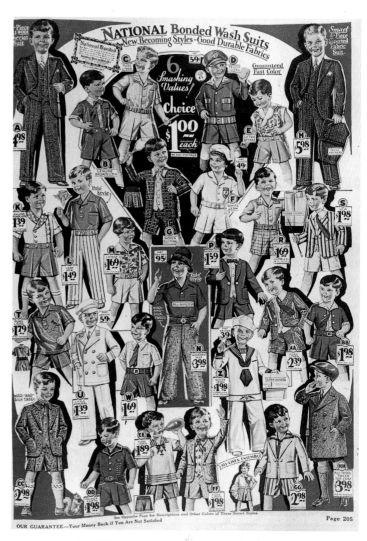

Bellas Hess ad (1930) for a variety of boy's clothing, including: three-piece "longie" suits (long pants), two-piece broadcloth "wash suits" with short knee pants, lumberjack suit, sailor suits, long pants, polo shirt, and top coat.

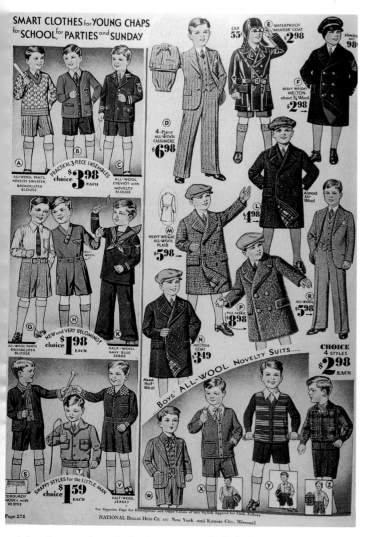

Advertisement from Bellas Hess (1931) for little boy's fashions, including short pants with coordinating shirts, sweaters, jackets, three-piece suits, overcoats, aviator-style jacket and helmet.

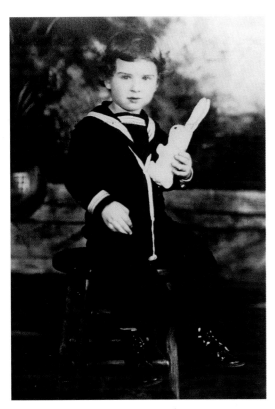

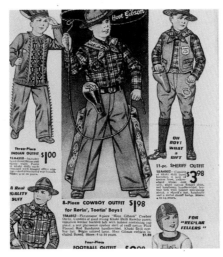

**Above:** Bellas Hess advertisement (1931) featuring Cowboy and Indian dress-up outfits.

**Right:** Boy's wool-plaid coat with matching belt and hat, short pants, hose, and high-top shoes, c. 1938-39. *Courtesy of Rose Jamieson.*

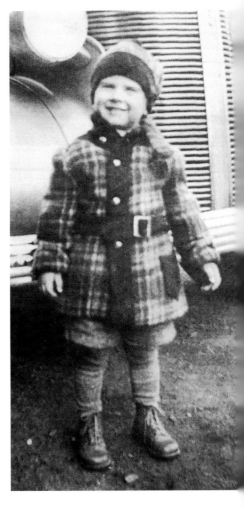

Sailor suit trimmed with white braid, worn with a bosun's whistle, and high-top shoes, c. 1938-39. *Courtesy of Rose Jamieson.*

*Knickers.* School-age boys wore knickers for sport with Argyle knee socks. They were made of cotton or wool and came in browns, blues, and grays.

*Sunsuits, Overalls, and Playsuits.* For these three styles, refer to the description under girls' clothing. Boys' versions of these styles were generally more severe with top-stitching and piping as their only form of ornamentation. Playsuits for boys resembled coveralls worn by auto mechanics.

*Ties.* Sears mail-order catalogs offered young boys' whimsical silk ties printed with cartoon characters such as Mickey Mouse, Dick Tracy, Skippy, and Popeye.

*Pullover Sweaters.* Crew-neck and V-neck sweaters were offered throughout the decade in solids, stripes, and various textures. Mickey Mouse sweaters were a perennial favorite. Turtleneck sweaters were offered during the second half of the decade.

*"Dress-up" Clothes.* Boys found it exciting to dress up like grown men and mail-order companies capitalized on this idea by carrying a line of dress-up clothes especially for boys. The would-be cowboy was outfitted with a ten-gallon hat, western shirt, bandanna, chaps, and holsters. Wanna-be Indians were offered feathered headdresses and fringed buckskin-style shirts and pants. For the future baseball player, a big league pin-striped shirt and knickers topped by a baseball cap. With the growing interest in air travel, Sears also offered the future pilot a sheepskin-lined leather jacket with matching aviator helmet and goggles.

## Sleep Wear

Boys' and girls' sleepers and bathrobes were remarkably similar, with the possible exception of color or fabric design.

## Outerwear

*Coats.* Double-breasted reefers and sailor coats with a navy insignia on the sleeve were worn for dressy occasions. For coldest weather, coats with matching aviator hats and zippered leggings were in order.

*Snowsuits.* Worn for play, snowsuits consisted of a double-breasted jacket (often plaid) with coordinating solid-color collar, belt, and loose-fitting bib-style pants. The rib-knit cuffs on the sleeves and pants were added protection against the cold. Head-hugging aviator or hockey-style caps completed the outfit.

## Accessories

*Hats.* There were many hat styles offered for young boys, including the aviator's helmet (wool fabric for young lads, leather with goggles for older boys), wool-knit hockey caps with a center pompon, white "gob" or middy sailor hat with up-turned brim, peaked jockey cap (similar to a baseball cap), wool golf cap, and the peaked ski cap with pull-down ear flaps. Ear muffs were also available.

*Shoes.* Leather oxfords and high-top boots (a carry-over from the previous decades) were worn by boys. Also popular were two-toned moccasin-style oxfords, T-strap sandals, and saddle shoes.

*Jewelry.* Boy's jewelry was primarily limited to wrist watches which were available with Buck Rogers, Dick Tracy, and Boy Scout faces.

# Glossary

Capital letter = Long vowel sound

| | |
|---|---|
| A = say | O = toe |
| E = see | U = true |
| I = tie | OO = food |

Lower case letter = Short vowel sound

| | |
|---|---|
| a = hat | o = lot |
| e = net | u = but |
| i = pig | oo = cook |

There are some French words on this list which have become commonplace in the English language. These words were often given an English pronunciation. In such cases both the French and the English pronunciations are listed.

**Adrian, Gilbert**
As head costume designer for MGM studios, he influenced fashion through the styles he designed for stars like Joan Crawford, Jean Harlow, Norma Shearer, Katherine Hepburn, and Greta Garbo.

**Agnès** Fr. (ah-nyes)
French milliner who specialized in tailored sporty hats. She is remembered for her use of Cubist-style fabrics designed by such renowned artists as Piet Mondrian and Sonia Delaunay.

**Alençon lace** Fr. (a-lon-son)
This needlepoint lace was originally made in Alenc,*on, France in the early 17th century. Floral designs were created on a fine net ground and outlined with heavy thread called *cordonnet* (cor-dO-nA).

**appliqué**
A technique involving decorative pieces of fabric which are cut and either stitched or glued to a larger piece of fabric or a garment. This technique can also apply to leather. Origin: French - "applied to."

**armseye**
Arm's eye or armhole of a garment.

**Art Deco**
A decorative art movement introduced to the world at the *Parisian Exposition International des Arts Décoratifs et Industriels Modernes* in 1925. Art Deco was characterized by geometric shapes, parallel lines, concentric circles, step patterns, sunbursts, waterfalls, fountains, stylized flowers (i.e. the Deco rose), and other abstract motifs. This style was replaced c. 1935 by Retro Modern.

**Art Nouveau** Fr. (art new-vO)
A decorative art movement (c. 1895-1915) characterized by fluid lines, i.e. flowers with long swirling tendrils, and women with long flowing hair. The width of these undulating lines also fluctuated creating a very graceful look. Origin: French - *nouveau* - "new."

**Arts and Crafts Movement**
Introduced in the late 19th century, this movement promoted handmade decorative arts, as apposed to machine-made mass-produced items.

**ascot**
Long narrow scarf attached to the neck of a blouse in back. The ends are brought around, looped under the chin, and held in place with a scarf pin. Origin: race track at Ascot Heath, England.

**asterism**
Star-like figure produced by reflected light from cabochon-cut sapphires.

**Astrakhan cloth**
Astrakhan cloth was a heavy knitted or woven fabric with a deep curly pile in imitation of Persian lamb.

**atelier** Fr. (a-tu-lEA)
A couturier(e)'s workshop or studio.

**Augustabernard**
Born Augusta Bernard in Provence, France. Combined her two names when she opened her own shop in 1919. She designed clothing for the custom departments at Henri Bendel and Bergdorf Goodman. She is known for her simple timeless bias-cut crepe and satin evening gowns of the late 1920s through 1934 (when she retired).

**avant-garde** Fr. (a-von gard)
An unconventional new style. Origin: French - "leading part of an army."

**baguette** Fr. (ba-get)
A diamond, emerald, or rhinestone cut in a long, narrow rectangle. Origin: French - "long leaf of bread."

**Bakelite**
The trade name for a synthetic resin or plastic named after its inventor, Belgian chemist L.H. Baekeland. It reached the height of popularity in the late '20s and '30s, when it was molded or carved into colorful jewelry, buttons, and buckles.

**bandoulière** Fr. (bon-dOO-lE-Ar) / Eng. (ban-du-lEr)
Name used by Schiaparelli for her shoulder-strap bags. Origin: French - "shoulder strap."

**basque bodice**
A snug fitting woman's bodice which extends below the waist.

**batiste** Fr. (ba-tEst)
A sheer, light-weight woven fabric of linen or fine quality mercerized cotton. It was used for blouses, dresses, lingerie, and men's shirts.

**baton** Fr. (ba-ton)
The *baton*-link carrying chain was used for handbags and vanity cases. It contained alternate links which resembled slender metal bars. Origin: French - "stick."

**beadlite**
Introduced in the late 20s, beadlite was a variation of armor mesh containing small dome-shaped links resembling beads. Beadlite purses were often enameled.

**beauvais bags** Fr. (bO-vA)
Small evening bags featuring pastel chain-stitch embroidery (usually flowers) surrounded by white, pearl, or black seed beads. Origin: Beauvais - city in France.

**bezel**
A metal rim which surrounds a stone (usually cabochon cut) securing it in its setting.

**bias cut**
A method of cutting garment pieces developed by French couturiere Madeleine Vionnet. Instead of placing the pattern pieces so that the warp threads run vertically and the weft threads run horizontally, pattern pieces are turned slightly so that the warp and weft threads are both on the diagonal. This gives the fabric a natural elasticity causing it to cling to the contours of the body. The bias-cut dresses of the 30s required soft supple fabrics such as silk satin, silk velvet, crepe de chine, and chiffon.

**bishop sleeve**
A long full set-in sleeve which was gathered into a short cuff at the wrist or a longer cuff extending from the wrist to the elbow. This longer cuff was often decorated with a row of closely spaced buttons. Origin: a bishop's ecclesiastical garment.

**boat neckline**
A shallow, slightly curved neckline resembling the hull of a boat. Also called a *bateau* (bah-tO) neckline, which means boat in French.

**bouffant** Fr. (bOO-fon) / Eng. (bOO-font)
Puffed out or full, as in *bouffant* skirt.

**boutonnière** Fr. (bOO-tu-nE-Ar) / Eng. (bOO-tun-nEr)
A single fresh flower placed in the buttonhole of a man's lapel. Origin: French - "buttonhole."

**brocade**
A luxurious fabric with a raised pattern woven in, created on the Jacquard loom. The pattern is produced by the incorpora-
tion of several different weaves which include the satin, rib, plain, and twill weaves. This fabric is not reversible as it has "floats" or loose threads running across the reverse side.

**brogue** (brOg)
Men's sturdy low-heeled oxford with small perforations called broguings arranged in decorative patterns. Origin: Irish/Scotch country shoe.

**bugle beads**
Small tubular glass beads produced in various lengths. They can be opaque, transparent, silver-lined, or pearlized.

**cabochon** Fr. (ka-bo-shon)
A jewelry term for an shiny unfaceted dome-shaped stone. It could be round, oval, square, rectangular, or triangular. Origin: French - *caboche* "knob."

**calotte** Fr. (ka-lot)
A small round skullcap originally worn by the ancient Greeks, adopted by women during the 1930s.

**cartouche** Fr. (kar-tOOsh)
Small smooth area (often slightly raised) on the surface of a metal object designed for an engraved monogram.

**celluloid**
A semisynthetic thermoplastic made of pyroxylin and camphor. This highly flammable substance was often dyed to look like ivory, tortoise shell, coral, or amber.

**challis** Fr. (shal-E)
This light-weight plain-weave worsted has a soft brushed surface. It was a popular fabric for dresses and is usually printed in a mini floral or geometric pattern. Also spelled **challie**, **challys**, or **challi**. Origin: Anglo-Indian - "*shalee.*"

**chambray** (shom-brA)
Cotton fabric with a linen finish made by weaving white weft threads through colored warp threads. Origin: Cambrai, France where it was first produced.

**chamois** Fr. (sha-mwah) / Eng. (sha-mE)
Buff colored skin from the chamois antelope of the European mountains.

**champlevé** Fr. (shom-luh-vA) / Eng. (shom-plu-vA)
An enameling technique in which a design is carved or routed out of the surface of a metal object to form a shallow cavity. This cavity is then filled with enamel.

**Chanel, Gabrielle "Coco"**
Chanel was the most influential fashion designer of the 1920s. She is noted for her classic suits, jersey dresses, costume jewelry, cardigan sweaters, beach pajamas, Chanel No 5 perfume, and her "little black dress."

**Chelsea collar**
A long pointed collar attached to a deep V-neckline.

**chenille** Fr. (shun-nE-yah) / Eng. (shu-nEl)
Soft fuzzy yarn with the feel of velvet. This two-ply yarn is twisted with short fluffy 1/8 inch threads caught between the plies and protruding from them to form a pile. A favorite fabric for bathrobes and bedspreads. Origin: French - "caterpillar."

*chiné* Fr. (shEn-A)
A French term for the Chinese textile printing technique in which the warp threads are printed before the weft threads are woven in. This creates a design with a soft blurred effect. Also called "warp print."

*chou* Fr. (shOO) pl. choux (shOO).
A large fabric flower used as a trimming. Origin: French - "cabbage or rosette."

*cloche* Fr. (klush) / Eng. (klOsh)
Bell-shaped hat with deep snug fitting crown and narrow brim. It covered the forehead in front and the hair to the nape of the neck in back. Origin: French - "bell."

**clogs**
Clogs were a sport shoe with thick wood or cork soles and leather uppers. They were derived from the French *sabot* (sa-bO) or Dutch *klompen* worn by peasant farmers.

**coney** (kOO-nE)
A term used in the fur trade for rabbit fur. Rabbit was often dyed to resemble more expensive furs such as beaver-dyed coney or chinchilla-dyed coney.

*couture* Fr. (kOO-tOOr)
Original styles created by fashion designers from the finest fabrics. Origin: French - "sewing, needlework."

**couture house** Fr. (kOO-tOOr)
The headquarters of a French fashion designer which could include show rooms, fitting rooms, and an *atelier* or workroom.

*couturier* Fr. (kOO-tOOr-E-A)
French term for male fashion designer.

*couturiere* Fr. (kOO-tOOr-E-Ar)
French term for female fashion designer.

**cowl neckline**
The soft bias-cut fullness of the bodice was draped in graceful U-shaped folds over the bust. To encourage this draping, a small nickel-sized metal weight was often suspended on a cord from the edge of the neck fabric on the inside of the bodice.

**crepe** Fr. (krep) / Eng. (krape)
A fabric with a pebbly surface made from highly twisted threads.
**crepe de chine** Fr. (krep-duh-shEn) / Eng. (krape duh shEn)
Fine light-weight low-luster crepe fabric made of raw silk with highly twisted weft threads. Used for lingerie, dresses, and blouses. Origin: French - "crepe of China."

**Cubism**
An art movement of the early 20th century, in which the subject was reduced to the simplest geometric forms. Shapes were used in abstract arrangements rather than realistic representations of nature. Cubism had a profound influence on the Art Deco movement.

**cummerbund**
A wide cloth band worn around the waist of a dress or men's tuxedo pants. Origin: Hindi/Persian - *kamarband* "loin band."

*de rigueur* Fr. (duh rE-ger)
Necessary, compulsory, a must.

**debutante**
A young woman from a wealthy family who, at age 18, is introduced into polite society for the first time at a series of fancy parties and balls. Origin: French - "beginner."

*dirndl* skirt (durn-dl)
A full skirt which is gathered into a waist band. Origin: Tyrolean peasant costume.

**doll hat**
Small hat, of the late '30s, held over the right eye by a back strap.

*d'Orsay* slippers
A woman's slipper which is cut away to the sole at the sides forming a broad V.

**dotted Swiss**
A crisp, often sheer fabric with rows of tiny raised dots which can be woven, embroidered, or flocked.

**double-clip brooch**
A brooch which can be converted to two dress clips.

**dress clips**
Jeweled ornaments worn singly or in pairs to adorn a neckline or a lapel. They were fastened to a garment by means of a hinged clamp on the underside of the clip.

**dressmaker bathing suit**
A swimsuit resembling a short dress.

**engine turnings**
Decorative machine engraving on metal objects such as jewelry, compacts, vanities, cigarette cases, and lighters. Typical patterns were rows of dots, circles, squares, waves, and stripes. Also popular were sunrays, basket weaves, concentric circles, and kaleidoscopes.

**espadrilles** Fr.
A canvas shoe with a rope sole, laced across the instep and up the leg.

**fagoting** (also **faggoting**) Fr.
Fancy crisscross embroidery stitches (like tiny connecting bridges) which stretch across a 1/4 inch gap between the parallel edges of two pieces of fabric. Fagoting provided a decorative, more supple alternative to the common seam. Origin: French - *fagot* "bundles of sticks."

**faille** Fr. (fl-yah) / Eng. (file)
Ribbed fabric of silk or rayon. It was used for women's dresses, suits, and coats; as well as the lapels and trouser stripes of men's tails and tuxedos.

**Fauvisme** Fr. (fOv-Esmu) **Fauvism** Eng. (fOv-ism)
An expressionist art style characterized by bold distortions and bright colors. Henri Matisse and André Derain were noted French fauvist painters. Origin: French - *Les Fauves* "the wild beasts."

**faux** Fr. (fO)
French term meaning false, fake, or synthetic.

**filigree**
Jewelry made of fine wire twisted into delicate lacy openwork resembling lace. By the 1930s, filigree work was die cast from such metals as platinum, white gold, sterling, brass, and base metal. Origin: French - *filigrane*.

**flounce**
Strip of fabric, gathered at the top and stitched to a bodice or skirt (often at the hem). Can be single or multiple rows.

**frou-frou** Fr. (frOO frOO)
1. Rustling sound of lady's skirts or petticoats. 2. An abundance of ruffles, ribbons, and laces.

**full-fashion marks**
Small desirable dots or marks in the knit along the seams of hosiery caused by increasing or decreasing stitches.

**fur clip**
A jeweled ornament with two sharp needle-like prongs hinged to the under side. These prongs were pushed into and then out of the fur or fabric to hold the clip in place.

**galoshes**
Waterproof mid-calf boots worn over shoes. Also spelled galoshe or golosh. Origin: French.

**gauntlet**
A glove with a wide flared cuff reminiscent of gloves worn by 17th century Musketeers. Origin: French - *gant* "glove."

**georgette**
A sheer loose-weave fabric with a pebbly surface similar to crepe. It was popular for evening wear during the 1920s and early 1930s.

**gilet** Fr. (zhE-lA)
A sleeveless bodice front, "plastron," or "dickey" worn under a suit jacket in place of a blouse. Derived from the French word for a man's 19th century vest.

**gillie oxford**
This Scottish dancing shoe, originally worn with a kilt, was introduced in the United States by the Prince of Wales and was often referred to as the "Prince of Wales shoe." It had no tongue and was laced through leather loops rather than eyelets. (Also spelled ghillie.)

**glacé kid** Fr. (gla-sA)
A smooth glossy finish applied to goatskin by the use of a glass roller. This soft leather was used for gloves, shoes, and handbags. Also called "glazed kid." Origin: French - "frozen."

**godet** Fr. (gO-dA)
Triangular or arch-shaped pieces of fabric inserted into the hem of a dress to create a flare.

**Glen Urquhart Plaid**
Suit material having narrow intersecting lines in soft subdued shades of gray, tan, brown, black, or navy in white. Also called a glen check, it was named for the Glen Urquhart valley in Scotland.

**grosgrain** (grO-grAn)
Ribbon with a width-wise rib or corded effect created by placing filling or weft threads together in groups. Origin: French.

**guilloché enameling** Fr. (gE-yO-shA)
Decorative treatment applied to metal objects. Engine turnings (machine engraved patterns) were covered with a layer of translucent enamel which allowed the engraved patterns to show through.

**halter**
A strap which encircles the neck and supports the front of a sundress, evening gown, blouse, or bathing suit leaving bare shoulders and back.

**hand-tooled leather**
Leather that has been stamped by hand with a metal die (tool) producing an impressed design.

**haute couture** Fr. (O-tuh kOO-tOOr)
High fashion. Origin: French - feminine form of *haut* - "high."

**huaraches** (wah-rah-cha)
A shoe made of narrow, closely-woven strips of leather. Origin: Mexican - "woven low-heeled sandals."

**ingénue** Fr. (an-zhe-nOO)
An innocent, inexperienced young woman.

**jabot** Fr. (zha-bO)
Decorative vertical ruffle suspended from the center of the neckline on a lady's blouse or dress. Origin: French - "frill."

**jersey**
Soft knitted cloth featuring the V-shaped knit stitch. Chanel was the first to use lowly wool jersey as dress fabric. Origin: the British Isle of Jersey in the English Channel where it was first produced.

**jodhpurs** Fr. (jod-perz)
Riding pants which flared out over the hips, then fit snugly from the knees down. Origin: Jodhpur - a city in India.

**Juliet (Juliette) cap**
A Renaissance-style openwork mesh skull cap which was often decorated with jewels or pearls, from the costume of Shakespeare's heroine.

**Juliet sleeve**
A long Renaissance-style fitted sleeve surmounted by a round puffed portion at the top, named for Shakespeare's heroine.

**kiltie oxford**
Sport shoe with tasseled laces which tie over a large turned-over fringed tongue. Origin: adaptation of a Scottish shoe.

**lamé** Fr. (la-mA)
Woven fabric of gold or silver metallic thread.

**lapis lazuli** Fr. (la-pEs la-zOO-lE) / Eng. (la-pis la-zOO-lE)
An opaque gemstone of deep-blue color, often with white mottlings.

**Lastex**
Elastic fabric which is knit or woven from yarn made of a rubber core wrapped with silk, cotton, or rayon thread. It was used during the 1930s for foundation garments and bathing suits.

**lava-lava**
A wrap-around skirt made of colorful printed fabric worn by men and women in Polynesia. Worn as a swimsuit coverup during the 1930s.

**layette**
Garments and accessories assembled for the newborn including diapers, nightgowns, kimonos, *sacques*, booties, bibs, undershirts, blankets, towels, and washcloths.

**lingerie** Fr. (lan-zha-rE)
Ladies intimate apparel including undergarments and sleepwear. Origin: French - *linge*, "linen."

**lisle** hose Fr. (lEl)
Fine cotton hosiery worn by men, women, and children throughout the 19th and early 20th centuries. Origin: Early spelling of Lille, France.

**lorgnette** Fr. (lor-nyet)
Eyeglasses with an articulated handle in place of temples. Origin: French - "opera glasses."

**Louiseboulanger** Fr. (lOO-Ez-bOO-lon-zhA)
Louiseboulanger combined her first and last names and opened a couture house in Paris in 1923. She is known for her ultra-chic bias-cut styles and sophisticated bi-level gowns. She closed her house in 1939 at the outbreak of World War II.

**maillot** Fr. (my-yO) / Eng. (mA-low)
A woman's one-piece bathing suit without a skirt.
**maison de couture** Fr. (mA-zOn du kOO-tOOr)
House of fashion.

**marabou**
Soft fluffy under plumage from the wings and tail of the African marabou stork. It was used to trim negligees and boudoir slippers during the 1920-'30s.

**marcasite** (mar-ku-zIt)
A silver-color iron pyrite used as an inexpensive substitute for diamonds. It is opaque and obtains its sparkle from the light reflected from its facets.

**matelassé** Fr. (mat-las-A)
A luxurious fabric, often made of silk, with a raised design in a heavy double-cloth weave.

**minaudiére** Fr. (mE-nO-dE-Ar)
Elegant jeweled box with compartments for a woman's lipstick, powder, cigarettes, keys, and other essentials designed by the jewelry firm, Van Cleef and Arpels. Origin: French "to put on airs to get attention."

**mirror-image clasp**
A two-part belt clasp with one side the reverse reflection of the other.

**moiré** Fr. (mwa-rA) / Eng. (mor-A)
Fabric with a watery-effect produced by the use of heated pressure rollers.

**Molyneux, Edward** Fr. (mOl-E-nu)
This English-Irish designer is noted for his tailored wool and printed silk suits, and matching ensembles.

**mousquetaire** Fr. (mOOs-ku-tAr)
Long formal gloves with a buttoned slit at the wrist. They could be worn smooth or crushed to the wrist.

**négligée** Fr. (neg-lE-zhA) / Eng. (neg-luh-zhA)
Flowing robe of satin fabric trimmed with feathers, usually worn over a matching nightgown. Also called a "dressing gown".

**Norfolk jacket**
Men's sport jacket featuring four box pleats (two in front and two in back). A matching belt was slipped through slits under each pleat. It was worn with knickers or long pants.

**nosegay**
A small round bouquet, the stems of which are often placed through the center of a white doily.

**nutria**
South American water-dwelling rodent with short soft brown fur, and webbed feet. Origin: Spanish.

**organdy**
A light-weight, sheer, stiff fabric usually made of cotton. A popular fabric for ingénue dresses.

**ombré** Fr. (Om-brA)
A fabric in which the colors blend into one another. Origin: French - "shaded."

**page boy**
Shoulder-length hair with the ends turned under all around.

**passementerie** Fr. (pas-mon-tu-rE)
Decorative braid which has been stitched to a garment creating a pattern or design.

**Patou, Jean** Fr. (pa-tOO, zhon )
French designer who, in 1929, lowered the hemline to mid-calf for day and the instep for evening. He returned the waist to its natural position that same year.

**pavé** Fr. (pa-vA)
For optimum sparkle, stones were set so close together that very little of the surface of the object was visible.

**peplum**
A small (often flared) skirt on a jacket extending below the waist.

**percale**
Light-weight plain-weave fabric made of fine combed cotton.

**Peter Pan collar**
Flat round collar with round ends.

**petit point** Fr. (pe-tE pwan) / Eng. (pe-tE point)
Embroidery which consists of rows of diagonal stitches on a grid-work canvas is called "needlepoint." Petit point contains as many as 1850 stitches to the square inch.

**Pierrot collar** Fr. (pE-ehr-O)
Large ruffled collar attached to a round neckline. Origin: costume of *Pierrot*, the French pantomime clown.

**pince-nez** Fr. (pans-nA)
Eyeglasses without temples, held in place by a spring-tension nose piece. Origin: French - "pinch nose."

**piqué** Fr. (pE-kA)
Crisp fabric made with cords causing a raised rib or grid effect.

**placket**
An opening at the neck, waistband, or wrist designed for ease in dressing and undressing.

**platinum blonde**
Hair which was bleached to a silvery white, introduced by actress Jean Harlow, the "blonde bombshell" of 1930s movies.

**pochette** Fr. (posh-et)
A flat rectangular handbag which reached its peak of popularity during the late '20s and '30s. It had a zipper top, flap top, or a metal frame with a clasp. *Pochettes* contained either a short horizontal top strap, or a vertical back strap. These bags were either carried by the top strap, tucked under the arm (called an underarm bag), or clutched in the hand (called a clutch bag). Origin: French - "small pocket."

**pongee**
A plain-weave fabric made from wild silk usually in its natural ecru color. The weft threads are irregular in thickness creating slubs. Origin: Chinese - *pen-chi* "home loom."

**prêt-à-porter** Fr. (pret-u-por-tA)
Ready-to-wear or off-the-rack clothing.

**princess line**
A garment with two long seams running from neck (or bust) to hem in front and back and no waist seam.

**rayon**
A synthetic fiber made from cellulose. Originally called artificial silk, it was renamed rayon in 1924. It draped well and accepted dye readily, but wrinkled easily and often shrunk with washing.

**Reboux** Fr. (re-bOO), **Caroline**
Leading French milliner who introduced the *cloche* hat (c. 1923), the gigolo hat (c. 1925), and elegant lamé turbans. She died in 1927.

**revers** Fr. (ru-vAr) Eng. (ri-vers or ri-vErz)
Lapels of a coat or jacket. Origin: French - "reverse or facing".

**reverse carved**
Carving on the back side of clear Bakelite jewelry or buttons which produces a 3-D image on the front side.

**rouleaux loops** Fr. (rOO-lO)
*Rouleaux* loops were used with closely-spaced covered buttons to fasten the backs of many 1930s gowns. They were created from a narrow tunnel of the dress fabric with or without a cord for filler.

**ruching** Fr. (rOO-shing)
Trim which resembles a ruffle. It consists of a strip of fabric, lace, ribbon, or net which is pleated width-wise and stitched down the center to a garment.

**sabot** Fr. (sa-bO)
See clogs.

**sacque** Fr. (sak) / sack Eng. (sak)
A loose fitting garment which hangs from the shoulders. Also infant's cardigan sweater.

**sans-serif** Fr. (son-su-rEf)
French term which refers to printed type or letters which have no serifs or fine lines projecting from the main stroke of the letter.

**satin**
Type of weave which produces fabric with a smooth glossy sheen.

**Schiaparelli** (Skap-a-rel-E), **Elsa**
Italian-born designer who began her career, in 1928, with the creation of *trompe l'oeil* (trick-of-the-eye) sweaters. Her 1930s fashions often featured surrealistic ideas contributed by such artists as Dali, Cocteau, and Vertès.

**scoop neckline**
Broad, round, open neckline.

**self fabric**
The same fabric as the garment.

**selvage**
The side edges of a piece of fabric where the weft thread wraps around the end warp thread to prevent fraying. Origin: formerly "self edge."

**serge**
A smooth durable fabric made with worsted yarns in the twill weave. Used for suits, skirts, and trousers.

**shantung**
A silk fabric with an uneven surface made of thread with elongated slubs. Origin: Shantung, China where it was first produced.

**shawl collar**
A long gently-curved one-piece collar without notches. It is attached to a V-neckline and tapers to a point at the bottom.

**shirring**
Parallel rows of gathering stitches.

**snood**
Bag-like hair net designed to retain the hair at the back of a woman's neck. Also called *résille* Fr. (rA-zE-yah).

**spats**
Protective covering for shoes and hose made of felt or linen. Fastened with buttons on the outside of the leg and a strap under the instep. Origin: Shortened version of "spatterdashes."

*stephane*
Crescent-shaped headdress worn by ancient Greek women.

**surplice** Fr. (sur-plEs) Eng. (sur-plis)
A crisscrossed bodice front consisting of two overlapping sides with diagonal upper edges which create a V-neckline when closed. Origin: French.

**Surrealism**
Surrealism was a hallucinatory form of modern art based on an artist's wild imagination and the bizarre manifestations of his/her subconscious. It was introduced shortly after World War I, but did not reach its height of popularity until the mid-1930s. Atypical effects were created by displacing a familiar object from its customary surroundings to a totally foreign environment or juxtaposing it with a dissimilar object. Familiar objects were also altered to resemble something totally unrelated, i.e. Schiaparelli's bird cage hat.

**swagger coat**
Woman's coat with a full flared back.

**sweetheart neckline**
Neckline containing two arches, one over each breast resembling the top of a heart.

**taffeta**
A crisp stiff plain-weave fabric made of silk or rayon with an iridescent luster. Its stiffness made it an ideal fabric for the full-skirted styles of the late '30s. Origin: Persian - *taftan* "to weave."

**tap pants**
Wide-leg underpants which ended just above the mid-thigh. They resembled the short pants worn by tap dancers featured in 1930s movies.

**toque** (tOk)
Small round brimless hat, perched on the top of the head. Origin: French - "jockey's cap."

*toile* Fr. (twal)
A muslin garment pattern.

**trapunto**
A form of quilting used as decoration for garments and hand bags during the late '30s and '40s.

*tremblant* Fr. (trom-blon)
A brooch which contained an element fastened to it by the use of a spring, thus causing the element to jiggle as the wearer moved about. It is also called a "trembler," "nodder," "springer," or "bobber."

*tricorne* **hat** Fr. (trE-korn) / Eng. (trI-korn)
This hat was worn by men in the 18th century and adopted for women during the 1930s. It featured a wide brim, cocked on three sides forming three points. Also spelled *tricorn*. Origin: French - *corne* "horn."

*trompe-l'oeil* Fr. (tromp loy)
Any design element or detail which is deceiving to the eye, i.e. the trompe l'oeil sweaters designed by Elsa Schiaparelli. Origin: French - "trick of the eye."

**tulle** Fr. (tool)
Fine net with hexagonal holes. It was left unstarched for bridal veils and starched for bouffant skirts. Origin: the city of Tulle, France where it was made.

**tuxedo collar**
Similar to the shawl collar, but retaining the same width down the full length of the garment.

*vicuña* Sp. (vI-kOOn-yah)
The soft strong fiber of the South American *vicuña*, a member of the llama family. Dark brown or fawn in color, it was used for coats, jackets, and suits. Origin: Spanish.

*vieux* **rose** Fr. (vEyu)
The color "old rose" or "dusty rose". Origin: French - *vieux* - "old".

**Vionnet** (vE-O-nA), **Madeleine**
One of the most influential French designers, Vionnet set the trend for bias-cut dresses and other garments in the late '20s and '30s. She introduced the cowl and halter necklines.

**voile** Fr. (vwal) / Eng. (voil)
Fine sheer open-weave cotton fabric of tightly-twisted threads, used for blouses and dresses. Origin: French "veil."

**velour felt**
Felt made of fur which has a soft velvety feel, used for better-quality hats.

**wing sleeves**
Sleeves made of large stiff ruffles which are gathered into the armseye.

# Bibliography

## BOOKS

Baker, Lillian. *Art Nouveau and Art Deco Jewelry*. Paducah, Kentucky: Collector Books, 1981.

Baker, Lillian. *100 Years of Collectible Jewelry*. Paducah, Kentucky: Collector Books,1978

Baker, Lillian. *Twentieth Century Fashionable Plastic Jewelry*. Paducah, Kentucky: Collector Books, 1992.

Ball, Joanne Dubbs. *The Art of Fashion Accessories*. Atglen, Pennsylvania: Schiffer Publishing Ltd., 1993.

Ball, Joanne Dubbs. *Costume Jewelers, The Golden Age of Design*. Atglen, Pennsylvania: Schiffer Publishing, 1990.

Battle, Dee and Alayne Lesser. *The Best of Bakelite and Other Plastic Jewelry*. Atglen, Pennsylvania: Schiffer Publishing Ltd., 1996.

Batterbury, Michael and Ariane. *Fashion the Mirror of History*. New York: Greenwich House, 1977.

Baudot, François. *Elsa Schiaparelli*. New York: Universe Publishing, 1997.

Becker, Vivienne. *Fabulous Costume Jewelry, History of Fantacy and Fashion in Jewels*. Atglen, Pennsylvania: Schiffer Publishing Ltd., 1993.

Bell, Jeanenne. *Old Jewelry*. Florence, Alabama: Books Americana Inc., 1985.

Black, J. Anderson, and Madge Garland. *A History of Fashion*. London: Orbis, 1975.

Blum, Stella. *Everyday Fashions of the Twenties*. New York: Dover Publications, Inc., 1981.

Boardman, Michelle. *All That Jazz: Printed Fashion Silks of the '20s and '30s*. Allenotwn, Pennsylvania: Allentown Art Museum, 1998.

Carter, Alison. *Underwear, The Fashion History*. New York: Drama Book Publishers, 1992.

Carter, Ernestine. *The Changing World of Fashion*. New York: G.P.Putnam's Sons, 1977.

Cera, Deanna Farneti. *Jewels of Fantasy: Cotume Jewelry of the 20th Century*. New York: Harry N. Abrams, Inc., 1992.

Cera, Deanna Farneti. *The Jewels of Miriam Haskell*. Milan, Italy: Ideal Books, 1997.

Costintino, Maria. *Men's Fashion in the Twentieth Century*. New York: Costume & Fashion Press, 1997.

Davidov, Corune and Dinny Redington Dawes. *The Bakelite Jewelry Book*. New York: Abbeville Press, 1988.

De Castelbajac, Kate. *The Face of the Century: 100 Years of Makeup and Style*. New York: Rizzoli, 1995.

Dooner, Kate. *A Century of Handbags*. Atglen, Pennsylvania: Schiffer Publishing Ltd., 1993.

Ewing, Elizabeth. *Dress and Undress, A History of Women's Underwear*. London: Bibliophile, 1978.

Ewing, Elizabeth. *History of 20th Century Fashion*. New York: Costume & Fashion Press, 1985.

Ettinger, Roseann. *Compacts and Smoking Accessories*. Atglen, Pennsylvania: Schiffer Publishing Ltd., 1991.

Ettinger, Roseann. *Handbags*. Atglen, Pennsylvania: Schiffer Publishing Ltd., 1991.

Ettinger, Roseann. *Popular Jewerly 1840-1940*. Atglen, Pennsylvania: Schiffer Publishing Ltd., 1990.

Folledore, Guiliano. *Men's Hats*. Modena: Zanfi Ediori, 1989.

Gaston, Mary Frank. *Collector's Guide to Art Deco*. Paducah, Kentucky: Collector Books, 1997.

Gerson, Roselyn. *Vintage Ladies' Compacts*. Paducah, Kentucky: Collector Books,1996.

Gerson, Roselyn. *Vintage Vanity Bags & Purses*. Paducah, Kentucky: Collector Books, 1994.

Giles, Stephen. *Jewelry Antiques Checklist*. London: Reed International Books, Limited, 1997.

Glynn, Prudence. *In Fashion, Dress in the Twentieth Century*. New York: Oxford University Press, 1978.

Grasso, Tony. *Bakelite Jewelry*. London: Quintet Publishing Limited, 1996.

Jargstorf, Sibylle. *Baubles, Buttons and Beads, The Heritage of Bohemia*. Atglen, Pennsylvania: Schiffer Publishing, 1993.

Kelly, Lyngerda and Nancy Schiffer. *Costume Jewelry, The Great Pretenders*. Atglen, Pennsylvania: Schiffer Publishing Ltd., 1987

Kelly, Lyngerda and Nancy Schiffer. *Plastic Jewelry*. Atglen, Pennsylvania: Schiffer Publishing Ltd., 1987.

Kennett, Frances. *The Collector's Book of Fashion*. New York: Crown Publishers, Inc., 1983.

Kirke, Betty. *Madeleine Vionnet*. San Francisco: Chronicle Books, 1998.

Lansdell, Avril. *Seaside Fashions 1860-1939*. Buckinghamshire, England: Shire Publications Ltd., 1990.

Martin, Richard. *Fashion and Surrealism*. New York: Rizzoli, 1987.

Martin, Richard. *Flair*. New York: Rizzoli, 1992.

Martin, Richard. *Haute Couture*. New York: Harry N. Abrams, Inc., 1995.

Martin, Richard and Harold Koda. *Splash! A History of Swimwear*. New York: Rozzoli, 1990.

Miller, Harrice Simmons. *Costume Jewelry*. New York: Avon Books, 1994.

Mueller, Laura M. *Collector's Encyclopedia of Compacts, Carry-alls, and Face Powder Boxes, Volume I.* Paducah, Kentucky: Collector Books, 1994.

Mueller, Laura M. *Collector's Encyclopedia of Compacts, Carryalls, and Face Powder Boxes, Volume II.* Paducah, Kentucky: Colleator Books, 1997.

Mulvagh, Jane. *Costume Jewelry in Vogue.* New York: Condé Nast Publishing Ltd.

McDowell, Colin. *Hats: Status, Style and Glamour.* London: Thames and Hudson Ltd., 1992.

McDowell, Colin. *McDowell's Directory of Twentieth Century Fashion.* New York: Prentice Hall Press, 1987.

McDowell, Colin. *Shoes, Fashion and Fantasy.* New York: Rizzoli, 1989.

Menkes, Suzy. *The Windsor Style.* Topsfield, Massachusetts: Salem House Publishers, 1988.

Milbank, Caroline Rennolds. *Couture, The Great Designers.* New York: Stewart, Tabori & Chang, Inc., 1985.

Milbank, Caroline Rennolds. *New York Fashion, The Evolution of American Style.* New York, Harry N. Abrams, Inc., 1989.

Newman, Harold. *An Illustrated Dictionary of Jewelry.* London: Thames and Hudson, 1981.

Osborne, Peggy Ann. *Button Button.* Atglen, Pennsylvania: Schiffer Publishing Ltd., 1997.

Probert, Christina. *Lingerie in Vogue.* New York: Abbeville Press, 1981.

Probert, Christina. *Swimwear in Vogue, Since 1910.* New York: Abbeville Press, 1981.

Reilly, Maureen and Mary Beth Detrich. *Women's Hats of the 20th Century.* Atglen, Pennsylvania: Schiffer Publishing Ltd., 1997.

Robins, Bill. *An A-Z of Gems and Jewelry.* New York: Arco Publishing, 1982.

Romero, Christie. *Warman's Jewelry.* Radnor, Pennsylvania: Wallace-Homesstead Book Company, 1995.

Romero, Christie. *Warman's Jewelry (2nd edition).* Iola, Wisconsin: Krause Publications, 1998.

Ross, Josephine. *Society in Vogue, The International Set Between the Wars.* New York: Vendome Press, 1992.

Rudoe, Judy. *Cartier 1900-1939.* New York: Harry N. Abrams, Inc., 1997.

Schiaparelli, Elsa. *Shocking Life.* New York: E.P.Dutton & Co., Inc., 1954.

Schiffer, Nancy. *Handbook of Fine Jewelry.* Atglen, Pennsylvania: Schiffer Publishing Ltd., 1991.

Schoeffler, O.E. and William Gale. *Esquire's Encyclopedia of 20th Century Men's Fashion.* New York: McGraw-Hill Book Company, 1973.

Shields, Jody. *All That Glitters, The Glory of Costume Jewelry.* New York: Rizzoli, 1987.

Shields, Jody. *Hats, A Stylish History and Collector's Guide.* New York: Clarkson Potter Publishers, 1991.

Simonds, Cheri. *Collectible Costume Jewelry 1925-1975.* Paducah, Kentucky: Collector Books, 1986.

Smith, Pamela. Vintage Fashion & Fabrics. New York: Alliance Publishers, 1995.

Steele, Valerie. *Women of Fashion, Twentieth-Century Designers.* New York: Rizzoli, 1991.

Stegemeyer, Anne. *Who's Who In Fashion.* New York: Fairchild Publications, 1980.

Swann, June. *The Costume Series, Shoes.* London: B.T. Batsford Ltd., 1982.

Tortora, Phyllis and Keith Eubank. *Survey of Historic Costume.* New York: Fairchild, 1994.

Tolkien, Tracy and Henrietta Wilkinson. *A Collector's Guide to Costume Jewelry.* Ontario: Firefly Books Ltd., 1997.

Tranquillo, Mary D., *Styles of Fashion, A Pictorial Handbook.* New York: Van Nostrand Reinhold Company, 1984.

Trasko, Mary. *Daring Do's: A History of Extraordinary Hair.* New York: Flammarion, 1994.

Trasko, Mary. *Heavenly Soles, Extraordinary Twentieth-Century Shoes.* New York: Abbeville Press, 1989.

White, Palmer. *Elsa Schiaparelli: Empress of Paris Fashion.* New York: Rizzoli, 1986.

Wilcox, R. Turner. *The Dictionary of Costume.* New York: Charles Scribner's Sons, 1969.

Willett C. and Phillis Cunnington. *The History of Underclothes.* London: Faber & Faber Limited, 1981.

Zimmerman, Catherine S. *The Bride's Book, A Pictorial History of American Bridal Gowns.* New York: Arbor House, 1985.

## CATALOGS

Berth Robert - 1934
Fifth Avenue Modes - 1935
Hamilton Garment Co. - 1930
Hardy & Hayes Jewelry - 1931
Howard Clothes (for men) - 1937
Jason Weiler-Baird North Co. (Wholesale Jewelry) 1930
Lane Bryant - 1938-39
Marshall Field & Company - 1932
Matthews Beautifit Lingerie - 1937-38
L. & C. Mayers Co. - (Wholesale Jewelry) 1933
L. & C. Mayers Co. (Wholesale Jewelery) 1939
Montgomery Ward - 1935, 1937.
National Bellas Hess - 1930-31, 1934.
E.L. Rice & Company (Wholesale Jewelery) 1931
S.Kind & Sons (Wholesale Jewelry) 1930
Sears, Roebuck and Co. - 1929-30, 1931, 1933-34, 1935-36, 1936, 1937, 1939-40.

## PERIODICALS

Art Needlework - 1936-37
Butterick Fashion News - December 1934.
Cosmopolitan - 6/33
Delinator - 1/30, 4/30, 7/30, 9/31, 9/32, 12/32, 6/33, 12/34, 4/35, 6/35, 7/35, 8/35, 4/36, 5/36, 7/36, 12/36, 2/37.
Deutfche Moden-Beitung - 12/35, 7/36, 11/36, 12/37, 12/38
Harper's Bazaar - 2/37, 7/37, 11/37, 12/37, 1/38, 3/1/38, 3/15/38.
Ladies' Home Journal - 11/35, 3/36.
Photoplay - 5/33.
McCall's - 1/30, 10/32, 12/32, 4/34, 5/34, 8/34, 10,34, 5/35, 9/35, 10/35, 7/37, 11/37, 1/38, 6/38, 4/39,
McCall's Fashion Book - summer 1935.
Needlecraft - The Home Arts Magazine - 10/33, 8/34, 10/34, 1/35, 5/35, 7/35, 11/35, 2/36, 4/36, 5/36, 8/36, 6/37, 7/37, 8/37.
Pictorial Review Combined with Delineator - 2/39, 3/39.
Pictorial Fashion Book - 7/35.
Pictorial Preview of Paris Fashions - 4/35.

Pictorial Review - 2/32, 2/35, 4/35, 8/35, 4/36, 5/38.
Simplicity Fashion Forcast 10/37
Woman's Home Companion - 6/35, 6/37, 7/37, 9/41, 10/37, 11/38, 12/39.
You (Holiday Number - 1938-39.
Vogue Pattern Book - 10 & 11/34.

## ARTICLES FROM PERIODICALS

Boehlke, Heidi L. "Ruth M. Kapinas, Munsingwear's Forgotten 'Foundettes' Designer." *Dress* 20 (1993): 45-52.

Bryant, Nancy O. "Insights Into the Innovative Cut of Madeleine Vionnet." *Dress* 12 (1986): 73-86.

Cunningham, Patricia. "Swimwear in the Thirties: The B.V.D. Company in the Decade of Innovation." *Dress* 12 (1986): 11- 27.

Martin, Richand, Harold Koda, Laura Sinderband. "Three Women: Madeleine Vionnet, Claire McCardell, and Rei Kawakubo." *Fashion Institute of Technology* (1987).

Perlingieri, Ilya Sandra. "Born to Shock, Elsa Schiaparelli's Clothing Designs from the 1930s Are Innovative Today." *Threads* 16 (April/May 1988): 38-43.

Shaeffer, Claire. "At the Lesage Embroidery Ateliers." *Threads* 16 (April/May 1988): 43-45.

# Index

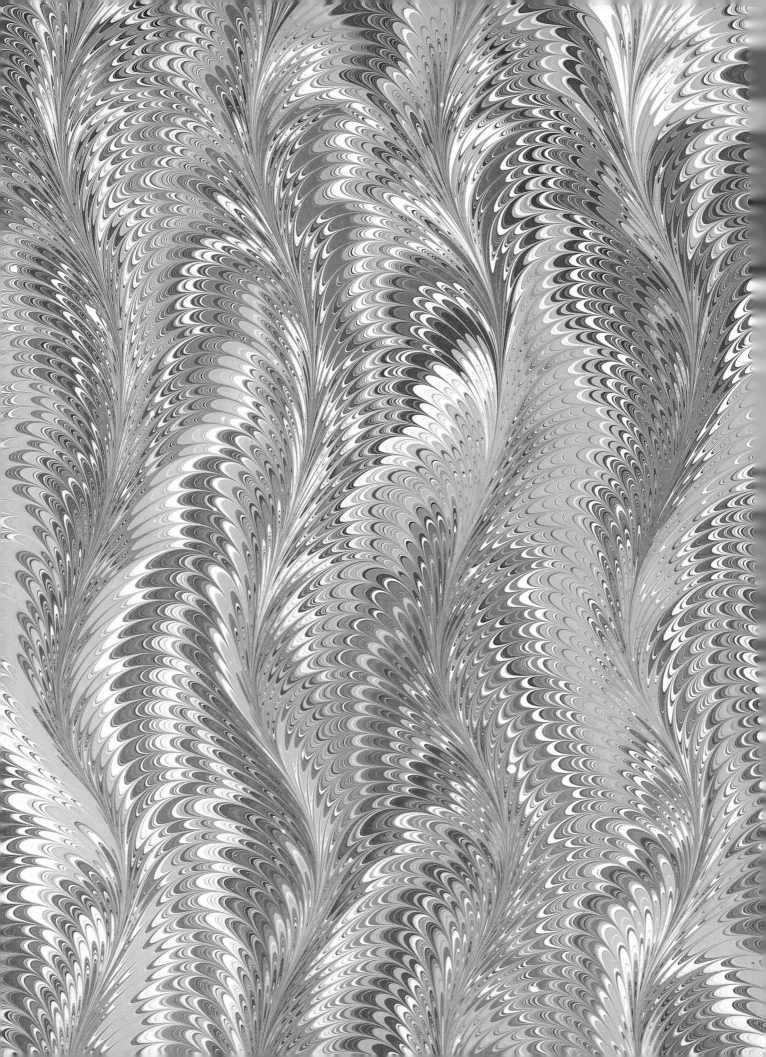